AF412805

Frontiers in Diabetes

Vol. 26

Series Editor

Massimo Porta Turin

The Diabetic Foot Syndrome

Volume Editors

Alberto Piaggesi Pisa
Jan Apelqvist Lund

36 figures, 14 in color, and 12 tables, 2018

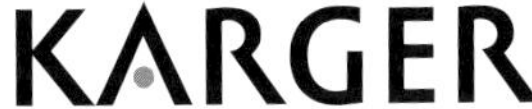

Basel · Freiburg · Paris · London · New York · Chennai · New Delhi · Bangkok · Beijing · Shanghai · Tokyo · Kuala Lumpur · Singapore · Sydney

Frontiers in Diabetes

Founded 1981 by F. Belfiore, Catania

Alberto Piaggesi, MD
Diabetic Foot Section
Department of Medicine
University of Pisa, Pisa, Italy

Jan Apelqvist, MD
Department of Endocrinology
University Hospital of Skåne, Malmö, Sweden
and
Division for Clinical Sciences
University of Lund, Lund, Sweden

Library of Congress Cataloging-in-Publication Data

Names: Piaggesi, Alberto, editor. | Apelqvist, Jan, editor.
Title: The diabetic foot syndrome / volume editors, Alberto Piaggesi, Jan
 Apelqvist.
Other titles: Frontiers in diabetes ; v. 26. 0251-5342
Description: Basel ; New York : Karger, 2017. | Series: Frontiers in
 diabetes, ISSN 0251-5342 ; vol. 26 | Includes bibliographical references
 and indexes.
Identifiers: LCCN 2017042611| ISBN 9783318061444 (alk. paper) | ISBN
 9783318061451 (e-ISBN)
Subjects: | MESH: Diabetic Foot--therapy | Diabetic Foot--complications |
 Diabetic Foot--surgery
Classification: LCC RD781 | NLM WK 835 | DDC 617.5/85--dc23
LC record available at https://lccn.loc.gov/2017042611

© Copyright 2018 by S. Karger AG, P.O. Box, CH–4009 Basel (Switzerland)
www.karger.com
Printed on acid-free and non-aging paper (ISO 9706)
ISSN 0251–5342
e-ISSN 1662–2995
ISBN 978–3–318–06144–4
e-ISBN 978–3–318–06145–1

Contents

Preface

In recent years, the "diabetic foot" (DF), has become a common name to describe the chronic complications of diabetes mellitus in the lower limb; it has also rapidly increased its relevance among various specialties such as diabetology, podiatry, vascular surgery, interventional cardiology and radiology, infectious diseases, orthopaedic surgery and others that are involved in its management both from a clinical and a scientific point of view: in 1971, 15 papers were indexed in PubMed under the heading "DF" compared to 785 in 2016, with a constantly increasing trend along the years, covering a variety of aspects, from pathogenesis to local and systemic management, from revascularization to Charcot foot surgery.

A substantial number of guidelines and consensus documents have been released and regularly adjourned over the years, and study groups, and even scientific societies, have been created with DF as the subject of interest and focus for research [1–3].

This interest in the DF has been prompted mainly by its increasing prevalence. It has been estimated that 1 out of 3 individuals with diabetes is likely to develop a DF ulcer during his or her lifetime, and going by the characteristics of the pathology, DFU is known to be a progressive condition affecting the lower limb with dramatic consequences, both for the limb and for the individual [4].

Once every 20 s, a limb is being lost globally because of diabetes, and patients with DF have mortality rates that are higher than those of many forms of cancer [5, 6].

The DF is a complex disease, with a multifactorial pathogenesis and with multidimensional clinical patterns, ranging from a prevalently ischaemic condition progressively evolving towards a critical end stage to a pure neuropathic disease with an alternance of chronic stable phases and reacutization alongside mixed neuro-ischaemic forms, all leading to ulcerations and eventually getting complicated with infections [7].

This pathogenetic and clinical complexity, which develops during a long and usually almost asymptomatic pre-clinical course, dramatically turning into a hyperacute phase, evolving frequently into a chronic condition with a high risk of recurrence, should be identified with the more appropriate definition of diabetic foot syndrome (DFS), encompassing all the aspects of the disease [8].

During the recent 10 years, thanks to some studies that re-shaped the knowledge and clinical evidence on DFS – one for all the EURODIALE study, which has so far produced 15 original papers and 2 reviews – the scientific and clinical profile of this pathology has significantly changed, leading to the understanding that DFS is an organ manifestation of a systemic chronic disease and not just a simple and local ulceration [9, 10].

New diagnostic, therapeutic and organizational tools have been put into practice to improve our adequacy to fight the disease; as a consequence, the number of major amputations is decreasing in some countries like the United Kingdom and the United States, and also, life expectancy is increasing [11].

In this volume of *Frontiers in Diabetes*, dedicated to the DFS, we collected 16 contributions from some of the most experienced and qualified scientists and clinicians who are experts in the different aspects of the disease, trying to give an up-to-date picture of the clinical scenario, the more recent acquisitions in the understanding of the mechanisms at the base of the pathology, the current standards of therapy and the organizational tasks that a modern approach to such a complex pathology deserves.

We asked all the contributors to submit a paper that should be as much informative and straight-to-the point as possible, including not only their own experience in the field, in any case relevant for the issues for which they have been selected, but also a wider picture that could link each section to the other, so as to produce a volume of *Frontiers in Diabetes* that would be more than the sum of the single contributions, and which could make worthwhile reading not only to the specialists but also to a wider audience comprising all the caregivers involved in the management of the patients at risk for developing the pathology, those affected and those who are at risk of recurrences.

This DF syndrome volume opens with a section on the general aspects of the disease: from an epidemiological survey point of view of what is actually considered a global pandemia to the different insights on the pathogenesis of the disease, including a very interesting original review by Nina Petrova on the recent findings in the pathogenesis of Charcot foot and their links to the clinical presentation, and a review made by Coppelli et al. on the role of microangiopathy in the determinisms of DFS, not to forget the weight that co-morbidities have from a clinical and prognostic point of view, analyzed by Meloni et al.

A relevant section of the volume has been dedicated to the clinical forms of the pathology, with a special emphasis on infections, treated in the contributions of Carlo Tascini and Eric Senneville, and on ischaemia, for which Ferraresi et al. reviewed the indications to revascularization, while Mike Edmonds correlated the pathogenesis of the diabetic macroangiopathy to its clinical presentation.

The therapeutic approach has been developed giving to surgery a wider significance than in other settings dealing with DFS, because it has gained an important place in the therapeutic strategy for this pathology. Javier Aragòn – Sanchez developed a section on the surgical management of DF infections, while Dalla Paola et al.

did the same for the surgery of the Charcot foot including other crucial aspects of therapy, such as offloading, written by Sicco Bus, and local care, by Fran Game.

Last but certainly not least, the organizational features, with a discussion on the role of a dedicated network in the management of the DFS, the importance of an integrated approach for the successful management of the ischaemic foot on the structured dedicated program that Prof. Joseph Mills implemented at the Bylor College of Medicine in Houston, and the re-evaluation of the outcomes made by Clerici et al., are all integrated in this volume because of their importance and current relevance.

After having read all these worthwhile contributions, we are immensely satisfied of having accomplished a major task of creating the needed awareness about DFS among the community of specialists and caregivers and sincerely hope that this volume will find its place on every desk of those interested and committed to the management of the DFS.

Alberto Piaggesi, MD, Pisa
Jan Apelqvist, MD, Lund

References

1 Sanders LJ, Robbins JM, Edmonds ME: History of the team approach to amputation prevention: pioneers and milestones. J Am Podiatr Med Assoc 2010;100:317–334.

2 Formosa C, Gatt A, Chockalingam N: A critical evaluation of existing diabetic foot screening guidelines. Rev Diabet Stud 2016;13:158–186.

3 Schaper NC, Van Netten JJ, Apelqvist J, Lipsky BA, Bakker K; International Working Group on the Diabetic Foot (IWGDF): Prevention and management of foot problems in diabetes: a summary guidance for daily practice 2015, based on the IWGDF guidance documents. Diabetes Metab Res Rev 2016; 32(suppl 1):7–15.

4 Boulton AJM: The diabetic foot; in De Groot LJ, Chrousos G, Dungan K, Feingold KR, Grossman A, Hershman JM, Koch C, Korbonits M, McLachlan R, New M, Purnell J, Rebar R, Singer F, Vinik A (eds): Endotext [Internet]. South Dartmouth, MDText.com, Inc., 2000–2016.

5 Zhang P, Lu J, Jing Y, Tang S, Zhu D, Bi Y: Global epidemiology of diabetic foot ulceration: a systematic review and meta-analysis [†]. Ann Med 2017;49:106–116.

6 Armstrong DG, Wrobel J, Robbins JM: Guest Editorial: are diabetes-related wounds and amputations worse than cancer? Int Wound J 2007;4:286–287.

7 Edmonds M: A natural history and framework for managing diabetic foot ulcers. Br J Nurs 2008; 17:S20, S22, S24–S29.

8 Jeffcoate WJ, Chipchase SY, Ince P, Game FL: Assessing the outcome of the management of diabetic foot ulcers using ulcer-related and person-related measures. Diabetes Care 2006;29:1784–1787.

9 Prompers L, Huijberts M, Apelqvist J, Jude E, Piaggesi A, Bakker K, Edmonds M, Holstein P, Jirkovska A, Mauricio D, Ragnarson Tennvall G, Reike H, Spraul M, Uccioli L, Urbancic V, Van Acker K, van Baal J, van Merode F, Schaper N: High prevalence of ischaemia, infection and serious comorbidity in patients with diabetic foot disease in Europe. Baseline results from the Eurodiale study. Diabetologia 2007;50:18–25.

10 Schaper NC: Lessons from Eurodiale. Diabetes Metab Res Rev 2012;28(suppl 1):21–26.

11 Lombardo FL, Maggini M, De Bellis A, Seghieri G, Anichini R: Lower extremity amputations in persons with and without diabetes in Italy: 2001–2010. PLoS One 2014;9:e86405.

Piaggesi A, Apelqvist J (eds): The Diabetic Foot Syndrome.
Front Diabetes. Basel, Karger, 2018, vol 26, pp 1–18 (DOI: 10.1159/000480040)

The Diabetic Foot Syndrome Today: A Pandemic Uprise

Jan Apelqvist

Department of Endocrinology, University Hospital of Skåne, Malmö, and Division for Clinical Sciences, University of Lund, Lund, Sweden

Abstract

Diabetes mellitus is growing at epidemic proportions worldwide; currently 415 million adults are estimated to have diabetes and by 2040, this number is estimated to increase to 642 million. As a consequence, the prevalence of diabetes-related complications is bound to increase. Diabetic foot disorders are common throughout the world, resulting in major medical, social and economic consequences for the patients, and a public health problem. The risk for ulceration and amputation is much higher in individuals with diabetes compared to that of the non-diabetic population: it is estimated that every 20 s an amputation is performed on an individual with diabetes somewhere in the world. Foot ulceration is the commonest major end point among diabetic complications. More than 5% of diabetic patients have a history of foot ulceration and the cumulative lifetime incidence may be as high as 25%. Incidence and prevalence figures related to both foot ulcerations and lower extremity amputations have been reported worldwide. There is a substantial global variation in the incidence and prevalence of amputation and diabetic foot ulcer (DFU). The variation may be partially explained by differences in the measurement of amputation and DFU, as well as the ascertainment of diabetes, demographic factors, setting or other confounders. There is an urgent need to determine a standardized way to report the incidence and prevalence of diabetes-related amputation and foot ulcer in order to be able to be used as a marker of quality of care.

Background

Diabetes is now one of the most common non-communicable diseases at the global level. It is the fourth or fifth leading cause of death in most of the developed countries and is epidemic in many developing and newly industrialized nations. It is estimated that today approximately 415 million adults have diabetes. Around 80% of these people live in developing countries. By 2030, the global estimate is expected to rise to about 642 million type 1 diabetes accounts for a small percentage of the total burden of diabetes in the population. Type 2 diabetes constitutes about 85–90% of all diabetes in developed countries and accounts for an even higher percentage in developing countries as it is reported in the last edition of the Diabetes Atlas of the International Diabetes Federation (http://www.eatlas.idf.org). The diabetic foot defined as infection, ulceration and/or destruction of deep tissues associated with neurological abnormalities and various degrees of peripheral vascular disease in the lower limb present a particularly troubling picture and it has been claimed that every 20 s, a lower limb is amputated due to diabetes. It is estimated that 50–70% of all lower extremity amputations are related to diabetes. Of all amputations in diabetic patients, 85% are preceded by a foot ulcer, which subsequently deteriorates to a severe infection or gangrene. Four out of five ulcers are claimed to be preceded by external trauma. The epidemiology of the diabetic foot is presented focusing on lower extremity ulcers and amputations. Diabetic foot complications result in huge costs for both society and people living with diabetes. Foot problems use 12–15% of the healthcare resources available for treating diabetes. In developing countries, figures up to 40% have been reported [1–4]. All these considerations make the diabetic foot syndrome a challenging health issue with clinical, social and economical implications, which should be at the top of the agenda of physicians, health care providers and policymakers.

Frequent Statements Regarding Diabetes-Related Lower Leg Amputations
- 50–70% of all non-traumatic amputations in persons with diabetes
- 85% of diabetes-related amputations precipitated by a foot ulcer
- 15–40 higher risk of a lower extremity amputation in persons with diabetes
- 0.9–2.4% annual incidence of lower leg amputations
- 1.3–7% prevalence of diabetes-related amputations

Incidence and Prevalence of Diabetes-Related Lower Leg Amputation

A major adverse outcome for diabetic foot problems is the amputation of the lower leg. Amputations remain common and serious complications of both types of diabetes and are associated with significant mortality [3–5].

The study of the epidemiology of diabetic foot disease has been beset by numerous problems relating to diagnostic tests and population selection [1, 5]. With regard to the incidence and prevalence of amputations, the numerator is usually the number of new major amputations (definition of "major" usually includes operations at or above the ankle), minor amputations (amputations below the ankle, which usually but not always may include amputations limited to digits), or all amputations (major and minor combined).

In most studies, irrespective of design and study population excluding amputations due to trauma and tumour, the annual incidence the incidence of a lower-leg amputation in people with diabetes has been estimated to range from 7 to 206 per 100,000, inhabitants per year [3, 4]. This wide variation was confirmed in a systematic review conducted by Moxey et al. [6] of data from 1989 to 2010, which reported that the incidence of all forms of lower extremity amputation ranges from 46.1 to 960 per 10^5 in the population with diabetes and major amputation ranging from 5.6 to 600 per 10^5.

Corresponding marked geographical variation in amputation rates has been reported within specific regions of an individual country and between countries such as the United Kingdom and North America [7–10]. According to the Diabetes Atlas, the middle 50% of amputation prevalence ranged between 0.9 and 2.4%, with a corresponding incidence of amputation of between 181 and 463 per 100,000 people with diabetes.

Most data from the last decade using which the incidence of major amputation is expressed in terms of the "at risk" (i.e., those with diabetes), but otherwise more or less unselected, populations are derived from Europe and the United States. Incidences of total amputations (lower extremity amputation; LEA) reported in the last 15 years and expressed in terms of people with diabetes have ranged from 1.76 to 3.44 per 1,000 patient-years in Europe, and was 2.2 per 1,000 in the United States [11].

Europe

Eastern Europe

A nationwide study (2004–2012) of major Lower Limb Amputation in Hungary reported that 50.4% of the amputees were diabetic [12]. The annual crude and age-adjusted major amputation rates exhibited no significant long-term pattern over the observation period. The major lower limb amputation incidence for the overall period was 317.9/105 among the diabetic population. In Rumania, a dramatic increase in the rates of amputations in persons with type 2 diabetes during 2006–2010 has been reported [13].

France

In France, the incidence of diabetes-related amputations varied between 1.84 and 3.45/1,000 individuals. In metropolitan France, the incidence of lower-limb amputation was approximately 2 per 1,000 but with marked regional differences [14, 15].

Germany

Using data of a nationwide statutory health insurance, the incidences of amputations (per 100,000 person years) in 2005–2007 was 121.2 in diabetic subjects in Germany. When the incidence of amputations in diabetic subjects was standardized to the estimated German diabetic population, the incidence was 278.9. The age-gender adjusted risk of having an amputation was 7.4-fold (6.3–8.7) in the diabetic compared to the non-diabetic population [16]. Between 2006 and 2012, in a corresponding study conducted by Heyer et al. [17], the amputation rates per patient in Germany have remained stable in the overall population and show a slight decline in patients with diabetes mellitus and in individuals with arterial occlusive disease.

Scandinavia

In a study from Finland [18], the incidence of LEA amputations done during the period 1990–2002 analyzed retrospectively was 94.6–73.2/1,000,000 individuals with diabetes. Incidence reported from Trondheim [19] were 2.4 per 1,000 patient-years (0.23). A Swedish population-based study conducted during 1982–2001 reported an incidence of major amputations at baseline 16 and an end-of-period incidence of 6.8/10.5; the same study reported an incidence of minor amputations at baseline and end-of-period incidence of 4.7 and 6.5, respectively, [20] after the introduction of a multidisciplinary specialist diabetic foot clinic.

In a retrospective study for the years 1981–1995 in a central district hospital in Copenhagen, Denmark [21], involving a catchment area population of about 178,000, the incidence of major amputations decreased from 27.2 to 6.9/100,000 population.

Italy

A recent study, evaluating nationwide data from the National Institute of Health database, on lower extremity amputation rates between 2001 and 2010, showed how the crude rates of amputations, which in 2001 were 296.6 × 100,000 persons with diabetes, and 8.5 × 100,000 for persons without diabetes, in 2010 fell to 247.2 × 100,000 in diabetic patients but did not change (8.6 × 100,000) in persons without diabetes. The reduction in amputations rates in diabetic patients over this 10-year period was of – 30.7% for major amputations and of – 4.6% for minor amputations, suggesting an earlier and more diffuse approach aimed at limb salvage [22].

Spain

Incidences reported from Andalusia (Spain) were 3.4 per 1,000 patient-years [23], and in Madrid 46.1/10.5 including all lower extremity amputations by diabetes [24]. In a study based on Spanish national hospital discharge data in patients with type 1 diabetes, the incidence of minor and major amputations decreased significantly from 2001 to 2008 (0.88–0.43 per 100,000 inhabitants and 0.59–0.22 per 100,000 inhabitants, respectively). In patients with type 2 diabetes, the incidence of minor and major LEAs increased significantly (9.23–10.9 per 100,000 inhabitants and 7.12–7.47 per 100,000 inhabitants) [25].

United Kingdom and Ireland
The incidences of major (above the ankle) amputation per 1,000 patient-years were reported to be 1.11 and 0.97 in Scotland and England, respectively, and as low as 0.76 and 0.67 in particular towns in the United Kingdom: Middlesbrough and Ipswich [1, 26–28]. Incidences reported from Tayside (Scotland) and Ireland were 2.4 and 1.76 per 1,000 patient-years respectively [29, 30].

A study in 2012 by Holman et al. [8] demonstrated an eightfold variation in the rate of all amputations (LEA) and a tenfold variation in major amputations among the primary care trusts (PCTs) in England. The investigators also noted close correlations between PCTs in the incidences of major and of minor amputations in people with and without diabetes, indicating that geographic variation in the incidence of amputation was unrelated to diabetes. Variation was unlikely to be related to access to care, although it could be related in part to social deprivation and ethnicity.

United States
In the United States, diabetic foot complications are a major cause of hospital admission [2, 3]. In 1997, nearly 70% of all amputations were for people with diabetes. Hospitalizations for lower extremity amputations rose from 33,000 in 1980 to 71,000 in 2005; foot ulcers and amputations were more common among ethnic minority groups, especially among the Hispanic and black people who are less likely to have health insurance [3]. Other surveys from the United States have been restricted to populations for which reliable data on the prevalence of diabetes exist, principally those in the Veterans Health Administration and/or those receiving health care from Medicare or Medicaid. These populations are at greater risk, and the reported incidence of both major and total amputations (LEA) is correspondingly higher [31–36]. Variation in the incidence of amputation within the United States has been reported in several carefully conducted investigations. In 1996/1997, Wrobel et al. [36] found an 8.6-fold variation in the incidence of amputation in the Medicare population and suggested that the variation could be associated with regional variation in care. Margolis et al. [32] reported the annual incidence of lower extremity amputation to be on the order of 4–5 per 1,000 person-years in 5 million beneficiaries with diabetes in the US Medicare population between 2006 and 2008. They found a three- to fivefold geographic variation in the incidence of amputation, and that areas of higher and lower incidence appeared to cluster in specific geographic regions. The clustering was maintained after adjusting for variations in race, income, education, physician access, age of the population, incidence of diabetes and frequency of microvascular and macrovascular complications. It was assumed that variation in the incidence of amputation could be due to the disease process, implementation of guidelines, health care provider training and/or therapeutic preference or patient preference. These findings contradicted those of Tseng et al. [37] who demonstrated different outlier centres for high rates of incidence of major and of minor amputation in Medicare beneficiaries in the Veterans Health Administration system, both with and without diabetes.

Pacific, Middle East and Northern Africa

Most of these data are collected from western Europe and the United States, but there is an increasing concern regarding the development in other parts of the world especially the Pacific, Middle East and Northern Africa [37] with regard to the prevalence of diabetes-related amputation of 0.7–5%. There are substantial differences both with regard to the incidence and prevalence of diabetes-related amputations globally.

A total of 26 Organization for Economic Cooperation and Development (OECD) countries contributed to the OECD data collection for at least 1 year in the reference time frame, showing a decline in rates of over 40%, from a mean of 13.2 (median 9.4, range 5.1–28.1) to 7.8 amputations per 100,000 in the general population (median 9.9, range 1.0–18.4). Despite an overall significant reduction observed across 12 consecutive years, amputation rates among people with diabetes remain still high in most OECD countries. In 2011, one amputation every 7 min among subjects aged 15 years or over could be directly attributed to diabetes [38].

In the South-East Asia region, 24.2% of all live births are affected by the presence of high blood glucose during pregnancy. In the Middle East and North Africa regions, 2 out of 5 adults with diabetes go undiagnosed. In the South and Central America regions, the number of people with diabetes is likely to increase by 65% by 2040. It is estimated that between 9.5 and 29.3 million people live with diabetes in the Africa region. As a consequence, the prevalence of diabetes-related complications is bound to increase [39–44].

Asia: in view of the vast population of this continent, data about diabetic foot problems are sparse. India has more people with diabetes than any other country, and foot problems and amputations remain very common [45].

Africa: Sub-Saharan Africa Diabetic foot complications constitute an increasing public health problem and are a leading cause of admission, amputation and mortality in diabetic patients [43, 44]. A review of the epidemiology of diabetic foot problems in Africa highlighted not only the frequency of neuropathy but also the increasing frequency of peripheral vascular disease [46, 47].

A population-based study from Australia suggested that risk factors for foot ulceration might be lower than those in other Western countries, but a subsequent report showed that foot screening is poor, with less than half of the diabetic population reporting a regular foot examination [48]. In a study from New Zeeland published in 1998, the number of admissions for diabetic foot disease actually increased over a 13-year period [49]. A figure of 3.8 per 1,000 was reported from Western Australia, but this referred to amputations undertaken over a longer period from 1996 to 2005 [50]. Variation noted in Australia has been linked to the prevailing socioeconomic status.

In the Caribbean, diabetes prevalence is approaching a rate of 20% in many islands, and amputations in diabetic patients are among the highest in the world [51]. In South and Central America, the prevalence of diabetes is high, ranging from 5 to 20%, with an increasing awareness of the diabetic foot especially in Brazil [52, 53].

All these studies and reports illustrate not only the substantial impact of diabetes-related lower leg amputations but also a substantial global variation in the incidence and prevalence of lower leg amputations. Variation may be explained by differences in the methodology in measurement of amputation, type of amputation, as well as the ascertainment of diabetes. Variation may also be partially explained by race/ethnicity, treatment of diabetes, the management of diabetic foot disease, societal factors, patient behavior and mood, access to care, and aspects of specialist care [54]. Until proper population-based registers of people with diabetes are available, reliable data relating to accurate estimates of the prevalence and incidence of these late complications will be limited. It is clear, however, that foot ulcers and amputations remain common and serious complications, which are associated with significant mortality.

Factors Contributing to the Methodology of Registration as Well as Variation of Incidence and Prevalence of Diabetes-Related Amputations

- Diagnosis and prevalence of diabetes mellitus in the population
- Underreporting diabetes status
- Absence of uniform out-patient data describing major foot problems and the growing number of minor out-patient surgical procedures
- Study population – hospital/area based – hospital discharge data annual estimates of civilian, non institutionalized, hospitalized individuals
- Type of study survey/questionnaire/cross-sectional study/medical records/physical examination
- Registration-medical records-in hospital registration-continuous registration-national records
- Number of patients, extremities or number of procedures (re-amputation)
- Amputation level/definition-minor/major – including toe, transmetatarsal, Ray, Syme, below knee, above knee and hip disarticulation

Methodological Considerations with Regard to Incidence and Prevalence of Lower Leg Amputation

It is essential to know the extent of a clinical problem. Much effort has been undertaken to identify all diabetic foot problems around the world. Incidence and prevalence figures concerning both foot ulcerations and lower extremity amputations have been reported extensively worldwide.

Although amputation seems a clear defined endpoint, there are several methodological issues. The difficulty in evaluating epidemiological data with regard to the incidence of amputation is well recognized [5, 54, 55]. There are many important confounders explaining differences in data collection and reflecting the complexity of data involved in any detailed presentation of amputation epidemiology. Adequately performed population-based studies regarding the incidence of amputations in the lower-leg are limited.

When amputation rates have to be reported, a number of parameters are considered essential: which amputation in a sequence is used as the outcome measure (i.e., the first amputation, the number of amputations or the final amputation level)? Does the number reported indicate the number of individuals undergoing amputation or the number of limbs amputated? Are the results based on the number of hospitalizations?

People with diabetes have below-ankle amputations done more frequently than people without diabetes. As a consequence, studies that focus primarily on above-ankle amputations tend to underestimate the total number of diabetes-related amputations [4, 5]. In most countries, amputations are probably underestimated because a continuous registration system is not in place [3].

A fundamental methodological question to all epidemiological studies is the completeness of the material with regard to diabetes. Most amputation studies are based on central registers and subject to any shortfall inherent in such registers. The shortcomings of national registers are well known [4, 54]. An important issue is that the diagnosis of diabetes is not established or not recorded at the time of amputation.

The results are dependent on the estimates of the number of diabetic subjects in the general population. The definition of diabetes has been revised several times over the past years by country-specific professional societies as well as by world bodies. These changes in diagnostic criteria for diabetes have tended to increase the number of individuals diagnosed with the disease. There will be an inevitable reduction in the incidence on amputation in such an expanded, at-risk population [17]. An illustration of this potential phenomenon has presented both in the Netherlands [56] and in the United States [11]. Data from the Netherlands when expressed per 100,000 of the total population showed no decline in lower extremity amputations, but when expressed as a proportion of the rising population with diabetes, there was a clear downwards trend [56].

A number of subjects are likely to have undiagnosed diabetes. The diagnosis of diabetes is frequently defined as previously known diabetes usually identified as treatment with insulin or oral agents, and whether glycaemic status is evaluated on all individuals in the study population is frequently not established or established/recognized at the time of amputation. Corresponding underestimations have been reported from a number of areas. Potentially a misclassification could lead to an under- or overestimation. In most studies, amputations are lumped together. A single toe, a whole forefoot or an above-knee amputation all have different impacts. Not only has a patient 2 legs, but taking minor amputations into consideration, all 10 toes are potential subjects for amputation, simultaneously or on different occasions. Central registers do not usually differentiate the left from the right side or primary amputation from re-amputation. After one or more minor amputations, when complete healing happens, a major amputation on the same side may follow – perhaps years later – and thus several final amputation levels have to be considered in the same patient. Amputations may also have taken place before the time period of the study. All these are events that may influence incidence calculations. To reflect a true epidemiological picture, final amputation levels must have preference over primary amputation levels. Clear definitions with regard to all these aspects are mandatory to make comparisons between studies possible.

Another issue is if the study is a geographical defined area studied or hospital/clinic based. The setting as well as the information related to whether the hospital is a referral primary/secondary or tertial unit is of further importance. Amputations are frequently not performed in one hospital or one clinic only. A patient can undergo an amputation in another hospital or clinic in the surrounding areas. The health care structure and reimbursement routines have been reported to influence the reported amputation rate. All routine registers have a certain inherent shortfall. By systematic scrutiny of different independent registration systems, these pitfalls can be reduced (including data/records from both in and out hospital clinics involved in treating patients with diabetes and operation theatre records) [5, 57].

Additional Confounders When Comparing Amputation-Related Data
- Indication for amputation
- Selection of amputation level
- Co-morbidity
- Reimbursement
- Resource utilization
- The structure and effectiveness of health care services
- Treatment strategies
- Social, societal factors, race and ethnicity

Indications for Amputation

The most common indications for amputation described in the literature are gangrene, infection, and non-healing ulcers [58]. The indications most commonly cited are gangrene and infection frequently occurring simultaneously. It has to be emphasized that a non-healing ulcer in itself should not be considered an indication for amputation, since long duration is not an unfavourable factor with regard to amputation as long as the duration of ulcer in itself is not considered an indication [57]. There are very few studies with regard to the incidence or prevalence of amputation that report the indication for the surgical procedure as well as the selection of the amputation level. Those few studies state that the immediate indications for amputation in patients with diabetes are often multiple [4] of which progressive gangrene (50–70%) and infection (25–50%) are the most common and frequently in combination (25–50%).

Selection of Amputation Level

Most studies/reports regarding the incidence of lower amputations are focused on amputations at or above the ankle in people with or without diabetes. Studies that focus primarily on above-ankle amputations tend to underestimate the total number of diabetes-related amputations performed. There is still some controversy concerning the benefit of a primary minor amputation vs primary major amputation (below knee) [54, 57]. The advantages of primary major amputation are a lower re-amputation rate and shorter healing time. Minor amputations are associated with a higher re-amputation rate and as a consequence, longer wound healing time. However, in a prospective study, the long-term outcome after a healed index amputation in patients with diabetes and foot ulcer was evaluated and it was concluded that those subjects with an index major amputation had a higher mortality rate, an equal rate of new amputations irrespective of level, an increased rate of new contralateral amputations and a lower potential for rehabilitation than patients with an index minor amputation [4, 5, 57].

Ideally when evaluating diabetes-related amputations, the total amputation rate irrespective of the level should be reported along with indications and the rationale for level selection.

Common Statements Regarding Foot Ulcers in Individuals with Diabetes Mellitus
- 2.1–5.9% annual cumulative incidence of foot ulcer
- 1.5–8.3% prevalence of foot ulcers
- 7% one-year incidence of first foot ulcer in neuropathic feet
- 11–25% annual cumulative incidence of re-ulceration or new foot ulcer
- 30–50% new ulcers within 2 years after a healed foot ulcer
- 10% of ulcers in subjects with previously unknown diabetes

Incidence and Prevalence of Foot Ulceration (Diabetic Foot Ulcer) in Individuals with Diabetes Mellitus

The major adverse outcomes of diabetic foot problems are foot ulcers and amputations. Up to 85% of all amputations begin with an ulcer; every year, approximately 4 million more people develop a diabetic foot ulcer (DFU; International Diabetes Federation. Diabetes Atlas http://www.eatlas.idf.org).

A diabetic foot wound is caused by infection, ulceration and destruction of deep tissues associated with neurological abnormalities and various degrees of peripheral vascular disease in the lower limb. A foot ulcer is the general term used to describe a full thickness wound below the ankle in a diabetic patient, irrespective of duration. (International Working Group on the Diabetic Foot; international consensus on the diabetic foot and practical guidelines on the management and the prevention of the diabetic foot. Amsterdam, the Netherlands (2015; http://www.diabeticfoot.nl). Active foot disease may be of recent onset or due to a deteriorating chronic situation and refers to anyone with diabetes who presents with a foot lesion.

More information is available on the number of amputations than on the number of ulcers. As most of the information in the current literature comes from selected populations, and different definitions are used, it is difficult to evaluate the extent of foot problems worldwide. It is also likely that the type of ulcer varies around the world: in western countries, up to 60% of new ulcers are associated with peripheral arterial disease, so called neuro-ischaemic and ischaemic ulcers; in developing countries, neuropathic ulcers of various origins are more common.

The point prevalence of foot ulcers in developed countries varies between 1.5 and 10% in various populations [59–70]. In European countries such as France 1.8–6.0%, Greece 4.8%, Slovakia 0.9%, Sweden 3.0–8.3%, and the United Kingdom 1.3–7.4%. In the United States, a prevalence of foot ulcers of 9.5–10.5% have been reported in various populations. Corresponding prevalence figures from countries outside Europe/the United States have been reported from Algeria (11.9%), Bahrein (5.9%) and India (3.6%) [71–73].

Foot ulcers occur in both type 1 diabetes and type 2 diabetes. In elderly patients with diabetes type 2, the reported prevalence of foot ulcers has been 5–10%. In studies that focused on younger subjects with type 2 diabetes or individuals with diabetes type 1, the estimated prevalence was 1.7–3.3% (15.3). In community-based European studies, the prevalence varies between 1.4 and 8.3% and in clinic-based studies from developing countries, a prevalence of 3.6–11.9% was reported especially from Arab countries with a high prevalence of diabetes of 19.2–29.2%. In western countries, on average 2 out 100 individuals with diabetes have a foot ulcer [15]. The prevalence increases in populations in the presence of predisposing factors.

An incidence of foot ulcers in individuals with diabetes of 2.1–5.9% has been reported from studies in Western Europe and North America [15]. Two European countries reported the annual incidence of foot ulcers in the general population to be just more than 2% (Netherlands 2.1% and the United Kingdom 2.2) [66, 69]. The incidence of diabetic foot ulceration varies with the population studied, the criteria and definitions of foot lesions used, and with differences in study design.

Incidences of 2.5–7.2% have been reported in high-risk or selected populations compared to 0.6–2.2% in European community-based studies and 3–6% in clinic-based studies from developing countries [15, 45]. Ulceration is much more common in patients with predisposing risk factors; annual incidence rates in neuropathic individuals vary from 5 to over 7% [66, 68]. It is likely that the cumulative lifetime incidence of foot ulcers may be as high as 25% or even higher in individuals with diabetes and a previously healed ulcer 30–50% will have a new foot ulcer within 2 years [1, 66].

Studies from the United Kingdom suggest that foot ulcers and amputation are less common in Asian patients of Indian subcontinent origin [1, 6, 66]. Possible explanations for the findings in Asian patients relate to differences in limited joint mobility and to better foot care in certain religious groups. In North American studies, ulceration was more common in Hispanic Americans and in Native Americans than in non-Hispanic whites [3]. Foot ulceration also appears to be associated with social deprivation [3]. In most reports with regard to foot ulcers, there is male dominance [74, 75].

In many reports, prevalence data rely on hospital discharge or claims data [2, 3]. In US data based on the rate of hospital discharges for diabetic patients, the ulcer prevalence among persons aged 44 was 6.5/1,000 diabetics and it rose progressively to 10.3/1,000 diabetics in individuals aged 75 [3].

Factors Contributing to the Methodology of Registration as Well as Variation of Incidence and Prevalence of DFU in Individuals with Diabetes
- Definition and prevalence of diabetes mellitus
- Prevalence of diabetes established or unknown
- Foot ulcer-definition, etiology, classification, type and site
- Study population-hospital, clinic, community or area based
- Setting – university hospital, referral unit, primary care, home care
- Clinical investigation-screening-medical records-survey-questionnaire
- Drop out rate-clinical investigation-self reported-survey

Methodological Considerations with Regard to the Reporting of Incidence and Prevalence of Foot Ulcer

A substantial quantum of epidemiological data has been published on the diabetic foot, but they are difficult to interpret because of variability in the methodology and in the definitions used in these reports [3]. In general, there is lack of consistency in population characteristics (ethnicity, social level, accessibility to care), definitions and how results are presented.

As a consequence, adequately performed population-based studies regarding the incidence and prevalence of foot ulcer in the lower-leg are scarce. Most studies are performed from the perspective of patients attending a dedicated clinic or in a selected study population. The difference in the reported incidence and prevalence are in many cases, related to differences in the design of the study, demographic factors prevalence of diabetes and definition and classification of ulcer, as well as variations in registration systems. A major confounder is that a foot ulcer is frequently not reported or detected by the patient himself. In a study, 25% of the patients with a full-skin foot ulcer denied the presence of the ulcer at an interview followed by a physical examination [57]. In 10% of patients with an ulcer below the ankle, diabetes was not previously not diagnosed. In 50% of patients with diabetes mellitus and a foot ulcer, the treating physician was not aware of the ulcer and the ulcer was not recorded in the medical records. As a consequence, studies tend to underestimate the total number of foot ulcers. The study design and method are essential in that respect. If it is a survey with self-reported questionnaire, interview, analysis of medical records or cross sectional clinical study, then it will have a substantial influence on the outcome [3, 57]. In most countries, foot ulcers are underestimated, as a continuous registration system is not in place.

Foot Ulcer-Definition, Etiology, Classification, Type and Site

A DFU is usually defined as a lesion/wound through all layers of the skin located below the ankle in an individual with diabetes mellitus. In many studies regarding incidence and prevalence of foot ulcers, there is not any definition and the ulcers are not classified. DFUs represent a heterogeneous pathological entity, caused by a broad range of aetiological factors in a diverse patient population.

The most important factors related to the development of foot ulcers in individuals with diabetes are peripheral neuropathy, minor foot trauma, foot deformity and decreased tissue perfusion [54]. DFUs are frequently seen in patients with a combination of 2 or more risk factors occurring together [74, 75].

With regard to the etiology of foot ulceration, peripheral vascular disease and neuropathy are frequently present in the same patient. Although traditionally it is stated that the majority of foot ulcers are purely neuropathic, an increase in the incidence of neuroischaemic and/or ischaemic foot ulcers has been found. In large cohort studies in Europe, neuroischaemic or ischaemic ulcers accounted for 50–58% of all DFUs admitted to specialist care [74, 75].

Ulcers frequently result from external trauma to the insensitive foot, such as ill-fitting shoes, burns, walking bare foot and having foreign objects in shoes [57, 75]. However, an ulcer caused by increased mechanical stress due to disturbed biomechanics is usually localized to the metatarsal heads or the plantar area of the first digit, whereas decubitus ulcers are located at the heel. Plantar neuropathic foot ulcers constitute 18–23% out of foot ulcers in large European cohort studies [74, 75] but are substantial and more frequent in countries like the Middle East and North Africa [39–45].

The distribution of type, site and cause of ulcer can vary country by country depending on the climate, access and use of foot wear, physical activity and culture [39–45].

It should also be recognized that in many cases, the ulcer is a sign of an underlying multiorgan disease such as cardio cerebrovascular disease and nephropathy [74, 75]. Foot ulcer range in extent of tissue damage and wound characteristics. A classification system is essential not only for management but also for understanding the differences in different patient populations and countries in terms of the incidence and prevalence of the ulcer and the distribution of ulcer with regard to etiology, site and type [6].

Incidence and Prevalence of Diabetes-Related Amputations as a Marker of Quality of Care

The present review on the prevalence and incidence of DFU and amputation shows a marked variation worldwide in the rates of foot ulcer and amputation and emphasizes the fact that still one amputation every 20 s could be directly attributed to diabetes. In 1989, the St. Vincent Declaration launched by WHO Europe and IDF Europe triggered the attention of governments on the rate of limb amputations in individuals with diabetes mellitus. After over 25 years, there is still insufficient information available to monitor progress in this direction.

It can be concluded that lower extremity amputation continues to be a major source of morbidity and mortality worldwide, the extent of this burden cannot be accurately quantified because of international variation and lack of standardized reporting measures. Effective standardized reporting methods of major, minor and at-risk populations are needed.

Until proper population-based registers of people with diabetes are available, reliable data relating to accurate estimates of the prevalence and incidence of these late complications such as amputations and DFU will be limited to community-based studies or studies from dedicated centres or clinics.

Reports about a decrease in the incidence of amputations due to diabetes from usually unselected populations may have resulted to a very large extent simply from a restructuring of clinical services. A considerable number of reports and studies indicate a substantial decrease in the amputation rate in diabetic subjects. The general conclusion from these studies is that strategies including preventive measures and a multidisciplinary approach to established foot ulcers, strict amputation criteria and a continuous registration of amputations can bring a substantial decrease in amputation rate in patients with diabetes (49–85%).

Several population-based studies observed a significant reduction in major amputations over time, and after correction for the increasing number of people with diabetes, in some countries, a relative decrease was observed over a longer period of time in the number of lower-extremity amputations in people with diabetes [18–31].

Leg amputations are related to increased mortality in people with diabetes. By the time an amputation is necessary, people have usually had diabetes for many years and often have severe co-morbidity. Death around the time of the amputation occurs in up to 10% of cases. Death rates increase over the 5 years following amputation: 30% of patients die within 1 year, 50% die within 3 years and 70% die within 5 years [5]. In developing countries, these figures tend to be even higher because many people seek medical attention only when their foot problem is so far advanced that their limbs and their lives are threatened.

Given that the incidence of amputation can also be influenced by a wide variety of clinical and social factors, it is not surprising that considerable variation exists between published studies from different countries. The demonstration of wide variation within a single country or between countries or communities that have very similar populations, health care systems, and procedures for documenting amputation incidence is of a mayor concern. When eight- to tenfold variation exists within similar health care systems, it is essential that the reasons are explored. While race and social deprivation both make an important contribution to variation, another is likely to relate to aspects of the structure of care.

Social, economic and geographical factors linked to ethnicity may prevent certain individuals from accessing health care resources and the benefits of limb-salvaging interventions The structure and effectiveness of health care services' access to effective primary care will be reduced or absent in many nations or in poorer communities in others, and the incidence of amputation has been shown to drop dramatically when programs are introduced to correct this. The impact of race is complex because it overlaps with social and societal factors and also due to poverty, deprivation, and restricted access to health care services in developing countries and among ethnic minorities in developed countries.

When assessing the impact of an interventional program, a number of basic underlying factors, such as prevalence of diabetes, the age profile of the population, comorbidity and smoking habits must be considered. Such factors may mask the effect of intervention unless compared to a situation where such intervention is not applied and must be considered when assessing future incidence rates [54]. The difference in incidence results, has to be analyzed from the perspective of the design of the study, demographic factors, prevalence of diabetes, as well as variations in registration systems and differences in reimbursement of various procedures [8, 9, 54].

Amputation rate should therefore not be used as a quality indicator in diabetic foot disease, unless it can be corrected for the relevant characteristics of the patient, the leg and the foot [54]. There is an urgent need for a standardized way to report incidence and prevalence of diabetes-related amputation and foot ulcer and amputation and DFU which can be used as a marker of quality of care. Therefore, given the limitations of epidemiological research about the prevalence and incidence of foot-related complications, they still are the backbone of clinical research in the area of the diabetes-related foot complications.

References

1 Boulton AJM, Vileikyte L, Ragnarson-Tennvall G, Apelqvist J: The global burden of diabetic foot disease. Lancet 2005;366:1719–1724.

2 Driver VR, Fabbi M, Lavery LA, Gibbons G: The costs of diabetic foot: the economic case for the limb salvage team. J Am Podiatr Med Assoc 2010;100: 335–341.

3 Reiber GE, LeMaster JW: Epidemiology and economic impact of foot ulcers and amputations in people with diabetes; in Bowker JH, Pfeifer M (eds): Levin and O'Neals the Diabetic Foot, ed 7. Philadelphia, Mosby Elsevier, 2008, pp 3–22.

4 Larsson J, Apelqvist J: Towards less amputations in diabetic patients. Incidence, causes, cost, treatment, and prevention – a review. Acta Orthop Scand 1995; 66:181–192.

5 Larsson J, Eneroth M, Apelqvist J, Stenström A: Sustained decrease of major amputation in diabetic patients – an analysis of a 20-year period in a defined population (628 amputations in 461 patients). Acta Orth 2008;79:665–673.

6 Moxey PW, Gogalniceanu P, Hinchliffe RJ, et al: Lower extremity amputations – a review of global variability in incidence. Diabet Med 2011;28:1144–1153.

7 Connelly J, Airey M, Chell S: Variation in clinical decision making is a partial explanation for geographical variation in lower extremity amputation rates. Br J Surg 2001;88:529–535.

8 Holman N, Young RJ, Jeffcoate WJ: Variation in the recorded incidence of amputation of the lower limb in England. Diabetologia 2012;55:1919–1925.

9 Vamos EP, Bottle A, Edmonds ME, et al: Changes in the incidence of lower extremity amputations in individuals with and without diabetes in England between 2004 and 2008. Diabetes Care 2010;33:2592–2597.

10 van Houtum WH, Lavery LA: Regional variation in the incidence of diabetes-related amputations in The Netherlands. Diabetes Res Clin Pract 1996;31:125–132.

11 Li Y, Burrows NR, Gregg EW, et al: Declining rates of hospitalization for nontraumatic lower-extremity amputation in the diabetic population aged 40 years or older: U.S., 1988–2008. Diabetes Care 2012;35:273–277.

12 Kolossváry E, Ferenci T, Kováts T, Kovács L, Járai Z, Menyhei G, Farkas K: Trends in major lower limb amputation related to peripheral arterial disease in Hungary: a nationwide study (2004–2012). Eur J Vasc Endovasc Surg 2015;50:78–85.

13 Veresiu IA, Iancu SS, Bondor C: Trends in diabetes-related lower extremities amputations in Romania – a five year nationwide evaluation. Diabetes Res Clin Pract 2015;109:293–298.

14 Fosse S, Hartemann-Heurtier A, Jacqueminet S, Ha Van G, Grimaldi A, Fagot-Campagna A: Incidence and characteristics of lower limb amputations in people with diabetes. Diabet Med 2009;26:391–396.

15 Richard JL, Schuldiner S: [Epidemiology of diabetic foot problems]. Rev Med Interne 2008;29:S222–S230.

16 Icks A, Haastert B, Trautner C, Giani G, Glaeske G, Hoffmann F: Incidence of lower-limb amputations in the diabetic compared to the non-diabetic population. Findings from nationwide insurance data, Germany, 2005–2007. Exp Clin Endocrinol Diabetes 2009;117:500–504.

17 Heyer K, Debus ES, Mayerhoff L, Augustin M: Prevalence and regional distribution of lower limb amputations from 2006 to 2012 in Germany: a population based study. Eur J Vasc Endovasc Surg 2015;50:761–766.

18 Eskelinen E, Eskelinen A, Albäck A, Lepäntalo M: Major amputation incidence decreases both in non-diabetic and in diabetic patients in Helsinki. Scand J Surg 2006;95:185–189.

19 Witsø E, Lium A, Lydersen S: Lower limb amputations in Trondheim, Norway. Acta Orthop 2010;81:737–744.

20 Larsson J, Eneroth M, Apelqvist J, Stenström A: Sustained reduction in major amputations in diabetic patients: 628 amputations in 461 patients in a defined population over a 20-year period. Acta Orthop 2008;79:665–673.

21 Holstein P, Ellitsgaard N, Olsen BB, Ellitsgaard V: Decreasing incidence of major amputations in people with diabetes. Diabetologia 2000;43:844–847.

22 Lombardo FL, Maggini M, De Bellis A, Seghieri G, Anichini R: Lower extremity amputations in persons with and without diabetes in Italy: 2001–2010. PLoS One 2014;9:e86405.

23 Almaraz MC, González-Romero S, Bravo M, et al: Incidence of lower limb amputations in individuals with and without diabetes mellitus in Andalusia (Spain) from 1998 to 2006. Diabetes Res Clin Pract 2012;95:399–405.

24 Calle-Pascual AL, Redondo MJ, Ballesteros M, Martinez-Salinas MA, Diaz JA, De Matias P, et al: Nontraumatic lower extremity amputations in diabetic and non-diabetic subjects in Madrid, Spain. Diabetes Metab 1997;23:519–523.

25 López-De-Andrés A, Martínez-Huedo MA, Carrasco-Garrido P, Hernández-Barrera V, Gil-de-Miguel A, Jiménez-García R: Trends in lower-extremity amputations in people with and without diabetes in Spain, 2001–2008. Diabetes Care 2011;34:1570–1576.

26 Kennon B, Leese GP, Cochrane L, et al: Reduced incidence of lower-extremity amputations in people with diabetes in Scotland: a nationwide study. Diabetes Care 2012;35:2588–2590.

27 Canavan RJ, Unwin NC, Kelly WF, et al: Diabetes and non-diabetes related lower extremity amputation incidence before and after the introduction of better organized diabetes foot care: continous longitudinal monitoring using a standard method. Diabetes Care 2008;31:459–463.

28 Krishnan S, Nash F, Baker N, et al: Reduction in diabetic amputations over 11 years in a defined U.K. population: benefits of multidisciplinary team work and continuous prospective audit. Diabetes Care 2008;31:99–101.

29 Buckley CM, O'Farrell A, Canavan RJ, et al: Trends in the incidence of lower extremity amputations in people with and without diabetes over a five-year period in the Republic of Ireland. PLoS One 2012;7:e41492.

30 Schofield CJ, Yu N, Jain AS, et al: Decreasing amputation rates in patients with diabetes – a population-based study. Diabet Med 2009;26:773–777.

31 Margolis D, Malay DS, Hoffstad OJ, et al: Incidence of Diabetic Foot Ulcer and Lower Extremity Amputation among Medicare Beneficiaries, 2006 to 2008. Rockville, Agency for Healthcare Research and Quality, 2011.

32 Margolis DJ, Hoffstad O, Nafash J, et al: Location, location, location: geographic clustering of lower-extremity amputation among Medicare beneficiaries with diabetes. Diabetes Care 2011;34:2363–2367.

33 Goldberg JB, Goodney PP, Cronenwett JL, et al: The effect of risk and race on lower extremity amputations among Medicare diabetic patients. J Vasc Surg 2012;56:1663–1668.

34 Tseng CL, Rajan M, Miller DR, et al: Use of administrative data to risk adjust amputation rates in a national cohort of medicare-enrolled veterans with diabetes. Med Care 2005;43:88–92.

35 Tseng CL, Rajan M, Miller DR, et al: Trends in initial lower extremity amputation rates among Veterans Health Administration health care system users from 2000 to 2004. Diabetes Care 2011;34:1157–1163.

36 Wrobel JS, Mayfield JA, Reiber GE: Geographic variation of lower-extremity major amputation in individuals with and without diabetes in the Medicare population. Diabetes Care 2001;24:860–864.

37 Tseng CL, Helmer D, Rajan M, et al: Evaluation of regional variation in total, major, and minor amputation rates in a national health-care system. Int J Qual Health Care 2007;19:368–376.

38 Carinci F, Massi Benedetti M, Klazinga NS, Uccioli L: Lower extremity amputation rates in people with diabetes as an indicator of health systems performance. A critical appraisal of the data collection 2000–2011 by the Organization for Economic Cooperation and Development (OECD). Acta Diabetol 2016;53:825–832.

39 Laclé A, Valero-Juan LF: Diabetes-related lower-extremity amputation incidence and risk factors: a prospective seven-year study in Costa Rica. Rev Panam Salud Publica 2012;32:192–198.

40 Fei YF, Wang C, Chen DW, et al: [Incidence and risk factors of amputation among inpatients with diabetic foot]. Zhonghua Yi Xue Za Zhi 2012;92:1686–1689.

41 Zubair M, Malik A, Ahmad J: Incidence, risk factors for amputation among patients with diabetic foot ulcer in a North Indian tertiary care hospital. Foot (Edinb) 2012;22:24–30.

42 Li X, Xiao T, Wang Y, et al: Incidence, risk factors for amputation among patients with diabetic foot ulcer in a Chinese tertiary hospital. Diabetes Res Clin Pract 2011;93:26–30.

43 Tchakonté B, Ndip A, Aubry P, Malvy D, Mbanya JC: [The diabetic foot in Cameroon]. Bull Soc Pathol Exot 2005;98:94–98.

44 Kidmas AT, Nwadiaro CH, Igun GO: Lower limb amputation in Jos, Nigeria. East Afr Med J 2004;81:427–429.

45 Ramachandran A: Specific problems of the diabetic foot in developing countries. Diabetes Metab Res Rev 2004;20:S19–S22.

46 Abbas ZG, Archibald LK: Epidemiology of the diabetic foot in Africa. Med Sci Monit 2005;11:RA262–RA270.

47 Abbas ZG, Gill GV, Archibald LK: The epidemiology of diabetic limb sepsis: an African perspective. Diabet Med 2002;19:575–579.

48 Tapp RJ, Zimmet PZ, Harper CA, et al: Diabetes care in an Australian population: frequency of screening examinations for eye and foot complications of diabetes. Diabetes Care 2004;27:688–693.

49 Payne CB, Scott RS: Hospital discharges for diabetic foot disease in New Zealand 1980–1993. Diabet Res Clin Pract 1998;39:69–74.

50 Davis WA, Norman PE, Bruce DG, et al: Predictors, consequences and costs of diabetes-related lower extremity amputation complicating type 2 diabetes: the Fremantle Diabetes Study. Diabetologia 2006;49:2634–2641.

51 Gulliford MC, Mahabir D: Diabetic foot disease and foot care in a Caribbean community. Diabetes Res Clin Pract 2002;56:35–40.

52 Pedrosa HC, Leme LA, Novaes C, et al: The diabetic foot in South America: progress with the Brazilian save the diabetic foot project. Int Diab Monitor 2004;16:10–16.

53 Jimenez JT, Palacios M, Cañete F, et al: Prevalence of diabetes mellitus and associated cardiovascular risk factors in an adult urban population in Paraguay. Diabet Med 1998;15:334–338.

54 Schaper NC, Apelqvist J, Bakker K: Reducing lower leg amputations in diabetes: a challenge for patients, healthcare providers and the healthcare system. Diabetologia 2012;55:1869–1872.

55 Jeffcoate WJ, van Houtum WH: Amputation as a marker of the quality of foot care in diabetes. Diabetologia 2004;47:2051–2058.

56 van Houtum WH, Rauwerda JA, Ruwaard D, Schaper NC, Bakker K: Reduction in diabetes-related lower-extremity amputations in The Netherlands: 1991–2000. Diabetes Care 2004;27:1042–1046.

57 Apelqvist J, Larsson J: What is the most effective way to reduce incidence of amputation in the diabetic foot? Diabetes Metab Res Rev 2000;16:S75–S83.

58 International Working Group on the Diabetic Foot 2015: International Consensus on the Diabetic Foot and Guidance on the Management and Prevention of the Diabetic Foot. The Hague, www.iwgdf.org (accessed September 1, 2015).

59 Rathur HM, Boulton AJM: The diabetic foot. Clin Dermatol 2007;25:109–120.
60 Walters DP, Gatling W, Mullee MA, Hill RD: The distribution and severity of diabetic foot disease: a community study with comparison to a non-diabetic group. Diabet Med 1992;9:354–358.
61 Moss SE, Klein R, Klein BE: The prevalence and incidence of lower extremity amputation in a diabetic population. Arch Intern Med 1992;152:610–616.
62 Borssén B, Bergenheim T, Lithner F: The epidemiology of foot lesions in diabetic patients aged 15–50 years. Diabet Med 1990;7:438–444.
63 de Sonnaville JJ, Colly LP, Wijkel D, Heine RJ: The prevalence and determinants of foot ulceration in type II diabetic patients in a primary health care setting. Diabetes Res Clin Pract 1997;35:149–156.
64 Malgrange D, Richard JL, Leymarie F: Screening diabetic patients at risk for foot ulceration. A multi-centre hospital-based study in France. Diabetes Metab 2003;29:261–268.
65 Fagot-Campagna A, Fosse S, Weil A, Simon D, Varroud-Vial M: Rétinopathie et neuropathie liées au diabète en France métropolitaine: dépistage, prévalence et prise en charge médicale, étude Entred 2001. Bull Epidemiol Hebd (Paris) 2005;12:48–50.
66 Detournay B, Cros S, Charbonnel B, Grimaldi A, Liard F, Cogneau J, et al: Managing type 2 diabetes in France: the ECODIA survey. Diabetes Metab 2000; 26:363–369.
67 Abbott CA, Carrington AL, Ashe H, Bath S, Every LC, Griffiths J, et al: The North-West Diabetes Foot Care Study: incidence of, and risk factors for, new diabetic foot ulceration in a community-based patient cohort. Diabet Med 2002;19:377–384.
68 Vozar J, Adamka J, Holeczy P: Diabetics with foot lesions and amputations in the region of Horny Zitmy Ostrov 1993–1995. Diabetologia 1997;40(suppl 1):A46.
69 Manes C, Papazoglou N, Sassidou E, Tzounas K: Prevalence of diabetic neuropathy and foot ulceration: a population-based study. Wounds 2002;14: 11–15.
70 Muller IS, de Grauw WJ, van Gerwen WH, Bartelink ML, van Den Hoogen HJ, Rutten GE: Foot ulceration and lower limb amputation in type 2 diabetic patients in Dutch primary health care. Diabetes Care 2002;25:570–574.
71 Ramsey SD, Newton K, Blough D, McCulloch DK, Sandhu N, Reiber GE, et al: Incidence, outcomes, and cost of foot ulcers in patients with diabetes. Diabetes Care 1999;22:382–387.
72 Al-Mahroos F, Al-Roomi K: Diabetic neuropathy, foot ulceration, peripheral vascular disease and potential risk factors among patients with diabetes in Bahrain: a nationwide primary care diabetes clinic-based study. Ann Saudi Med 2007;27:25–31.
73 Behhadj MA: La pace du pied diabetique [in French]. Diabetes Metab 1998;24(suppl):LXVII.
74 Pendsey S: Epidemiological aspects of the diabetic foot. Int J Diab Dev Countries 1994;2:37–38.
75 Gershater MA, Löndahl M, Nyberg P, et al: Complexity of factors related to outcome of neuropathic and neuroischaemic/ischaemic diabetic foot ulcers: a cohort study. Diabetologia 2008;52:398–407.

Jan Apelqvist, MD
Department of Endocrinology, University Hospital of Skåne
Jan Waldenströms gata 24, level 2
SE–205 02 Malmö (Sweden)
E-Mail Jan.Apelqvist@skane.se

Piaggesi A, Apelqvist J (eds): The Diabetic Foot Syndrome.
Front Diabetes. Basel, Karger, 2018, vol 26, pp 19–32 (DOI: 10.1159/000480041)

A Complication of the Complications: The Complexity of Pathogenesis and the Role of Co-Morbidities in the Diabetic Foot Syndrome

Marco Meloni · Valentina Izzo · Laura Giurato · Luigi Uccioli

Dipartimento di Medicina dei Sistemi, Università degli Studi di Roma Tor Vergata, Rome, Italy

Abstract

Diabetic foot syndrome (DFS) is considered the most severe and complicated framework of 2 diabetes-related long-term complications, peripheral neuropathy and peripheral arterial disease, and foot ulceration is usually their main clinical expression. Due to the presence of several co-morbidities, diabetic foot patients are often very fragile subjects and foot ulceration is usually only an aspect of a complex clinical condition. Diabetes-related chronic complications affecting other organs, mainly kidneys and heart, can deeply influence not only the patient's general health but also the outcomes of foot ulcers. Ulcer-related outcomes may be deeply influenced by co-morbidities associated with diabetic foot disease. Therefore, DFS not only requires a treatment plan addressing ulcers characteristics but also the assessment method of all co-morbidities that may influence the outcomes. A global approach is mandatory to reduce major amputations and increase survival among diabetic patients. The aim of this review is to describe the co-morbidities that influence the pathophysiology of the DFS and its outcomes. © 2018 S. Karger AG, Basel

Introduction

Diabetic foot syndrome (DFS) is considered the most severe consequence of 2 diabetes-related long-term complications, peripheral neuropathy (PN) and peripheral arterial disease (PAD), and foot ulceration is usually their main clinical expression. Diabetic foot ulcers (DFUs) affect up to 15% of the diabetic population along their life and represent the first reason for hospitalization, minor and major amputation among diabetic subjects [1, 2].

The prevalence of major amputation among diabetic subjects is approximately 4.8% involving more than 1 million people [3, 4] despite significant differences

existing between countries belonging to the Organization for Economic Cooperation and Development [5]. In more than 85% of cases, lower limb amputation is a complication of a foot lesion [6, 7].

Due to the presence of several co-morbidities, DFS patients are often very fragile and foot ulceration may only be a part of a very complex clinical condition. In these patients, long-standing diabetes may be responsible of chronic complications affecting other organs, that is, kidneys and heart. Kidneys and heart, by themselves, may deeply influence not only the general health of the patient but also the outcomes of foot ulceration.

DFS must be considered not only a local problem, characterized in many cases by a non-healing ulcer, but a complex systemic framework in which specific long-term complications (PN and PAD) are imbedded in the general health of the patient. Therefore, DFS requires not only an immediate recognition of ulcers aetiology to address the right therapeutic approach but also the assessment of all co-morbidities that may deeply influence the outcomes. The management of DFUs requires a global and multidisciplinary approach to reduce the risk of amputation and death.

Pathophysiology of Diabetic Foot

Diabetic foot is usually classified under neuropathic, ischaemic and neuro-ischaemic categories according to the prevalent chronic complication PN and/or PAD or coexistence of both. It is very important to make this differential diagnosis because the different conditions have different therapeutic approach and different outcomes [8]. In this review, we describe the pathophysiology of the 2 conditions, neuropathic and ischaemic foot, whereas in the clinical context, it is very difficult to find a pure neuropathic or a pure ischaemic foot, but it is very common to find the 2 chronic complications in a majority of the diabetic foot cases.

The neuropathic foot is the consequence of diabetic neuropathy and its 3 components: sensory, motor and autonomic. Motor neuropathy is responsible for the appearance of foot deformities related to the progressive atrophy of intrinsic muscles of the foot. The consequence of this is the protrusion of the metatarsal heads, the altered biomechanics of the walking cycle and the appearance of peak plantar pressures [9]. Sensory neuropathy is responsible for the reduced perception of pain during walking or even after a trauma [10, 11]. Furthermore, thermal discrimination can be lost with a high risk of burns [10]. Denervation of sweat glands due to autonomic neuropathy may cause dryness of the skin that may develop breaks and fissures [12]. In addition, autonomic neuropathy may be responsible of the impaired microcirculation response to cutaneous stimuli with the appearance of abnormal inflammatory responses to foot injuries [13]. PN is a risk factor for foot ulceration, and foot ulceration is the main clinical manifestation of neuropathic foot. Because of the specific pathophysiologic mechanisms, foot ulceration is localized in high-pressures areas, mainly at the level of

metatarsal heads; offloading is the treatment of choice and total contact cast is the gold standard. When a neuropathic lesion is adequately offloaded, it should heal in a reasonable time frame (4–6 weeks). The patient with a neuropathic lesion, in general, may be followed in an outpatient clinic setting unless an infection superimposes. In that case, the infection becomes the most important clinical condition, mainly if it is detrimental to the limb or life threatening.

Ischaemic foot is related to the presence of PAD, which is the most significant and independent risk factor for major amputation [8]. PAD in diabetic patients is usually very distal involving the area below the knee. It affects different arterial vessels and shows rapid progression [14, 15]. Lower limb ischaemia also increases the risk of foot infection [16]. Furthermore, diabetes per se increases the risk of infections [17–19].

Patients with ischaemic foot lesions have, in a majority of cases, very bad clinical conditions. PAD is accompanied by ischaemic heart disease in 50% of patients and by carotid disease in one fourth of these. Different levels of renal insufficiency may be present and the number of diabetic patients in dialysis treatment with critical limb ischaemia (CLI) is increasing.

These kinds of patients may not be followed as outpatient clinic patients, but they require hospitalization to be treated by revascularization, mainly in the presence of a non-healing ulcer or even worse, when an infection is superimposed and a gangrene has formed in part of the foot.

These patients are the most difficult to treat because of the presence of heart failure (HF) and/or renal insufficiency. Anaemia and malnutrition may also be present in many cases. In addition, a bad metabolic control may further complicate the clinical framework. Therefore, CLI in diabetic patients is not only detrimental to the limb but also threatening to the life, and its treatment may be crucial to patients' survival [20].

In the following sections, we describe separately these conditions, but the reader must have clear understanding that all these co-morbidities may be present at the same time in the same patient, leading to a condition that is very difficult to treat.

Impact of Co-Morbidities on DFS

Usually, literature related to diabetic foot focus on ulcer characteristics and their treatment, while very little space is dedicated to the impact of co-morbidities in patients with DFUs. Also, guidelines rarely deal with co-morbidities; when they do, they play a significant role in both the treatment and prognosis of DFU patients.

Only a few studies, to our knowledge, have systematically assessed the effects of patients' co-morbidities as well as foot and ulcer characteristics at baseline on DFU outcomes. Patients with DFUs are usually affected by several diabetes-related complications like visual impairment, neurological disorders, cardiovascular disease, PAD, cerebrovascular disease and chronic kidney disease. It is not simple to assess the incidence of different co-morbidities in patients affected by DFUs because different

studies have evaluated heterogeneous populations in terms of age, diabetes duration, etiology of ulcer and other cardiovascular risk factors.

Some interesting observations are reported by the EURODIALE study. It is an international collaborative network aimed to assess the major predictors of clinical outcome in a large sample of European patients with DFUs. One thousand two hundred two consecutive patients with a new foot ulcer were included in 14 diabetic foot clinics across Europe. The mean age of these patients was 64.7 and diabetes duration was >10 years in approximately 70% of patients. Polyneuropathy was present in 78.5% of cases, PAD in 47.5%, visual impairment in 15.3%, end-stage renal disease (ESRD) in 5.8% and HF in 10.9%. However, HF, ERSD and visual impairment showed a greater incidence in patients with PAD.

Furthermore, healing rates in patients with PAD were lower than those in patients without PAD. In addition, the presence of infection, which is generally considered a significant predictor of not healing and major amputation, was only predictive in individuals with PAD. Among the different co-morbidities, ESRD alone reduced the chance of healing [8].

Therefore, the first consideration that comes out from this close analysis is that patients with ischaemic DFUs show more co-morbidities than subjects with neuropathic DFUs and PAD reduces the chance of healing; therefore, the effect of infection on wound healing seems to be significant only in patients with PAD. Furthermore, renal impairment is a negative predictor of healing both in neuropathic and ischaemic ulcers.

Evidences about the role of co-morbidities can be extrapolated from a paper by Gershater et al. [21], where the complexity of factors related to the outcome of neuro-ischaemic/ischaemic DFUs was evaluated. Two thousand four hundred eighty patients were included and prospectively followed and treated until healing was achieved or death occurred. Among all predictors of healing, the absence of uraemia and heart disease was the clinical factor related to primary healing in all the population and in survivors. Nephropathy and uraemia were predictors of non-healing in survivor patients with ischaemic/neuroischaemic ulcers. Visual impairment and uraemia were related to minor and major amputations in neuropathic ulcers, while only uraemia was related to major amputation in ischaemic ulcers. This study highlights the role of co-morbidities in the outcomes of DFUs. Particularly, ESRD seems to negatively influence the outcome of each type of DFUs, increasing the risk of non-healing and minor or major amputation. Also, heart diseases increased the risk of non-healing of neuropathic and ischaemic DFUs. Furthermore, deceased patients showed more ischaemic ulcers and more co-morbidities than the other groups.

A recent paper of Alpeqvist highlights the potential role of co-morbidities in the outcomes of ischaemic DFUs. One thousand one hundred fifteen patients admitted to a multidisciplinary foot team because of ischaemic DFUs were prospectively followed until the final outcome (healing, amputation, death) was reached. Creatinine

values <130 µmol/L and the absence of congestive HF were positive predictors of primary healing. This analysis reinforces the role of renal impairment and HF in the prognosis of ischaemic DFUs [22].

Ghanassi et al. [23] reported the long-term outcomes of diabetic patients hospitalized for DFUs after 6.5 years of follow-up. Despite a satisfactory initial healing rate, the global long-term outcomes were poor. Approximately 52% of patients died and cardiovascular mortality was the main cause. Impaired renal function appeared to be an important marker of long-term prognosis, it being an independent predictor of healing failure, all-cause mortality and cardiovascular death. Nephropathy with albuminuria was associated with amputations.

Two interesting papers reported the long-term outcomes of diabetic patients with ischaemic foot ulcers and highlighted the role of co-morbidities as predictors of outcome. In the first one, Faglia et al., followed 554 patients with DFUs and CLI treated by revascularization. The mean follow-up after hospitalization was 6 years. With an annual incidence of 11.9%, 49.8% patients died; with an incidence per year of 3.7%, 13.4% patients received major amputation. Coronary artery disease (CAD) was the leading cause of death; dialysis and history of cardiac disease were predictors of death and were present among patients with cardiac disease; impaired ejection fraction was independently associated with death. Dialysis resulted also as an independent predictor of major amputation [24].

In a similar paper, our group followed 510 patients with DFUs and CLI treated by endovascular revascularization for a mean follow-up of 20 months. The rate of death and major amputation was, respectively, 16.2 and 15.7%. The overall analysis showed that dialysis and ischaemic heart diseases were more frequent among the deceased, amputees and not-healed patients than in healed patients. Furthermore, ischaemic heart disease was an independent predictor of non-healing [25].

Recently, we observed that our cohort of patients with ischaemic DFUs hospitalized from 2012 to 2016 showed high rates of co-morbidities: 80% had hypertension, 80% anaemia, 78% malnutrition, 76% dyslipidemia, 67% ischaemic heart disease, 48% nephropathy, 33% HF, and 32% ESRD under dialysis. We reported that patients with HF and dialysis had a very high risk of one-year mortality (56%) and the main causes of death were sepsis, high level of procalcitonin and congestive HF (unpublished data). The very interesting finding is that in the recent past, there was a significant increase in the number of patients with co-morbidities in comparison to the cohort of our patients evaluated less recently. We predominantly found a higher rate of ischaemic heart disease (68 vs. 41.8%) and dialysis (31.4 vs. 12.8%) in comparison to patients enrolled between 2002 and 2007 [25].

Therefore, the current patients show a more severe pattern of cardiovascular and renal disease than patients treated 10–15 years ago, and this new framework probably requires a greater effort for all clinicians working in the field of DFS.

Co-morbidities such as heart disease, CAD HF, and ESRD not only reduce the chance of healing and increase the risk of minor and major amputation, but also become independent predictors of mortality. Even if co-morbidities may be present in all DFU patients, they are more frequent in ischaemic/neuro-ischaemic patients than neuropathic patients, and ischaemic ulcers have worse outcomes in terms of amputation and death than not-ischaemic subjects. Therefore, renal function and heart function should always be assessed to ensure the correct treatment and guarantee the best prognosis of these fragile patients.

Impact of Dialysis on DFS

Renal disease and dialysis are independent strong factors for PAD [26]. The simultaneous presence of diabetes and dialysis significantly increases the risk of PAD. In diabetic-dialyzed patients, the prevalence of PAD reaches approximately 80% [27]. Furthermore, dialysis is an independent risk factor for foot ulceration, non-healing and amputation in diabetic subjects [8, 28–30]. A primary amputation rate of 44% has been reported in dialyzed diabetic patients with ischaemic foot lesions [31]. PAD in these patients is usually characterized by the involvement of the vessels below the knee and collateral vessels, widespread vascular calcification and impairment of microcirculation [32].

In a recent paper, our group confirmed that diabetic patients with ischaemic foot ulcers on dialysis have reduced chances of healing and higher risk of major amputation and death when compared to not-dialyzed patients [33].

The poor outcomes may be related to the complexity of vascular disease, the high risk of infection and the impairment mechanism of wound healing. We reported, in fact, 65% of limb salvage, 21% of mortality and 14% of major amputation after endovascular revascularization during a mean follow-up of 15 months, while the not-dialyzed patients had 78.2% of limb salvage, 10.8% of major amputation and 11% of death. In comparison to the not-dialysis group, patients on dialysis have a more severe vascular disease, more frequently a CAD, more heel ulcers, more steno-obstructions, higher risk of unsuccessful revascularization and were in need of more procedures to get limb salvage. However, it is hard to find a specific factor predictive of outcome in dialyzed subjects; therefore, we conclude that all diabetic-dialyzed patients with DFS have to be considered the highest risk patients as a whole.

In a large meta-analysis on diabetic-dialyzed patients with DFUs, Hinchliffe et al. [34] reports one-year limb salvage approximately of 70% among the survivors of a carefully selected group of patients to be revascularized. The long-term outcomes are poor: mortality, which is between 48 and 72% at 2 years, 56% at 3 years and 91% at 3 years.

Our results are similar to those reported by literature in terms of the percentage of limb salvage [33]. However, it must be highlighted that in these studies, the outcomes are referred only to patients revascularized after a careful selection, while the outcomes reported in our study refer to unselected consecutive patients. Dialysis and dialysis-related complications are able by itself to influence the prognosis, probably because of the severity of PAD, the impaired heart function and the impaired immune system with high risk of infection.

Impact of Heart Disease on DFS

Approximately 50% of diabetic patients with PAD show a simultaneous ischaemic heart disease [35]. Furthermore, in the last years, several papers have reported that the impairment of PAD in diabetic patients increases the risk of cardiovascular deaths [36].

The high rate of silent myocardial ischaemia in diabetic patients suggests for all patients with PAD the need of a cardiovascular screening to detect a possible CAD [37, 38].

Cardiac dysfunction appears to be common in DFUs patient, even in those without known heart disease. Löndahl et al. [39] reported that patients with chronic DFUs had in 69% of cases, myocardial infarction and/or hypertension and/or HF, in 78%, left ventricular dysfunction and/or hypertrophy and/or diastolic dysfunction and in 76%, echocardiographic signs of heart dysfunction in the absence of any history of cardiovascular disease.

To our knowledge, only one paper evaluated specifically the role of HF in hospitalized patients with DFUs. Xu et al. [40] documented that HF reduces the healing rate and increases the rate of ulcer recurrences, amputation and death. However, as reported earlier, the data recovered from different studies highlights the specific impact of CAD and HF in the prognosis of patients with DFUs, thereby becoming the main causes of death.

Therefore, it is clear that DFUs patients, mainly those with PAD, should be considered subjects with a high risk of CAD, left ventricular dysfunction and HF. Any pattern of cardiac disease has a significant influence on the outcome (non-healing, ulcer recurrence, major amputation) and increases obviously the risk of cardiovascular deaths in patients with DFS.

Impact of Nutritional Status on DFS

Extended wounds promote the loss of calories and proteins [41]. Poor nutritional status reduces regenerative capacity of tissues, and nutritional deficiency is related usually to poor clinical outcome.

Malnutrition is a common factor of wound chronicity [42]. Inadequate or excessive intake of calories, protein, fluid, or micronutrients is usually related to malnutrition. Old patients with severe co-morbidities, requiring continuous assistance, usually have a high risk of nutritional deficiency due to medical, psychological, social and economic aspects [43]. Weight loss, reduced subcutaneous fat and fluid accumulation are the first clinical signs of malnutrition as well as low or high values of body mass index [44].

Diagnostic markers of malnutrition in DFUs patients are not well defined, particularly in case of chronic inflammation or chronic ulcers. However, malnutrition should be always detected and adequate nutritional support ensured. Serum albumin, total lymphocytes, pre-albumin and transferrin <150 mg/dL are useful parameters to be evaluated [45, 46]. In particular, low values of albumin and weight loss are independent predictors of mortality and hospital complications [47].

Impact of Anaemia on DFS

Anaemia is common in patients with DFS. It can be related to age, diabetes, chronic kidney disease and chronic inflammatory status due to chronic wounds or infections. Low haemoglobin levels and low red blood cell count are found to be associated with major amputations [48]. Furthermore, mild or moderate anaemia has been associated with morbidity and mortality in patients with DFUs [49]. The role of anaemia is not completely clear. While the association between anaemia and diabetes is well known, its relationship and impact in DFS are less explained. It is probably a 2-way mechanism. DFUs are considered chronic inflammation and inflammation per se reduces myelogenesis. Infection can further reinforce this mechanism. On the other hand, it is possible that reduced levels of haemoglobin and peripheral oxygen can impair tissues repair. Iron has a beneficial action in wound healing due to its role as co-factor in collagen synthesis. Iron deficiency impairs T cells and phagocyte function in the inflammatory phase and decreased tensile strength and collagen synthesis during the proliferative phase [50]. Patients with iron deficiency-related anaemia benefit from iron supplementation. Patients with renal impairment and reduced erythropoiesis, mainly those on dialysis, usually need erythropoietin supplements.

Impact of Hyperglycemia on DFS

Persistent and uncontrolled hyperglycemia interferes with wound healing. The effect of hyperglycemia on the wound repair process is not referable to a single action. Endothelial dysfunction, proteins glycation, increased polyol pathway flux, negative nitrogen balance, increased activation of protein kinase C and increased hexosamine pathway flux may all play a significant role [51, 52].

It is well recognized that impaired glycaemic control in DFUs interferes with the hypoxia-inducible factor-1, a transcription factor able to adapt the cells' responses in case of hypoxia [53]. This abnormal condition can induce a pseudo-hypoxia influencing all the healing processes.

To our knowledge, currently, there are no studies to directly evaluate the impact of HbA1c on the outcomes of DFS. According to few studies, including ours, HbA1c is a predictor of major amputation [20, 25].

Hyperglycemia is also an independent risk factor for mortality in hospital patients with DFS. In fact, it promotes hospital infections, prothrombotic state and myocardial ischaemia [54]. In addition, it must be highlighted that superimposed infections of DFUs impair the metabolic control promoting hyperglycemia. Therefore, medical therapy, usually by insulin, should be adapted and in case of infection early debridement and antibiotic therapy have to be performed to remove the source infection and improve glycaemic control.

The Need of a Co-Morbidities Index in DFS

Several co-morbidities indexes have been developed to highlight the impact and severity of concomitant disease. They have been widely utilized by health researchers to measure burden of disease and case mix (i.e., Charlson Co-morbidity Index, Cumulative Illness Rating Scale, Index of Co-Existent Disease, Kaplan-Feinsten Index, ASA score). Among these, Charlson index is a valid prognostic indicator for mortality and it has also been used to define the risk of mortality in diabetic foot patients in some experimental cases (unpublished data). The preliminary results have shown its adaptability to be used also in these kinds of patients; however, it cannot be considered specific for DFS. However, the current co-morbidities indexes are not completely applicable to diabetic foot patients because they are usually related to cardiac risk in surgical patients. Furthermore, some specific parameters that influence the prognosis of diabetic foot patients are not completely analyzed in the majority of co-morbidities scores (i.e., ESRD, dialysis, infection).

Even if many variables can influence the outcomes of diabetic foot patients, we are of the opinion that it could be useful to develop a score for DFS to have an instrument able to define prognosis and consequently drive the treatment. Renal function, heart function, metabolic control, nutritional status and anaemia should be considered and evaluated in association with wound parameters such as infection and ischaemia, to roughly estimate the chance of limb salvage and the risk of major amputation and mortality.

A validated co-morbidities score could assist physicians in their selection of a suitable approach to treat patients with an infected-ischaemic foot. That is, this score helps physicians decide whether a limb salvage attempt is justified or whether primary amputation is preferred in order to reduce the risk of mortality due to high risk of sepsis or cardiac complications in fragile patients with several co-morbidities.

DFS and Mortality

Several observational studies have observed very high mortality rates in patients with DFUs [3]. It remains unclear if the excess of mortality observed reflects an increased cardiovascular risk or relates to ulcers consequences. Furthermore, long duration of diabetes is associated with greater risk foot ulceration [55] and adverse outcomes, including cardiovascular disease and all-cause mortality [56, 57].

While the cardiovascular deaths are higher in DFUs patients in comparison to diabetic patients without DFUs, the rate of cardiovascular mortality is similar in DFUs and diabetes-only patients [58]. Therefore, the excess of cardiovascular disease observed in DFS may only partly explain the reason behind the increased mortality rate. Probably, the high mortality in patients with DFUs may be explained by the advanced stage of diabetes, contextual co-morbidities and factors directly related to foot ulceration such as sepsis. Anyway, DFS should always be considered a strong risk factor for early-, middle- and long-term mortality. Particularly, ischaemic ulcers have shown a 5-year mortality approximately of 60% [59]. It is obvious that patients with DFUs are often fragile subjects and the appearance of foot ulceration could worsen their fragility.

Another aspect to be considered is the mortality status after a major amputation is performed. In fact, the rate of death in amputees is comparable to that observed in cancer patients [60].

A recent paper by Hoffstad et al. [61] confirms the increased mortality in a very large cohort of amputees, highlighting that co-morbidities may only partly justify this increased mortality. Also our group, evaluating the long-term outcomes related to a group of patients who underwent a limb salvage procedure, described a different mortality rate between amputee and healed patients [20]. Also, in this case, the co-morbidities could not explain the difference in amputation rates, suggesting that amputation by itself (because of unknown conditions, that is, lack of rehabilitation, depression, etc.) may explain the reason behind this increased mortality. Therefore, amputation never should be considered a fast solution for treating DFS, both by patients or health providers, unless a careful evaluation of the limb salvage options has been done [62].

Conclusion

On the basis of this overview, we highlight the following key points:

1. DFS is a complex condition characterized by the impairment of the peripheral nervous system and lower extremity blood perfusion that leads to foot ulcers and/or gangrene. Patients with DFS, particularly those with ischaemic ulcers, have several co-morbidities, mainly cardiovascular in nature.

2. The morbidity and mortality associated with diabetic foot lesions remain extremely high. Patients with DFUs have a higher risk of mortality than diabetic patients

without foot impairment. This greater mortality may be related to an advanced stage of diabetes with cardiovascular complications and to factors involved in foot ulceration such as sepsis and inflammation.

3. The role of co-morbidities in DFS is often underestimated even if it is well know that they can significantly influence both treatment patterns and outcomes of DFU patients. Usually, papers on DFUs report the outcomes according to ulcers' etiology but ulcer-related outcomes may underestimate the true morbidity and mortality associated with diabetic foot disease [63]. In a paper where ulcer- and person-related outcomes were compared, Jeaffcoate et al. found that almost 60% of ulcers healed at some stage, but only 45% of patients were alive and ulcer-free (with or without amputation) after 12 months of follow-up. Therefore, to evaluate the real impact of DFS on early- and long-term outcomes, a greater emphasis should be addressed to patient-related outcome measures.

4. Several complex factors are related to the outcomes of patients with DFUs: duration of disease, extent of tissue involvement and severity of PVD were strongly related to the probability of primary healing. However, data from different papers on DFUs showed that co-morbidities do play a key role in determining the outcomes of patients with DFS, particularly, the presence of ESRD and heart disease, increase in the risk of mortality and major amputation in all patients, more specially in subjects with ischaemic ulcers. These findings highlight that DFS should be recognized as a sign of underlying multi-organ disease.

5. Evidences suggest that nutritional status, anaemia and hyperglycemia deeply influence wound healing, major amputation and mortality in hospitalized patients.

6. In order to reduce the mortality associated to DFS, patients need an intensive global management and a multidisciplinary approach. Particularly, after revascularization of ischaemic foot ulcers, control of cardiovascular risk factors and medical management with dual antiplatelet therapy and statin is mandatory to both reduce the recurrence of CLI and improve survival [64]. In this context, a close follow-up is required. It has been reported that patients receiving clinical follow-up have better outcomes than patients who did not receive a periodical monitoring [20]. This may be related to improved control of all clinical factors: glycaemia, nutrition, renal functions, cardiovascular parameters. Therefore, a limb salvage protocol combined of surgical ulcers treatment, appropriate lower limb revascularization and close clinical follow-up appears to increase the rate of foot ulcer healing and improve long-term outcomes. Furthermore, prevention should be reinforced, particularly in highest risk patients. In this regard, guidelines should consider dialysis as an important risk factor for foot ulceration requiring intensive foot care.

7. A DFS co-morbidities index might be useful to highlight the individual risk and to help clinicians in the defining the best treatment. Obviously, personal experience on case by case basis should be the best guide for clinicians.

References

1 Reiber GE, Boyko EJ, Smith DG: Lower extremity foot ulcers and amputations in diabetes; in Diabetes in America, ed 2. Washington, US Government Printing Office, NIH Publication, 1995, Chapter 18, pp 409–428.

2 Frykberg RG, Haabershaw GM, Chrzan JS: Epidemiology of the diabetic foot: ulcerations and amputations; in Contemporary Endocrinology. Clinical Management of Diabetic Neuropathy, 1998, vol 7, pp 273–290.

3 Boulton AJ, Vileikyte L, Ragnarson-Tennvall G, Apelqvist J: The global burden of diabetic foot disease. Lancet 2005;336:1719–1724.

4 Johannesson A, Larsson GU, Ramstrand N, Turkiewicz A, Wiréhn AB, Atroshi I: Incidence of lower-limb amputation in the diabetic and nondiabetic general population: a 10-year population-based cohort study of initial unilateral and contralateral amputations and reamputations. Diabetes Care 2009;32:275–280.

5 Carinci F, Massi Benedetti M, Klazinga NS, Uccioli L: Lower extremity amputation rates in people with diabetes as an indicator of health systems performance. A critical appraisal of the data collection 2000–2011 by the Organization for Economic Cooperation and Development (OECD). Acta Diabetol 2016;53:825–832.

6 US Department of Health and Human Services: Diabetes Surveillance, 1997. Atlanta, Venters for Disease Control and Prevention, 1997.

7 American Diabetes Association: Diabetes Facts and Figures. Alexandria, American Diabetes Association, 2000.

8 Prompers L, Schaper N, Apelqvist J, Edmonds M, Jude E, Mauricio D, Uccioli L, Urbancic V, Bakker K, Holstein P, Jirkovska A, Piaggesi A, Ragnarson-Tennvall G, Reike H, Spraul M, Van Acker K, Van Baal J, Van Merode F, Ferreira I, Huijberts M: Prediction of outcome in individuals with diabetic foot ulcers: focus on the differences between individuals with and without peripheral arterial disease. The EURODIALE Study. Diabetologia 2008;51:747–755.

9 Boulton AJM: Peripheral neuropathy and the diabetic foot. The Foot 1992, vol 2, pp 67–72.

10 Litzelman DK, Marriott DJ, Vinicor F: Independent physiological predictors of foot lesions in patients with NIDDM. Diabetes Care 1997;20:1273–1278.

11 Macfarlane RM, Jeffcoate WJ: Factors contributing to the presentation of diabetic foot ulcers. Diabet Med 1997;14:867–870.

12 Edmonds ME: The neuropathic foot in diabetes. Part I: Blood flow. Diabet Med 1986;3:111–115.

13 Flynn MD, Tooke JE: Diabetic neuropathy and the microcirculation. Diabet Med 1995;12:298–301.

14 American Diabetes Association. Peripheral arterial disease in people with diabetes. Diabetes Care 2003;26:3333–3341.

15 Jude EB, Oyibo SO, Chalmers N, Boulton AJ: Peripheral arterial disease in diabetic and non diabetic patients: a comparison of severity and outcome. Diabetes Care 2001;24:1433–1437.

16 Shah BR, Hux JE: Quantifying the risk of infectious diseases for people with diabetes. Diabetes Care 2003;26:510–513.

17 Sato N, Shimizu H, Suwa K, Shimomura Y, Kobayashi I, Mori M: MPO activity and generation of active O2 species in leukocytes from poorly controlled diabetic patients. Diabetes Care 1992;15:1050–1052.

18 Marhoffer W, Stein M, Maeser E, Federlin K: Impairment of polymorphonuclear leukocyte function and metabolic control of diabetes. Diabetes Care 1992;15:256–260.

19 Muchová J, Liptáková A, Országhová Z, Garaiová I, Tison P, Cársky J, Duracková Z: Antioxidant systems in polymorphonuclear leucocytes of type 2 diabetes mellitus. Diabet Med 1999;16:74–78.

20 Giurato L, Vainieri E, Meloni M, Izzo V, Ruotolo V, Fabiano S, Pampana E, Lipsky B, Gandini R, Uccioli, L: Limb salvage in patients with diabetes is not a temporary solution but a life-changing procedure. Diabetes care 2015;38:e156–e157.

21 Gershater MA, Löndahl M, Nyberg P, Larsson J, Thörne J, Eneroth M, Apelqvist J: Complexity of factors related to outcome of neuropathic and neuroischaemic/ischaemic diabetic foot ulcers: a cohort study. Diabetologia 2009;52:398–407.

22 Apelqvist J, Elgzyri T, Larsson J, Löndahl M, Nyberg P, Thörne J: Factors related to outcome of neuroischemic/ischemic foot ulcer in diabetic patients. J Vasc Surg 2011;53:1582–1588.

23 Ghanassia E, Villon L, Thuan Dit Dieudonné JF, Boegner C, Avignon A, Sultan A: Long-term outcome and disability of diabetic patients hospitalized for diabetic foot ulcers: a 6.5-year follow-up study. Diabetes care 2008;31:1288–1292.

24 Faglia E, Clerici G, Clerissi J, Gabrielli L, Losa S, Mantero M, Caminiti M, Curci V, Quarantiello A, Lupattelli T, Morabito A: Long-term prognosis of diabetic patients with critical limb ischemia: a population-based cohort study. Diabetes care 2009;32:822–827.

25 Uccioli L, Gandini R, Giurato L, Fabiano S, Pampana E, Spallone V, Vainieri E, Simonetti G: Long-term outcomes of diabetic patients with critical limb ischemia followed in a tertiary referral diabetic foot clinic. Diabetes Care 2010;33:977–982.

26 Norgren L, Hiatt WR, Dormandy JA, Nehler MR, Harris KA, Fowkes FG; TASC II Working Group, Bell K, Caporusso J, Durand-Zaleski I, Komori K, Lammer J, Liapis C, Novo S, Razavi M, Robbs J, Schaper N, Shigematsu H, Sapoval M, White C, White J, Clement D, Creager M, Jaff M, Mohler E 3rd, Rutherford RB, Sheehan P, Sillesen H, Rosenfield K: Inter-society consensus for the management of peripheral arterial disease (TASC II). Eur J Vasc Endovasc Surg 2007;33(Suppl 1):S1–S75.
27 Schleiffer T, Hölken H, Brass H: Morbidity in 565 type 2 diabetic patients according to stage of nephropathy. J Diabetes Complications 1998;12:103–109.
28 Ndip A, Lavery LA, Boulton AJ: Diabetic foot disease in people with advanced nephropathy and those on renal dialysis. Curr Diab Rep 2010;10:283–290.
29 Jaar BG, Astor BC, Berns JS, Powe NR: Predictors of amputation and survival following lower extremity revascularization in hemodialysis patients. Kidney Int 2004;65:613–620.
30 Albers M, Romiti M, Braganca Pereira CA, Fonseca RL, da Silva Junior M: A meta-analysis of infrainguinal arterial reconstruction in patients with end-stage renal disease. Eur J Vasc Endovasc Surg 2001;22:294–300.
31 Lepäntalo M, Fiengo L, Biancari F: Peripheral arterial disease in diabetic patients with renal insufficiency: a review. Diabetes Metab Res Rev 2012;28:40–45.
32 Graziani L, Silvestro A, Bertone V, et al: Percutaneous transluminal angioplasty is feasible and effective in patients on chronic dialysis with severe peripheral artery disease. Nephrol Dial Transplant 2007;22:1144–1149.
33 Meloni M, Giurato L, Izzo V, Stefanini M, Pampana E, Gandini R, Uccioli L: Long term outcomes of diabetic haemodialysis patients with critical limb ischemia and foot ulcer. Diabetes Res Clin Pract 2016;116:117–122.
34 Hinchliffe RJ, Andros G, Apelqvist J, Bakker K, Friederichs S, Lammer J, Lepantalo M, Mills JL, Reekers J, Shearman CP, Valk G, Zierler RE, Schaper NC: A systematic review of the effectiveness of revascularization of the ulcerated foot in patients with diabetes and peripheral arterial disease. Diabetes Metab Res Rev 2012;28(suupl 1):179–217.
35 Ouriel K: Peripheral arterial disease. Lancet 2001;358:1257–1264.
36 Norman PE, Davis WA, Bruce DG, Davis TM: Peripheral arterial disease and risk of cardiac death in type 2 diabetes: the Fremantle Diabetes Study. Diabetes Care 2006;29:575–580.
37 Nesto RW, Watson FS, Kowalchuk GJ, Zarich SW, Hill T, Lewis SM, Lane SE: Silent myocardial ischemia and infarction in diabetics with peripheral vascular disease: assessment by dipyridamole thallium-201 scintigraphy. Am Heart J 1990;120:1073–1077.
38 Zellweger MJ: Prognostic significance of silent coronary artery disease in type 2 diabetes. Herz 2006;31:240–245.
39 Löndahl M, Katzman P, Fredholm O, Nilsson A, Apelqvist J: Is chronic diabetic foot ulcer an indicator of cardiac disease? J Wound Care 2008;17:12–16.
40 Xu L, Qian H, Gu J, Shi J, Gu X, Tang Z: Heart failure in hospitalized patients with diabetic foot ulcers: Clinical characteristics and their relationship with prognosis. J Diabetes 2013;5:429–438.
41 Langer G, Fink A: Nutritional interventions for preventing and treating pressure ulcers. Cochrane Database Syst Rev 2014;6:CD003216.
42 Thompson C, Fuhrman MP: Nutrients and wound healing: still searching for the magic bullet. Nutr Clin Pract 2005;20:331–347.
43 Pirlich M, Lochs H: Nutrition in the elderly. Best Pract Res Clin Gastroenterol 2001;15:869–884.
44 White JV, Guenter P, Jensen G, Malone A, Schofield M; Academy of Nutrition and Dietetics Malnutrition Work Group; A.S.P.E.N. Malnutrition Task Force; A.S.P.E.N. Board of Directors: Consensus statement of the academy of nutrition and dietetics/American society for parenteral and enteral nutrition: characteristics recommended for the identification and documentation of adult malnutrition (undernutrition). J Acad Nutr Diet 2012;112:730–738.
45 Yue DK, Swanson B, McLennan S, Marsh M, Spaliviero J, Delbridge L, Reeve T, Turtle JR: Abnormalities of granulation tissue and collagen formation in experimental diabetes, uraemia and malnutrition. Diabet Med 1986;3:221–225.
46 Raffaitin C, Lasseur C, Chauveau P, Barthe N, Gin H, Combe C, Rigalleau V: Nutritional status in patients with diabetes and chronic kidney disease: a prospective study. Am J Clin Nutr 2007;85:96–101.
47 Combe C, Chauveau P, Laville M, Fouque D, Azar R, Cano N, Canaud B, Roth H, Leverve X, Aparicio M; French Study Group Nutrition in Dialysis: Influence of nutritional factors and hemodialysis adequacy on the survival of 1,610 French patients. Am J Kidney Dis 2001;37:S81–S88.
48 Harwant S, Doshi HK, Moissinac K, Abdullah BT: Factors related to adverse outcome in inpatients with diabetic foot. Med J Malaysia 2000;55:236–241.
49 Chuan F, Zhang M, Yao Y, Tian W, He X, Zhou B: Anemia in patients with diabetic foot ulcer: prevalence, clinical characteristics, and outcome. Int J Low Extrem Wounds 2016;15:220–226.

50 Stechmiller J: Wound healing; in Mueller CM (ed). A.S.P.E.N. Adult Nutrition Support Core Curriculum. ed 2. Silver Spring, MD, American Society for Parenteral and Enteral Nutrition, 2012 pp 348–363.

51 McMurry JF Jr: Wound healing with diabetes mellitus. Better glucose control for better wound healing in diabetes. Surg Clin North Am 1984;64:769–778.

52 Hempel A, Maasch C, Heintze U, Lindschau C, Dietz R, Luft FC, Haller H: High glucose concentrations increase endothelial cell permeability via activation of protein kinase C alpha. Circ Res 1997;81:363–371.

53 Catrina SB, Okamoto K, Pereira T, Brismar K, Poellinger L: Hyperglycemia regulates hypoxia-inducible factor-1alpha protein stability and function. Diabetes 2004;53:3226–3232.

54 Owen RJ, Hiremath S, Myers A, Fraser-Hill M, Barrett BJ: Canadian association of radiologists consensus guidelines for the prevention of contrast-induced nephropathy: update 2012. Can Assoc Radiol J 2014;65:96–105.

55 Pham H, Armstrong DG, Harvey C, Harkless LB, Giurini JM, Veves A: Screening techniques to identify people at high risk for diabetic foot ulceration: a prospective multicenter trial. Diabetes Care 2000;23:606–611.

56 Silbernagel G, Rosinger S, Grammer TB, Kleber ME, Winkelmann BR, Boehm BO, März W: Duration of type 2 diabetes strongly predicts all-cause and cardiovascular mortality in people referred for coronary angiography. Atherosclerosis 2012;221:551–557.

57 Wannamethee SG, Shaper AG, Whincup PH, Lennon L, Sattar N: Impact of diabetes on cardiovascular disease risk and all-cause mortality in older men: influence of age at onset, diabetes duration, and established and novel risk factors. Arch Intern Med 2011;171:404–410.

58 Brownrigg JR, Davey J, Holt PJ, Davis WA, Thompson MM, Ray KK, Hinchliffe RJ: The association of ulceration of the foot with cardiovascular and all-cause mortality in patients with diabetes: a meta-analysis. Diabetologia 2012;55:2906–2912.

59 Armstrong DG, Wrobel J, Robbins JM: Guest editorial: are diabetes-related wounds and amputations worse than cancer? Int Wound J 2007;4:286–287.

60 Hoffmann M, Kujath P, Flemming A, Proß M, Begum N, Zimmermann M, Keck T, Kleemann M, Schloericke E: Survival of diabetes patients with major amputation is comparable to malignant disease. Diab Vasc Dis Res 2015;12:265–271.

61 Hoffstad O, Mitra N, Walsh J, Margolis DJ: Diabetes, lower-extremity amputation, and death. Diabetes Care 2015;38:1852–1857.

62 Uccioli L, Giurato L, Meloni M, Izzo V, Ruotolo V, Gandini R, Lipsky B: Comment on Hoffstad et al. diabetes, lower-extremity amputation, and Death. Diabetes Care 2016;39:e7.

63 Jeffcoate WJ, Chipchase SY, Ince P, Game FL: Assessing the outcome of the management of diabetic foot ulcers using ulcer-related and person-related measures. Diabetes care 2006;29:1784–1787.

64 De Martino RR, Eldrup-Jorgensen J, Nolan BW, Stone DH, Adams J, Bertges DJ, Cronenwett JL, Goodney PP; Vascular Study Group of New England: Perioperative management with antiplatelet and statin medication is associated with reduced mortality following vascular surgery. J Vasc Surg 2014;59:1615–1621, 1621.e1.

Prof. Luigi Uccioli
Dipartimento di Medicina dei Sistemi
Università degli Studi di Roma Tor Vergata
Viale Oxford 81
IT–00133 Rome (Italy)
E-Mail luccioli@yahoo.com

Piaggesi A, Apelqvist J (eds): The Diabetic Foot Syndrome.
Front Diabetes. Basel, Karger, 2018, vol 26, pp 33–47 (DOI: 10.1159/000480047)

Re-Evaluating the Outcomes in Diabetic Foot Management

Giacomo Clerici[a] · Elisabetta Iacopi[b] · Maurizio Santi Caminiti[a] ·
Andrea Casini[a] · Vincenzo Curci[a] · Ezio Faglia[c] · Alberto Piaggesi[b]

[a]Diabetic Foot Center, Humanitas University Hospitals, Bergamo and Milan, [b]Diabetic Foot Section,
Department of Medicine, University of Pisa, Pisa, [c]DEA Medica Onlus, Salerno, Italy

Abstract
The diabetic foot syndrome represents a relatively recent field of scientific interest: since the beginning the double origin of the disease has been evident: neuropathy and arteriopathy act together. In such a complex disease, the need for a "clinic" approach by a multidisciplinary team becomes evident. This approach requires the identification of goals for the creation and the development of a diabetic foot care network. Diabetic foot research and consensus organisms identified therefore three main targets: complete healing of the diabetic foot ulceration, limb salvage, and thus the possibility to walk without prosthesis, and, eventually, the improvement of life expectations. In recent years, these outcomes have been widely discussed. The complexity of patients, the wide variety of clinical conditions and the impact of diabetic foot on survival, quality of life and costs, let physicians move from an evidence-based medicine to a patient-oriented approach. Thus, new outcomes have been considered to take into account not only the evolution of the wound but also its impact on patient quality of life and independence status.   © 2018 S. Karger AG, Basel

Introduction

The International Diabetes Federation estimates that in 2040 one in 10 adults worldwide will be affected with diabetes mellitus [1]. It has been estimated that one limb is amputated every 20 s on the planet because of diabetes-related lower limb complications such as formation of gangrene, necrosis or ulcerations [2]. Diabetes can thus be considered the most frequent cause of lower extremity amputation (LEA) in the world, resulting in the loss of approximately 4,000 limbs every day [3].

One out of four of diabetic patients will develop a lower limb ulceration during their life and about one third of them will undergo an amputation with a relative risk of LEA 20-fold higher than general population [4]. The presence of diabetic foot is usually associated with the presence and higher severity of other chronic complications and of other important co-morbidities [5]. Furthermore, diabetic foot patients carry a mortality risk about two-fold higher compared to the general diabetic population. Diabetic foot should thus be considered not only a marker of severity in patients with diabetes but also a risk factor in terms of both LEAs and patient's life [6].

Despite its clinical relevance, which is so obvious today, foot disease and lower limb diabetes complications represent a relatively recent field of research [7]. The history of the diabetic foot has been built by far-sighted pioneers who have been able to see the way forward and have put some milestones in our approach to this pathology [8]. Since the very beginning, the double origin of the disease has been evident: in the fifties of the nineteenth century, Jean Martin Charcot began to focus on the damage that diabetes caused to nerve structures. In addition to motor impairment, he described tingling, burning and impaired sense of touch and heat. With the systematic study of diabetic neuropathy, the foot became a "target organ" with an increase in the development of plantar lesions; Charcot by analogy with its previously described "foot from tabe" would speak about "neuropathic foot" [9]. A few years later, some German scientists introduced the concept of diabetic gangrene. The dysvascular foot was considered a local manifestation of sclerotic macroangiopathy, whose clinical course can be accelerated by diabetes [10]. The diabetic foot patient appeared immediately as a rather complex patient who deserved to be managed, by a "multidisciplinary team" with an "integrated approach" [11]. The idea was that such a serious and fragile patient had to be managed by several professionals acting together in concert: not only physicians and nurses, but also podiatrists, surgeons, shoe-fitters. Along the following years, the concept became even more clear and detailed: different specialists had to be involved in the management of a diabetic foot patient: diabetologists, vascular surgeons, radiologists, infectious disease specialists, orthopedic surgeons, cardiologists. As a result, the "foot clinic" was born [12]. The clinic had to take care of all the aspects of patients' management: from the screening of the patients at an increased risk of ulceration, to the management of acute phases, up to the complete re-epithelialization and beyond, in the secondary prevention period. The aim of the clinic and of the multidisciplinary team is to consider the foot ulcer not just as a local manifestation but as a sign of a multi-organ disease in a chronic, fragile patient [13]. As Apelqvist [14] stated about the need to reach a holistic approach: "the assessment should be done at three different levels, each with the same relevance: the patient, the leg and the wound."

Although there has been much progress in our understanding of the etiopathogenesis and management of diabetic foot disorders over the last 30 years, a solid evidence-based thorough strategy is still missing. For this reason, International study groups involved in diabetes and wound management strongly recommend the planning and reporting of prospective randomized controlled trials in the prevention and management of diabetic foot lesions [15]. In such a complex and articulated setting, the identification of goals, even if very hard to reach, is a fundamental prerequisite to the

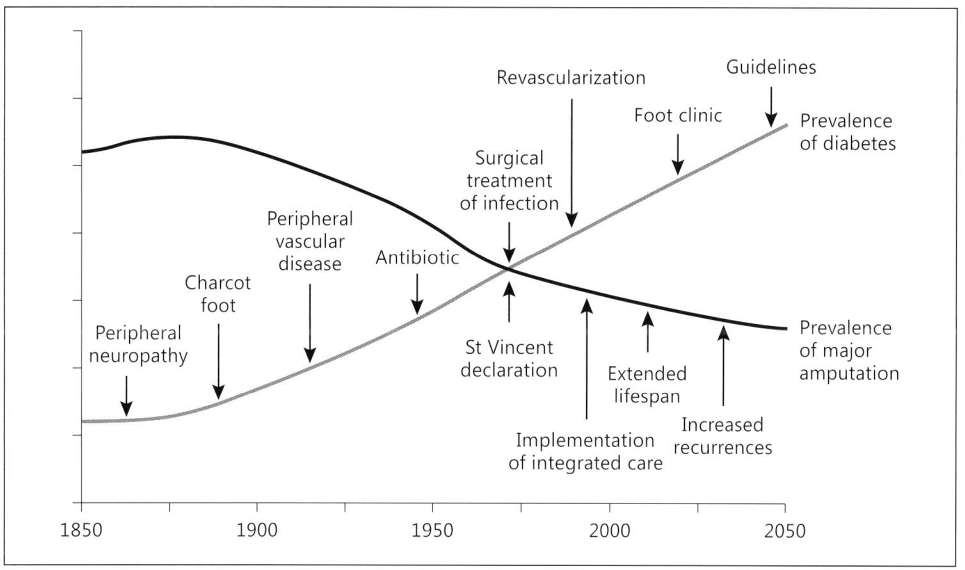

Fig. 1. Trends in the prevalence of diabetes and LEAs. The increasing prevalence of diabetes and its complications at the lower limb actually did not produce an increase of LEAs but actually a reduction due to the improvement of treatment strategies. More recently, the extension of lifespan and reduction in recurrences led to a "plateau" of LEAs.

creation and the development of a diabetic foot care network. This is in addition to considering that the larger study ever performed on diabetic foot disease, by the European Study Group on diabetes and the lower extremity (Eurodiale), demonstrated how a multidisciplinary approach, including prevention, patient and staff education, multidisciplinary treatment of ulcers, and close monitoring, could significantly improve the evolution of such patients. In particular, it ameliorated the limb salvage reducing amputation rates by 49–85% [16].

Diabetic foot research and consensus organisms identified therefore 3 main goals in the foot care: complete healing of the diabetic foot ulceration (DFU), limb salvage, and thus the possibility to walk without prosthesis, and eventually, the improvement of life expectations [17]. Perhaps, the time has come for a reappraisal of our action in trying to reach these outcomes and for an evaluation of their adequacy. In Figure 1, a schematic representation of the diabetic foot history and the limb outcome according to the evolution of our knowledge and technical possibilities can be observed.

The Limits of the Traditional Outcomes

Although they contributed very much in defining the quality of care and in setting the standards of care in diabetic foot management, the traditional outcomes in many cases do not reflect any more the reality of this pathology because of the chronicity of the disease, aging of the patients and the presence and severity of multiple co-morbidities, all factors that interfere with the management and outcomes of this patients with an increasing level of complexity.

Healing
The achievement and maintenance of complete healing of DFU (defined as complete and durable re-epithelization) can sometimes be very difficult to obtain and the time needed can be long and a rather stressful experience for the patient. As predictable, healing rates and healing times reported by many studies are very different according to the characteristics of the recruited patients [18]. Not only depending on the etiopathogenesis of the wound, in particular, the presence of critical limb ischaemia [19], but also, for example, on its localization within the foot: toes ulcers present a very different healing pattern when compared to midfoot ones, while the heel is very different from all the other regions for its peculiar characteristics [20, 21]. Furthermore, the different therapies performed had an impact on the chance to reach the healing target [22]. Eventually, the important impact of the infection, especially in case of deep infection, is that the expected healing rate is likely to decrease from 40 to 55% [23].

To achieve the healing of a lesion is obviously the main target that needs to be aspired. In recent years, many studies focused on the creation of a predictive model that would allow physicians to identify the characteristics associated with wound healing: from a successful revascularization procedure to infection control through early referral to third-level centres [24, 25].

When eventually the lesion heals, the patient begins a battle against the risk of recurrence [26]. Also in this area, our weapons are quite weak: different trials demonstrated an average prevalence of re-ulceration in about 40–60% of patients [27]. Since recurrences are so common after the healing of neuropathic or neuro-ischaemic DFU, it has been suggested that patients with a history of DFU should be described as having "a foot in remission" rather than healed. This might better communicate the risk of recurrence not only to the patient but also to other healthcare professionals [15].

The failure in achieving ulcer healing is associated with the worsening of the patient's health status, thereby reducing the quality of life and adherence to recommended self-care regimens [28]. Furthermore, it increases the long-term costs for patients' management [29]. Eventually, the presence of an ulcer, as predictable, represents the first risk factor for amputation, so its resolution has to be considered the main goal for physicians [30].

Life Expectation
It is nowadays well established that diabetic foot represents not only a local manifestation of disease, as a mirror of a systemic involvement, but rather a marker of a multiorgan complex and severe pathology. Diabetic patients with foot ulcers are at a higher risk of death, especially for cardiovascular causes, so that the foot disease can be considered a cardiovascular death risk marker [31].

During the previous years, several large trials tried to identify predictive factors that could stratify patients according to the risk of death: results are quite variable but some cornerstones have been detected [32]. The number and severity of co-morbidities are associated to an increased mortality risk, particularly regarding the history of cardiovascular disease [33, 34]. Despite this, surprisingly, there is still uncertainty about the influence of medical therapies on this cardiovascular death risk: according to some widely debated studies, coronary angioplasty would not be able to increase survival when performed in diabetic patients [35].

The presence of critical limb ischaemia is considered another important predictive factor, but luckily in this setting, our intervention can bring a significant improvement: a successful lower limb revascularization in these patients not only allows limb salvage but also is related to an increase in life expectation [36].

Eventually death and major amputation are indissolubly linked to each other and this linkage has been demonstrated by a wide range of literature data [37]. Patients submitted to major amputation are affected by an increased risk of death. This level of risk is directly correlated to the level of amputation, higher for more proximal intervention [37], and the risk curve fits suddenly after the intervention and remains high until 3 or 5 years after the procedure [38].

We are far from identifying parameters that would allow us to reduce, when correctly applied, the risk of death in our patients. The only evidence available underlines that our strongest weapon is the "holistic approach" to our patients, which takes into account all aspects of their management: from glycometabolic disturbances control to surgical management, through vascular assessment, control of infection, offloading strategies and co-morbidities evaluation [39].

A Paradigm Shift

In recent years, a different philosophy found its place in medicine: from an evidence-based practice, we are moving to a patient-oriented approach. From the search for medical golden standards adaptable to a patients' cohort as wide as possible, we are nowadays searching for targeted therapy guidelines. After the identification of the most useful therapeutic approaches to the different pathologies, medical science is now trying to understand when these approaches are more effective and when their use is not really the gold option for a patient [40]. Diabetic foot disease, as a paradigmatic multifactorial pathology, represents the typical environment in which, once the knowledge regarding the best treatments for different clinical pictures has been acquired, physicians have begun to ask themselves as to when these options were indeed the best choice to be given to patients [41].

In such a contest, it is important to understand whether the goals we have set ourselves for decades are truly to be pursued anyway. To do this, we have to reflect on our patients changing characteristics and on the methods we used to reach these goals.

Diabetic Foot Classification

Standardization of treatment has been for decades an unmet goal in diabetic foot management. Large studies had revealed the deep differences between centres and had related these discrepancies to a gap in obtaining good long-term outcomes [42]. To address this issue, diabetic foot specialists developed classification systems that could stratify patients in different groups according to the severity of the pathology to help homogenize the treatment strategies between the different centres.

As expected, the different classifications were based on various parameters, according to the expertise of the authors, and gave variable weightages to the different elements. A number of classifications thus became available for foot lesions overall, for osteomyelitis, critical limb ischaemia, local infection and nearly for all the characteristics related to diabetic foot disease [43].

Many of these classifications, related to a new field, such as diabetic foot has been for decades based on parameters developed among the general population, not always directly applicable to diabetic patients. These characteristics are typical of the classification for critical limb ischaemia. The concept of critical limb ischaemia was actually developed in the 1980s and its creator clearly stated that it would not apply to diabetic patients [44]. Despite this instruction, in the last 40 years, we have widely adopted these terms and classified diabetic patients according to this idea [45]. Furthermore, regarding peripheral arterial disease, some of the more ancient, widely adopted and apparently validated classifications are based on "pain" and this again is a flawed concept in diabetes [46]. Due to neuropathy, ischaemic patients are frequently insensitive: they rarely develop intermittent claudication and also rest pain, when present, appears during the very late phases of the disease, usually when foot lesions have developed [47].

The same can be said about diabetic foot infection classifications, which gave strong weightage to parameters such as fever, leukocytosis or increase in the number of inflammation parameters. It is well known, since almost 15 years, that due to concomitant immunodeficiency, just slightly less than half of diabetic patients in case of infection present with detectable systemic signs [48].

Therefore, rather than providing orientation, the classification may only confuse the clinician. Eventually, most of the classifications also showed other limits: first of all, they focused only on one of the different components of diabetic foot disease, disregarding the others; then they were aimed at stratifying patients rather than correlating the severity of the disease with the therapeutic approach and to the expected outcomes.

Patients' Evolution

Since the discovery of insulin, diabetic patients did not have to endure acute complications for long durations; however, they were affected by chronic complications of the disease, both micro and macrovascular, thereby changing a rapidly fatal acute disease into a chronic disabling condition. This happens within a population that is progressively getting older: the average age increased of a decade in just a generation [49]. Therefore, diabetologists today – and even more in the future – have to deal with a population

Table 1. Pros and cons of principal therapeutic options

Pros	Therapy	Cons
Potential toxicity on brain, heart, kidney, and liver	Antibacterial systemic therapy	Control of infection
Contrast medium nephropathy Acute cardiac failure Procedural risks	Revascularization procedures	Treat critical limb ischaemia
Neural damage Cardiorespiratory depression Gastrointestinal complications Worsening of renal failure	Chronic pain-killers	Control of pain
Procedural risks Bleeding and anaemia Anaesthesiology risks	Surgery	Arrest foot problems

who is aging. At the same time, our skills in managing diabetes chronic complications improved, implementing our ability to face chronic diseases typical of older population: cardiovascular disease, cerebrovascular illness, renal failure. The result of this evolution is that we have to manage patients getting not only older but also sicker, most often experiencing recurrences of the disease after recovering from the acute phase [50, 51].

Speaking about diabetic foot, it is well known that the pathogenetic elements of the disease – neuropathy, arteriopathy, immunopathy – exert a cumulative effect on the foot with aging. So the condition of diabetic foot patients progressively became more severe, both from a local and a systemic point of view, and therefore, they were in need of a more complex and integrated strategy of care [52].

Cost Analysis
Diabetic foot is doubtless a condition that would incur high personal, social, economic and medical costs. This has led to investigations focused on different cost components, thereby trying to correlate the cost factor to the different elements of diabetic foot and to reduce the high expenses involved. The costs vary greatly between different centres and are mainly related to hospitalization and infection control. All types of resource utilizations and related costs increased as the severity of the disease intensified [53].

Considering the economic health policy applied in recent years, cost analysis is becoming mandatory in diabetic foot care services. In view of the increasing number of diabetic patients, their higher level of co-morbidities and, eventually, the limitation to healthcare resource use, it is mandatory to prioritize health care expenses [54]. It is necessary for physicians to obtain data on treatment costs and their cost effectiveness to identify for each patient the more effective and cost-saving therapeutic option [55]. In Table 1, we report the main characteristics of these therapies.

The need to reduce major amputations has been clearly specified in the Saint Vincent Declaration, promulgated under the auspices of World Health Organization and International Diabetes Federation. Representatives of government, health ministers and diabetic patients all around the world signed in 1989 at Saint Vincent, a historical document, which is still the main international reference for the fight against diabetes and its complications. The experts who drafted the document identified 5 main goals to be achieved in diabetes management: to decrease of one third of blindness and kidney failure due to diabetes, to reduce morbidity and mortality related to coronary heart disease, to have no differences in pregnancy outcomes between diabetic and non-diabetic women, and to reduce the number of LEAs in those with diabetic gangrenes [74].

This goal has thereafter been confirmed by the International Diabetes Federation that has emphasized on how the achievement of increasing awareness regarding diabetes foot complications should be considered a key issue in diabetes management [75].

Since the Declaration of Saint Vincent, the reduction of major amputation was the main objective to pursue in diabetic foot care and the only hard outcome on which to evaluate the complexity and effectiveness of care.

Certainly, foot care specialists are of the opinion that major amputation is an event that has to be avoided at any cost, but this opinion is nowadays controversial if it should still be the only option of treatment [56].

In the daily setting of diabetic foot clinic, while working on a patient-centred approach and not just on a leg-centred one, major amputation can, in some cases, become a suitable therapeutic choice when some defined conditions are present [56].

The concept of limb saving is always mandatory, but it is anyhow secondary to the concept of saving life as a whole: when the local state of the limb is so severe that it is putting the patient's life to risk, the entire strategy must be re-evaluated [57]. In case of life-threatening conditions, such as a deep infected wound that is uncontrollable through antibiotic therapy and local surgical procedures, gas gangrene, abscesses and necrotizing fasciitis, or when sepsis occurs, a prompt major amputation could be the most ethical alternative [58, 59].

The same option should be considered for patients experiencing chronic rest pain due to critical limb ischaemia not, or not any more, revascularizable and at the same time not responsive to pain drugs. The quality of life of these patients may decrease to a point where the patients themselves feel that they require amputation [60].

In all other cases, limb saving has to be the priority. However, these attempts should be balanced considering the risk of performing therapies that are invasive or dangerous for patients. Prolonged multidrug antibacterial therapies, invasive procedures with administration of contrast medium and the use of chronic pain-killers may all worsen kidney and heart function of patients, putting them at risk of amodyalisis, cardiac failure and acute cardiovascular events [61–64].

In Table 1, the indications and potential adverse events of the components of the integrated approach to the management of diabetic foot are reported.

New Outcomes for a New Model of Care

Despite the importance of achieving healing of ulcers and avoiding major amputation and death, there is therefore the need to set new targets to achieve improved prognosis and quality of life in patients affected with DFU [65]. The identification of these goals passes through a wider analysis of patients' status and health care opportunities and is focused on therapeutic options rapidly evolving towards a patient-centred approach.

Quality of Life

The relationship between health-related quality of life (HRQoL) and ulcer healing has been extensively investigated during recent years. The impact of DFU on the quality of life is much heavier than the presence of diabetes itself [66]. The occurrence of a foot ulcer for the patient begins in him or her a nightmarish experience – the wound often does not heal through first home care and therefore, the patient has to seek medical attention. And so begins the sequence of hospital admission, surgical debridement or minor amputation, percutaneous angioplasty or by-pass in case of critical limb ischaemia, total contact cast or walker devices and an endless series of changing the dressings. All these traumatic events have to be endured abreast to the fear that if the ulcer does not heal, then the patient has to encounter the ghost of amputation with the associated risk of recurrences and negative consequences on family life and work habits [67].

Among diabetic foot patients, HRQoL is quite different based on the different stages of the disease and it is significantly poorer in patients with a non-healing DFU. While a major amputation and persistent ulceration bring a significant worsening of HRQoL, minor amputation does not. On the other hand, in diabetic patients, the level of HRQoL can predict better outcomes, both in terms of limb-saving and life-saving, and it is not related to healing [68]. This is the reason why HRQoL has become a strong predictor of outcomes in diabetic foot patients, and an aspect that should also be taken into account in any decision-making process about different therapeutic alternatives.

Healing Time

Healing time is one of the most controversial issues in the assessment of diabetic foot care. It is directly related to patients' quality of life because the longer the healing time, the stronger becomes the self-perception of the patient that he or she is "ill"; on the other hand, short healing time leads to a reduction in the risk of infections and increases the opportunity to achieve permanent and positive outcomes [69].

Wound care is aimed not only to increase healing rates but also to reduce the time needed to reach a condition of being completely healed [70].

Bilateral Secondary Prevention
Diabetic foot is considered by many physicians a relapsing-remitting disease. Since the first acute episode, the patient begins to lead a life that is characterized by treatment followed by healing if ever intervention made has been done correctly, and then when recurrence happens at a rate ranging from 40% to 60% [71]. Thus, reducing the incidence of re-ulcerations and recurrences is crucial to increase the quality of life of these patients. A number of studies evaluated the possible instruments that can be used to achieve this goal, and effective guidelines in this regard have been extensively published by IWGDF. The secondary prevention phase should be always put in place within the context of the same multi-disciplinary team who takes care of primary prevention and acute phases [72].

Secondary prevention has to be put in place also contralaterally: while we fight to save a limb, it is not less important to avoid contralateral ulceration or damage. Data from literature about the destiny of the contralateral limb in diabetic population is quite discouraging, especially in patients who have undergone major amputation. To preserve an intact contralateral limb in diabetic foot patients is more difficult because of the biomechanical consequences of the surgical procedure performed on the affected limb. Regular surveillance of the foot and limb allows early recognition of disease signs and the improvement of outcomes [73].

Minor and Major Amputations
Limb salvage represents a life-saving procedure: diabetic patients who had undergone a major amputation experienced an increased mortality risk when compared to non-amputated patients [76]. Death risk becomes even greater when the amputation level rises: recent trials showed a higher risk for thigh amputation versus leg amputation since the early post-operative years [77]. On the contrary, minor amputations, performed below the ankle, do not negatively impact survival chance of patients [78]. A similar effect can be observed on quality of life, usually severely affected by major amputations, while minor amputations have been demonstrated not to reduce HRQoL when compared to conservative treatment of foot lesions [79].

The advancements made in effective care tools for diabetic foot patients have led to a significant improvement in limb preservation as demonstrated recently by an increasing number of trials [80–83]. Surely an evolution of foot clinic network has been able to spread the correct management of diabetic foot according to international guidelines, thereby reinforcing the idea and the application of a multidisciplinarity approach in this field [84, 85]. Beyond their clinical means, LEAs have been identified as thorough markers of quality of care for diabetic patients and a proxy of adequacy of specialized care not only for lower limb complications but also for diabetes in general [86, 87]

Ability to Walk

In a patient who has undergone a major amputation up to the Chopart level, the ability to walk is preserved but often worsened, almost in the early post-operative period due to muscle weakness associated with a long illness period. However, in these patients, the wearing of customized shoes should be encouraged prior to beginning to walk again extensively in order to avoid recurrences. For major amputees, it is mandatory to guarantee the preservation of the walking ability [88]. A pre-procedural evaluation of the actual ability of the patient to recover based on his or her autonomy after the surgery should be carried out before any surgical procedure [89]. An early rehabilitation is associated with a better long-term walking ability [90]. The attempts made to preserve the ability to walk have to begin in a surgical room because it is here that the conditions that increase the possibility of creating a stump, which could constitute a good support for prosthesis – typically the type of surgical suture – become well known [91].

Conclusions

During the second half of the last century, medicine had focused itself on standardization, on searching for objective rules, based on evidence and literature. Physicians spoke about taking care of patients, but they took care of the disease instead. Classifications, schemes and algorithms were the bases of such a thought process. Even less space was given to personal initiative and to clinical evaluation because all patients had to receive optimal standard medical treatment, despite age, preferences, co-morbidities and status levels. The outcomes improved but not as much as expected; on the contrary, costs grew. Therefore, the necessity to re-evaluate the standards of care and outcomes in the management of chronic diseases, and of diabetic foot syndrome among them, emerged in the specialist community, to include patients' point of view and cost/effectiveness into the decision-making process. Formulating new therapeutic strategies – tailored to the clinical conditions of the patients, not to substitute old goals but to understand that parameters such as quality of life, patients' ability to walk and thus making them independent are as relevant as the correctness of diagnosis and implementation of guidelines – has to become the cornerstone of the diabetic foot care management. All efforts and steps to cure the patient as a whole and not just the leg have to be identified and implemented.

References

1 International Diabetes Federation: IDF Diabetes Atlas, ed 7. Brussels, Belgium: International Diabetes Federation, 2015.

2 Stuck RM, Sage R, Pinzur M, Osterman H: Amputations in the diabetic foot. Clin Podiatr Med Surg 1995;12:141–155.

3 Boulton AJ, Vileikyte L, Ragnarson-Tennvall G, Apelqvist J: The global burden of diabetic foot disease. Lancet 2005;366:1719–1724.

4 Matsuda A: Gangrene and ulcer of the lower extremities in diabetic patients. Diabetes Res Clin Pract 1994;24(suppl):S209–S213.

5 Singh N, Armstrong DG, Lipsky BA: Preventing foot ulcers in patients with diabetes. JAMA 2005;293: 217–228.

6 Benotmane A, Mohammedi F, Ayad F, Kadi K, Azzouz A: Diabetic foot lesions: etiologic and prognostic factors. Diabetes Metab 2000;26:113–117.

7 Markakis K, Bowling FL, Boulton AJ: The diabetic foot in 2015: an overview. Diabetes Metab Res Rev 2016;32(suppl 1):169–178.

8 Sanders LJ, Robbins JM, Edmonds ME: History of the team approach to amputation prevention: pioneers and milestones. J Vasc Surg 2010;52(3 suppl):3S–16S.

9 Kirby T: Solomon Tesfaye: preventing complications of diabetic neuropathy. Lancet Diabetes Endocrinol 2014;2:865.

10 Edmonds ME, Blundell MP, Morris ME, Thomas EM, Cotton LT, Watkins PJ: Improved survival of the diabetic foot: the role of a specialized foot clinic. Q J Med 1986;60:763–771.

11 Bakker K, Dooren J: [A specialized outpatient foot clinic for diabetic patients decreases the number of amputations and is cost saving]. Ned Tijdschr Geneeskd 1994;138:565–569.

12 Faglia E, Favales F, Aldeghi A, Calia P, Quarantiello A, Barbano P, Puttini M, Palmieri B, Brambilla G, Rampoldi A, Mazzola E, Valenti L, Fattori G, Rega V, Cristalli A, Oriani G, Michael M, Morabito A: Change in major amputation rate in a center dedicated to diabetic foot care during the 1980s: prognostic determinants for major amputation. J Diabetes Complications 1998;12:96–102.

13 Van Netten JJ, Price PE, Lavery LA, et al: Prevention of foot ulcers in the at-risk patient with diabetes: a systematic review. Diabetes Metab Res Rev 2016; 32(suppl 1):84–98.

14 Apelqvist J: The foot in perspective. Diabetes Metab Res Rev 2008;24(suppl 1):S110–S115.

15 Boulton AJM: The diabetic foot, 2016; in De Groot LJ, Chrousos G, Dungan K, Feingold KR, Grossman A, Hershman JM, Koch C, Korbonits M, McLachlan R, New M, Purnell J, Rebar R, Singer F, Vinik A (eds): Endotext [Internet]. South Dartmouth, MDText. com, Inc., 2000. http://www.ncbi.nlm.nih.gov/books/NBK409609/.

16 Schaper NC: Lessons from Eurodiale. Diabetes Metab Res Rev 2012;28(suppl 1):21–26.

17 Andersen CA: Diabetic limb preservation: defining terms and goals. J Foot Ankle Surg 2010;49:106–107.

18 Gershater MA, Löndahl M, Nyberg P, Larsson J, Thörne J, Eneroth M, et al: Complexity of factors related to outcome of neuropathic and neuroischaemic/ischaemic diabetic foot ulcers: a cohort study. Diabetologia 2009;52:398–407.

19 Margolis DJ, Kantor J, Berlin JA: Healing of diabetic neuropathic foot ulcers receiving standard treatment. A meta-analysis. Diabetes Care 1999;22:692–695.

20 Zimny S, Schatz H, Pfohl M: Determinants and estimation of healing times in diabetic foot ulcers. J Diabetes Complications 2002;16:327–332.

21 Pickwell KM, Siersma VD, Kars M, Holstein PE, Schaper NC; Eurodiale consortium: Diabetic foot disease: impact of ulcer location on ulcer healing. Diabetes Metab Res Rev 2013;29:377–383.

22 Lavery LA: Effectiveness and safety of elective surgical procedures to improve wound healing and reduce re-ulceration in diabetic patients with foot ulcers. Diabetes Metab Res Rev 2012;28(suppl 1): 60–63.

23 Pickwell K, Siersma V, Kars M, Apelqvist J, Bakker K, Edmonds M, et al: Predictors of lower-extremity amputation in patients with an infected diabetic foot ulcer. Diabetes Care 2015;38:852–857.

24 Caruana L, Formosa C, Cassar K: Prediction of wound healing after minor amputations of the diabetic foot. J Diabetes Complications 2015;29:834–837.

25 Wise J: Early referral for foot ulcers is vital, finds audit of diabetes care. BMJ 2016;352:i1820.

26 Apelqvist J, Larsson J, Agardh CD: Long-term prognosis for diabetic patients with foot ulcers. J Intern Med 1993;233:485–491.

27 Bus SA, Waaijman R, Arts M, de Haart M, Busch-Westbroek T, van Baal J, et al: Effect of custom-made footwear on foot ulcer recurrence in diabetes: a multicenter randomized controlled trial. Diabetes Care 2013;36:4109–4116.

28 Peikes D, Chen A, Schore J, Brown R: Effects of care coordination on hospitalization, quality of care, and health care expenditures among Medicare beneficiaries: 15 randomized trials. JAMA 2009;301:603–618.

29 Apelqvist J, Ragnarson-Tennvall G, Larsson J, et al: Long-term costs for foot ulcers in diabetic patients in a multidisciplinary setting. Foot Ankle Int 1995;16: 388–394.

30 Dubský M, Jirkovská A, Bem R, Fejfarová V, Skibová J, Schaper NC, et al: Risk factors for recurrence of diabetic foot ulcers: prospective follow-up analysis in the Eurodiale subgroup. Int Wound J 2013;10:555–561.

31 Boyko EJ, Ahroni JH, Smith DG, Davignon D: Increased mortality associated with diabetic foot ulcer. Diabet Med 1996;13:967–972.

32 Singh RK, Prasad G: Long-term mortality after lower-limb amputation. Prosthet Orthot Int 2016;40: 545–551.

33 Winkley K, Stahl D, Chalder T, Edmonds ME, Ismail K: Risk factors associated with adverse outcomes in a population-based prospective cohort study of people with their first diabetic foot ulcer. J Diabetes Complications 2007;21:341–349.

34 Leibson CL, Ransom JE, Olson W, Zimmerman BR, O'fallon WM, Palumbo PJ: Peripheral arterial disease, diabetes, and mortality. Diabetes Care 2004;27: 2843–2849.

35 BARI 2D Study Group, Frye RL, August P, Brooks MM, Hardison RM, Kelsey SF, MacGregor JM, Orchard TJ, Chaitman BR, Genuth SM, Goldberg SH, Hlatky MA, Jones TL, Molitch ME, Nesto RW, Sako EY, Sobel BE: A randomized trial of therapies for type 2 diabetes and coronary artery disease. N Engl J Med 2009;360:2503–2515.

36 Faglia E, Clerici G, Clerissi J, Gabrielli L, Losa S, Mantero M, et al: Long-term prognosis of diabetic patients with critical limb ischemia: a population-based cohort study. Diabetes Care 2009;32:822–827.

37 Morbach S, Furchert H, Gröblinghoff U, Hoffmeier H, Kersten K, Klauke GT, Klemp U, Roden T, Icks A, Haastert B, Rümenapf G, Abbas ZG, Bharara M, Armstrong DG: Long-term prognosis of diabetic foot patients and their limbs: amputation and death over the course of a decade. Diabetes Care 2012;35: 2021–2027.

38 Wukich DK, Raspovic KM: What Role Does Function Play in Deciding on Limb Salvage versus Amputation in Patients With Diabetes? Plast Reconstr Surg 2016;138(3 suppl):188S–195S.

39 Wukich DK, Armstrong DG, Attinger CE, Boulton AJ, Burns PR, Frykberg RG, Hellman R, Kim PJ, Lipsky BA, Pile JC, Pinzur MS, Siminerio L: Inpatient management of diabetic foot disorders: a clinical guide. Diabetes Care 2013;36:2862–2871.

40 Schaper NC: Diabetic foot ulcer classification system for research purposes: a progress report on criteria for including patients in research studies. Diabetes Metab Res Rev 2004;20(suppl 1):S90–S95.

41 Apelqvist J, Elgzyri T, Larsson J, Löndahl M, Nyberg P, Thörne J: Factors related to outcome of neuroischemic/ischemic foot ulcer in diabetic patients. J Vasc Surg 2011;53:1582–1588.e2.

42 Prompers L, Huijberts M, Apelqvist J, Jude E, Piaggesi A, Bakker K, Edmonds M, Holstein P, Jirkovska A, Mauricio D, Tennvall GR, Reike H, Spraul M, Uccioli L, Urbancic V, Van Acker K, Van Baal J, Van Merode F, Schaper N: Delivery of care to diabetic patients with foot ulcers in daily practice: results of the Eurodiale Study, a prospective cohort study. Diabet Med 2008;25:700–707.

43 Armstrong DG, Bharara M, White M, Lepow B, Bhatnagar S, Fisher T, Kimbriel HR, Walters J, Goshima KR, Hughes J, Mills JL: The impact and outcomes of establishing an integrated interdisciplinary surgical team to care for the diabetic foot. Diabetes Metab Res Rev 2012;28:514–518.

44 Brownrigg JR, Davey J, Holt PJ, Davis WA, Thompson MM, Ray KK, et al: The association of ulceration of the foot with cardiovascular and all-cause mortality in patients with diabetes: a meta-analysis. Diabetologia 2012;55:2906–2912.

45 Mills JL Sr, Conte MS, Armstrong DG, Pomposelli FB, Schanzer A, Sidawy AN, Andros G; Society for Vascular Surgery Lower Extremity Guidelines Committee: The Society for Vascular Surgery Lower Extremity Threatened Limb Classification System: risk stratification based on wound, ischemia, and foot infection (WIfI). J Vasc Surg 2014;59:220–234.e1–e2.

46 Becker F: Exploration of arterial function with non-invasive technics. Results in chronic arterial occlusive disease of the lower limbs according to Leriche and Fontaine classification. Int Angiol 1985;4:311–322.

47 Edmonds ME: The diabetic foot: pathophysiology and treatment. Clin Endocrinol Metab 1986;15:889–916.

48 Edmonds ME, Foster AV: Diabetic foot ulcers. BMJ 2006;332:407–410.

49 Jiang Y, Ran X, Jia L, Yang C, Wang P, Ma J, Chen B, Yu Y, Feng B, Chen L, Yin H, Cheng Z, Yan Z, Yang Y, Liu F, Xu Z: Epidemiology of type 2 diabetic foot problems and predictive factors for amputation in China. Int J Low Extrem Wounds 2015;14:19–27.

50 Thomson FJ, Masson EA: Can elderly diabetic patients co-operate with routine foot care? Age Ageing 1992;21:333–337.

51 Emerging Risk Factors Collaboration, Sarwar N, Gao P, Seshasai SR, Gobin R, et al: Diabetes mellitus, fasting blood glucose concentration, and risk of vascular disease: a collaborative meta-analysis of 102 prospective studies. Lancet 2010;375:2215–2222.

52 Gibson TB, Driver VR, Wrobel JS, Christina JR, Bagalman E, DeFrancis R, Garoufalis MG, Carls GS, Gatwood J: Podiatrist care and outcomes for patients with diabetes and foot ulcer. Int Wound J 2014;11: 641–648.

53 Prompers L, Huijberts M, Schaper N, Apelqvist J, Bakker K, Edmonds M, Holstein P, Jude E, Jirkovska A, Mauricio D, Piaggesi A, Reike H, Spraul M, Van Acker K, Van Baal S, Van Merode F, Uccioli L, Urbancic V, Ragnarson Tennvall G: Resource utilisation and costs associated with the treatment of diabetic foot ulcers. Prospective data from the Eurodiale Study. Diabetologia 2008;51:1826–1834.

54 Apelqvist J: Wound healing in diabetes. Outcome and costs. Clin Podiatr Med Surg 1998;15:21–39.

55 Ragnarson Tennvall G, Apelqvist J: Health-economic consequences of diabetic foot lesions. Clin Infect Dis 2004;39(suppl 2):S132–S139.

56 Game F: Choosing life or limb. Improving survival in the multi-complex diabetic foot patient. Diabetes Metab Res Rev 2012;28(suppl 1):97–100.

57 Lipsky BA, Berendt AR, Cornia PB, Pile JC, Peters EJ, Armstrong DG, et al: Infectious Diseases Society of America clinical practice guideline for the diagnosis and treatment of diabetic foot infections. Clin Infect Dis 2012;54:e132–e173.

58 Adam DJ, Raptis S, Fitridge RA: Trends in the presentation and surgical management of the acute diabetic foot. Eur J Vasc Endovasc Surg 2006;31:151–156.

59 Clerici G, Faglia E: Saving the limb in diabetic patients with ischemic foot lesions complicated by acute infection. Int J Low Extrem Wounds 2014;13:273–293.

60 Siersma V, Thorsen H, Holstein PE, Kars M, Apelqvist J, Jude EB, Piaggesi A, Bakker K, Edmonds M, Jirkovska A, Mauricio D, Ragnarson Tennvall G, Reike H, Spraul M, Uccioli L, Urbancic V, van Acker K, van Baal J, Schaper NC: Importance of factors determining the low health-related quality of life in people presenting with a diabetic foot ulcer: the Eurodiale study. Diabet Med 2013;30:1382–1387.

61 Akbari R, Javaniyan M, Fahimi A, Sadeghi M: Renal function in patients with diabetic foot infection; does antibiotherapy affect it? J Renal Inj Prev 2016;6:117–121.

62 Ndip A, Lavery LA, Boulton AJ: Diabetic foot disease in people with advanced nephropathy and those on renal dialysis. Curr Diab Rep 2010;10:283–290.

63 Nabuurs-Franssen MH, Huijberts MS, Nieuwenhuijzen Kruseman AC, Willems J, Schaper NC: Health-related quality of life of diabetic foot ulcer patients and their caregivers. Diabetologia 2005;48:1906–1910.

64 Kim NY, Lee KY, Bai SJ, Hong JH, Lee J, Park JM, Kim SH: Comparison of the effects of remifentanil-based general anesthesia and popliteal nerve block on postoperative pain and hemodynamic stability in diabetic patients undergoing distal foot amputation: a retrospective observational study. Medicine (Baltimore). 2016;95:e4302.

65 Moulik PK, Mtonga R, Gill GV: Amputation and mortality in new-onset diabetic foot ulcers stratified by etiology. Diabetes Care 2003;26:491–494.

66 Feng X, Astell-Burt T: Impact of a type 2 diabetes diagnosis on mental health, quality of life, and social contacts: a longitudinal study. BMJ Open Diabetes Res Care 2017;5:e000198.

67 Sehlo MG, Alzahrani OH, Alzahrani HA: Illness invalidation from spouse and family is associated with depression in diabetic patients with first superficial diabetic foot ulcers. Int J Psychiatry Med 2016;51:16–30.

68 Siersma V, Thorsen H, Holstein PE, Kars M, Apelqvist J, Jude EB, Piaggesi A, Bakker K, Edmonds M, Jirkovská A, Mauricio D, Ragnarson Tennvall G, Reike H, Spraul M, Uccioli L, Urbancic V, van Acker K, van Baal J, Schaper NC: Health-related quality of life predicts major amputation and death, but not healing, in people with diabetes presenting with foot ulcers: the Eurodiale study. Diabetes Care 2014;37:694–700.

69 Fiordaliso F, Clerici G, Maggioni S, Caminiti M, Bisighini C, Novelli D, Minnella D, Corbelli A, Morisi R, De Iaco A, Faglia E: Prospective study on microangiopathy in type 2 diabetic foot ulcer. Diabetologia 2016;59:1542–1548.

70 Game FL, Apelqvist J, Attinger C, Hartemann A, Hinchliffe RJ, Löndahl M, et al: Effectiveness of interventions to enhance healing of chronic ulcers of the foot in diabetes: a systematic review. Diabetes Metab Res Rev 2016;32(suppl 1):154–168.

71 Golomb BA, Dang TT, Criqui MH: Peripheral arterial disease: morbidity and mortality implications. Circulation 2006;114:688–699.

72 Dorresteijn JA, Kriegsman DM, Assendelft WJ, Valk GD: Patient education for preventing diabetic foot ulceration. Cochrane Database Syst Rev 2014;1:CD001488.

73 Faglia E, Clerici G, Mantero M, Caminiti M, Quarantiello A, Curci V, et al: Incidence of critical limb ischemia and amputation outcome in contralateral limb in diabetic patients hospitalized for unilateral critical limb ischemia during 1999–2003 and followed-up until 2005. Diabetes Res Clin Pract 2007;77:445–450.

74 The Saint Vincent declaration. Acta Ophtalmol Scand 1997;appendix II:63.

75 Bloomgarden ZT: International Diabetes Federation meeting, 1997. Neuropathy, information technology, cost of diabetes care, and epidemiology. Diabetes Care 1998;21:1198–1202.

76 Hoffstad O, Mitra N, Walsh J, Margolis DJ: Diabetes, lower-extremity amputation, and death. Diabetes Care 2015;38:1852–1857.

77 Ploeg AJ, Lardenoye JW, Vrancken Peeters MP, Breslau PJ: Contemporary series of morbidity and mortality after lower limb amputation. Eur J Vasc Endovasc Surg 2005;29:633–637.

78 Evans KK, Attinger CE, Al-Attar A, Salgado C, Chu CK, Mardini S, et al: The importance of limb preservation in the diabetic population. J Diabetes Complications 2011;25:227–231.

79 Pickwell K, Siersma V, Kars M, Apelqvist J, Bakker K, Edmonds M, Holstein P, Jirkovská A, Jude EB, Mauricio D, Piaggesi A, Reike H, Spraul M, Uccioli L, Urbancic V, van Acker K, van Baal J, Schaper N: Minor amputation does not negatively affect health-related quality of life as compared with conservative treatment in patients with a diabetic foot ulcer: an observational study. Diabetes Metab Res Rev 2017; 33.

80 Trautner C, Haastert B, Mauckner P, Gätcke LM, Giani G: Reduced incidence of lower-limb amputations in the diabetic population of a German city, 1990–2005: results of the Leverkusen Amputation Reduction Study (LARS). Diabetes Care 2007;30: 2633–2637.

81 Lombardo FL, Maggini M, De Bellis A, Seghieri G, Anichini R: Lower extremity amputations in persons with and without diabetes in Italy: 2001–2010. PLoS One 2014;9:e86405.

82 López-de-Andrés A, Martínez-Huedo MA, Carrasco-Garrido P, Hernández-Barrera V, Gil-de-Miguel A, Jiménez-García R: Trends in lower-extremity amputations in people with and without diabetes in Spain, 2001–2008. Diabetes Care 2011;34:1570–1576.

83 Kennon B, Leese GP, Cochrane L, Colhoun H, Wild S, Stang D, Sattar N, Pearson D, Lindsay RS, Morris AD, Livingstone S, Young M, McKnight J, Cunningham S: Reduced incidence of lower-extremity amputations in people with diabetes in Scotland: a nationwide study. Diabetes Care 2012;35:2588–2590.

84 Morbach S, Kersken J, Lobmann R, Nobels F, Doggen K, Van Acker K: The German and Belgian accreditation models for diabetic foot services. Diabetes Metab Res Rev 2016;32(suppl 1):318–325.

85 Owings TM, Woerner JL, Frampton JD, Cavanagh PR, Botek G: Custom therapeutic insoles based on both foot shape and plantar pressure measurement provide enhanced pressure relief. Diabetes Care 2008;31:839–844.

86 Brooke BS, Kraiss LW, Stone DH, Nolan B, De Martino RR, Reiber GE, Goodman DC, Cronenwett JL, Goodney PP: Improving outcomes for diabetic patients undergoing revascularization for critical limb ischemia: does the quality of outpatient diabetic care matter? Ann Vasc Surg 2014;28:1719–1728.

87 Jeffcoate WJ, van Houtum WH: Amputation as a marker of the quality of foot care in diabetes. Diabetologia 2004;47:2051–2058.

88 Brown BJ, Crone CG, Attinger CE: Amputation in the diabetic to maximize function. Semin Vasc Surg 2012;25:115–121.

89 Larsson J, Agardh CD, Apelqvist J, Stenström A: Long-term prognosis after healed amputation in patients with diabetes. Clin Orthop Relat Res 1998;350: 149–158.

90 Dillingham TR, Pezzin LE: Rehabilitation setting and associated mortality and medical stability among persons with amputations. Arch Phys Med Rehabil 2008;89:1038–1045.

91 Attinger CE, Brown BJ: Amputation and ambulation in diabetic patients: function is the goal. Diabetes Metab Res Rev 2012;28(suppl 1):93–96.

Alberto Piaggesi, MD
Diabetic Foot Section
Department of Medicine, University of Pisa
Via Paradisa 2, IT–56124 Pisa (Italy)
E-Mail piaggesi@immr.med.unipi.it

Piaggesi A, Apelqvist J (eds): The Diabetic Foot Syndrome.
Front Diabetes. Basel, Karger, 2018, vol 26, pp 48–59 (DOI: 10.1159/000480045)

The Charcot Foot Revisited: How the New Pathogenetic Findings Explain the Clinical Course of the Disease

Nina L. Petrova

Diabetic Foot Clinic, King's College Hospital NHS Foundation Trust, and Division of Diabetes and Nutritional Sciences, King's College London, London, UK

Abstract

Charcot neuropathic osteoarthropathy (CN) is one of the most debilitating complications of diabetic neuropathy. It classically presents as a red hot swollen foot, precipitated by trauma. The latter leads to fracture, bone fragmentation and ultimately foot deformity. Recent advances in imaging modalities have enabled the detection of initial signs of inflammation and pathological osteolysis before overt bone and joint destruction has occurred. Moreover, advances in cellular biology and molecular biology have helped to elucidate the mechanisms of increased osteoclastic activity in acute CN and its interaction with inflammation and neuropathy. This paper summarizes how new pathogenetic findings explain the clinical presentation of the disease. In particular, it revists how classical theories, related to the development of Charcot joints, have laid the foundation of a novel understanding of the pathogenesis of pathological bone destruction in the diabetic neuropathic foot.

Introduction

Charcot neuropathic osteoarthropathy (CN) or Charcot foot is one of the most challenging foot complications occurring in those with diabetes. The condition bears the name of the French neurologist, Jean Marie Charcot (1825–1893), who initially reported the neuropathic bone and joint disease in tabes dorsalis in 1868. Its association with diabetes was described by Jordan in 1936. The true prevalence of CN in diabetes is unknown and it is largely recognised that the condition is very much underreported. Charcot joints have been described in other peripheral neuropathies, including leprosy, congenital sensory neuropathy, familial amyloid neuropathy, alcohol neuropathy and more recently in human immunodeficiency virus-induced neuropathy [1–4]. However, in the 21st century, CN is most frequently seen in patients with diabetes. With the predicted global increase in the prevalence of diabetes (http://www.idf.org/sites/default/files/Atlas-poster-2014_EN.pdf), the burden of neuropathy and its related adverse complications including CN is also expected to rise (http://www.idf.org/diabetesatlas/5e/mortality).

In diabetes, CN is characterised by varying degrees of bone and joint disorganization, secondary to underlying peripheral neuropathy and trauma leading to fracture, bone fragmentation and ultimately foot deformity. The latter can be further complicated by an ulcer, which can become infected, and if not promptly managed it can lead to amputation [5].

In the last 20 years, considerable progress has been made in the early recognition of the acute Charcot foot when the X-ray is still negative (grade 0 or incipient Charcot foot) [6, 7]. Recent advances in imaging modalities have enabled the detection of initial signs of inflammation and pathological osteolysis before overt bone and joint destruction has occurred. Moreover, advances in cellular biology and molecular biology have helped to elucidate the mechanisms of increased osteoclastic activity in acute CN and its interaction with inflammation and neuropathy. This paper summarizes how new pathogenetic findings explain the clinical presentation of the disease. In particular, it revists how classical theories, related to the development of Charcot joints, have laid the foundation of a novel understanding of the pathogenesis of pathological bone destruction in the diabetic neuropathic foot.

The Classical Approach to the Charcot Foot – Classical Theories of the Pathogenesis of This Condition

Historically, 2 fundamental theories have been put forward to explain the aetiopathogenesis of CN. The first one, formulated by Charcot himself, known as the French theory, or the "neuro-trophic theory," suggests that the bone and joint changes seen in tabes dorsalis are a result of a spinal cord lesion. He believed that the impaired nutritive trophic regulation alters the sympathetic tone, leading to vasodilation and increased blood flow. Charcot also highlighted the importance of inflammation. He postulated that hyperaemia (inflammation) due to abnormal neurovascular control leads to increased bone resorption and osteopenia ultimately resulting in bone and joint destruction [8].

The second theory, known as the German theory or the "neuro-traumatic theory", was proposed by Volkman and Virchow. They attributed the joint destruction to external trauma and repetitive stress, which is quite often unperceived by the patient due to loss of proprioception and pain sensation. The patient continues to traumatise the bones and soft tissue. This can lead to joint swelling and ligament stretching, resulting in joint laxity [9]. Ultimately, the inflammatory response to injury leads to hyperaemia, soft tissue swelling and bone and joint destruction [8].

Although previously, these 2 classical theories have been perceived as conflicting with each other (disputing) [10, 11], it is now generally accepted that neither of them can fully explain the modern presentation of CN in diabetes. Common precipitating factors delineated in these theories are present in varying degrees in patients with this condition. For example, in type 1 diabetes, underlying osteopenia secondary to increased blood flow and autonomic neuropathy is a frequent forerunner to pathological fractures and CN as described in the neurovascular theory. In contrast, in type 2 diabetes, repetitive trauma in the insensitive foot with elevated plantar pressure as a result of the increased body mass index and profound neuropathy can lead to stress fractures and CN in the absence of osteopenia in accordance to the neurotraumatic theory [12]. Thus, the contribution of each of the theories to the pathogenesis of Charcot foot is now well appreciated. Moreover, knowledge from these 2 classical theories is fundamental to the modern approach of the pathogenesis of CN in diabetes.

Modern Hypothesis of the Pathogenesis of CN – Bridging Classical Factors with Cellular Pathways

The main features of CN in the diabetic neuropathic foot include exaggerated inflammatory response to trauma and pathological bone destruction. Advances in the understanding of the mechanisms of osteoclastogenesis and osteoclastic activity as well as the interaction between inflammation and bone have become central to the modern hypothesis of the pathogenesis of CN. It encompasses well-established characteristic factors of CN (neuropathy – abnormal loading – trauma – increased force – dislocation/fracture) together with current achievement in cellular biology. Two cellular pathways have been put forward as possible drivers of the extensive bone destruction that occurs in the diabetic neuropathic foot [13].

These include uncontrolled release of cytokines in the neuropathic foot and activation of the receptor activator of nuclear factor-kβ (RANK) ligand (RANKL)/osteoprotegerin (OPG) signalling pathway. What advances have we made to underpin the increased osteoclastic activity and the enhanced inflammatory response to trauma in the past few years?

Increased Osteoclastic Activity Is a Key Driver of Pathological Bone Destruction in the Acute Charcot Foot

There is a strong body of evidence to show that the pathological bone destruction of the acute Charcot foot is associated with increased osteoclastic activity. In CN, the serum concentrations of bone resorption markers are raised [14, 15] and there is evidence of osteopenia in the acute Charcot foot of both type 1 and type 2 diabetes [12, 16]. Moreover, computed tomography imaging in patients with active CN indicates

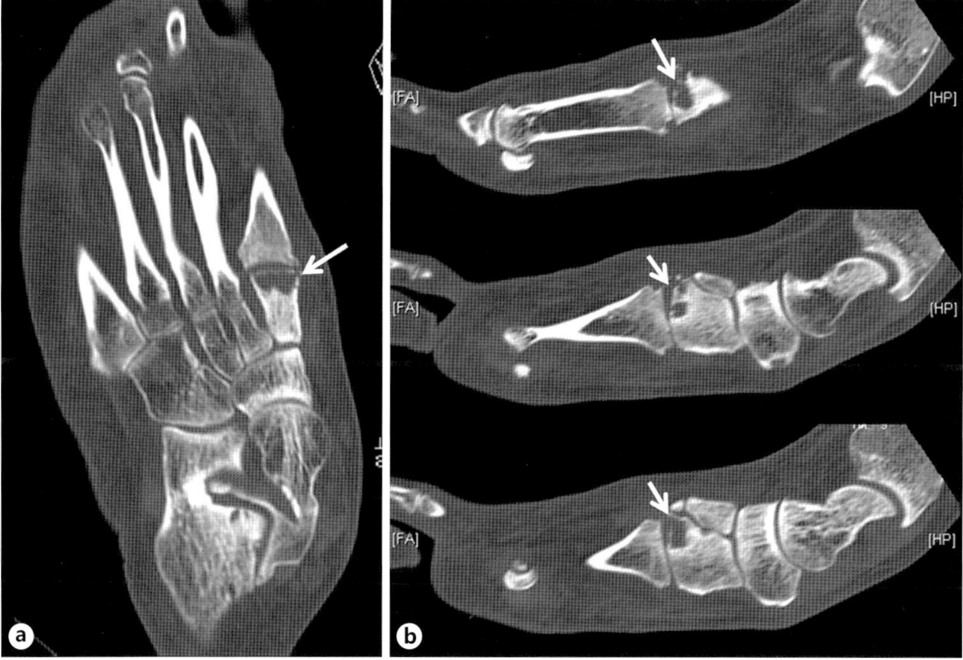

Fig. 1. Pathological osteolysis in stage 0 Charcot foot. Computed tomography shows subchondral cyst in the medial cuneiform on axial view (**a**) with erosions and bone fragmentation on sagittal views (**b**).

that pathological osteolysis is present not only in patients with extensive bone destruction (grade 1 Charcot Foot) but also in patients presenting with essentially normal radiographs (grade 0 Charcot foot; Fig. 1). These clinical observations indicate that in CN there is increased osteoclastic activity with a potential role of activated osteoclasts as key drivers of the pathological bone destruction in acute CN.

Mechanisms of Osteoclastogenesis

Recent advances in the cellular biology have enhanced our understanding of osteoclast function in both physiological and pathological conditions. Osteoclasts have been shown to be the principal cell type responsible for bone resorption [17]. These tissue-specific multi-nucleated cells are derived from differentiation of monocyte/macrophage precursor cells at or near the bone surface [18]. Osteoclastic precursors circulate in the blood in the monocytic fraction [19]. Subtypes of monocytes, which express the cluster of differentiation (CD) markers CD14, CD11b and CD61, exhibit 90-, 30-, and 20-fold higher osteoclast formation capacity in contrast to CD15+ and CD169+ monocytes that can hardly generate osteoclasts [20]. Two cytokines are both necessary and sufficient for osteoclastogenesis: RANKL, and macrophage-colony stimulating factor (M-CSF).

RANKL, a cytokine from the tumour necrosis factor (TNF)-ligand superfamily, is expressed on a variety of cell types (bone-forming osteoblasts, T lymphocytes, dendritic cells, endothelial cells and fibroblasts). RANKL binds to its target RANK, expressed on mononuclear osteoclastic precursors, induces NF-κβ signalling, resulting in NF-κβ translocation to the nucleus and drives osteoclastogenesis [21]. RANKL has been shown to stimulate the fusion of pre-osteoclasts, the attachment of the osteoclasts to the bone, and it is also an important factor for their activation and survival [22]. M-CSF, a hematopoietic growth factor, is an essential cytokine required for proliferation and survival of mononuclear cells and it acts via its receptor c-fms [23].

In the presence of RANKL and M-CSF, osteoclast precursors undergo various stages of proliferation, fusion and differentiation before they become fully functionally active, mature osteoclasts. These large multi-nucleated cells express a series of osteoclast markers, including tartrate-resistant acid phosphatase (TRAP), cathepsin K, calcitonin receptor and β_3-intergrin [18, 24]. To degrade mineralised matrix, these cells have a unique cytoskeleton. When in contact with the bone, they form a ruffled membrane and actin rings, characteristic of actively resorbing osteoclasts [25]. RANKL stimulates osteoclast activation by inducing the secretion of protons and lytic enzymes into a sealed resorption zone formed between the basal surface of the osteoclast and the bone surface [18]. The secreted protons in the resorption lacuna activate TRAP and cathepsin K which are essential for the degradation of bone mineral and collagen matrix [18]. The resorbed material is then removed by uptake and transcytosis through the osteoclasts. After completing the resorption, osteoclasts undergo apoptosis or migrate and perform a further round of resorption.

Osteoclast Formation and Osteoclast Function in CN – Evidence from in vitro Studies

The breakthrough discovery of RANKL in 1998, which was identified as osteoblast–produced, ligand-promoting osteoclast differentiation, has facilitated the establishment of an in vitro system to generate functional bone-resorbing osteoclasts without the need of co-culture of osteoblasts or stromal cells and haematopoietic cells [26, 27]. The technique to generate functional human osteoclasts from peripheral blood monocytes in the presence of M-CSF and soluble RANKL [19, 28] has been well recognised as a useful tool to determine the cellular mechanisms involved in the process of osteoclast formation and resorption in physiological and pathological conditions.

Recent studies using this technique have underscored the role of RANKL, as an osteoclastic activator in the pathogenesis of pathological bone destruction in CN [29]. In vitro studies have shown that the osteoclast formation from monocytes was similar between CN patients, diabetic patients and healthy controls. However, the newly formed osteoclasts derived from Charcot patients exhibited increased resorbing activity as demonstrated by large areas of resorption on bovine slices after toluidine blue staining in response to M-CSF + RANKL treatment [29]. The resorption was blocked by the addition of excess concentrations of OPG, confirming the role of RANKL as an activator of osteoclastic activity in acute CN [8, 29]. These observations suggest that osteoclasts from CN patients have increased resorbing potential and are in a higher activated state as compared to those from the diabetic or healthy control groups. This enhanced resorbing activity has been further reiterated by a novel application of surface profilometry [30]. This technique revealed a notable difference in the way newly formed osteoclasts generated from monocytes from Charcot patients and controls exert their resorbing activity. Resorption pits on bovine slices were significantly wider and deeper in Charcot patients compared with controls and more frequently appeared as multi-dented pits. Overall, surface profilometry unmasked the aberrant erosion profile of bovine bone discs resorbed by osteoclasts derived from patients with CN in the presence of M-CSF + RANKL [30]. These studies confirm that activated osteoclasts are key drivers of pathological bone resorption in CN and RANKL is the main osteoclast regulator.

RANKL Up-Regulation in CN – Does Neuropathy Play a Role?

Neuropathy is the common denominator of all conditions presenting with Charcot joints. The association between bone and nerve in CN is not fully understood. It is possible that in CN, the upregulation of RANKL could be triggered by the loss of nerve-derived peptides, for example, calcitonin gene-related peptide (CGRP) [31]. The latter is a neuropeptide that acts as a neurotransmitter in small fibres (C-fibres) [32]. Local innervation plays a modulating role in bone growth, repair and remodelling. The terminal structure of the osseous CGRP-containing nerves directly contact osteoblasts, osteoclasts, and the periosteal lining cells, and are a source of local CGRP, which can act as a local modulator of bone metabolism. CGRP increases osteoblastic cyclic adenosine monophosphate via its action on bone-specific CGRP receptors [33] thus stimulating osteogenesis [34]. Osseous CGRP-containing fibres are also involved in pathologic events in bone. The density of CGRP fibres is increased near sites of post-fracture osteogenesis (healing callus) and is decreased at the stumps of non-union [35]. Evidence from bone marrow macrophage cultures has shown that CGRP inhibits RANKL induced NF-κB activation, downregulates osteoclastic genes like TRAP and cathepsin K and decreases the number of TRAP-positive cells and RANKL-mediated bone resorption [36].

Thus, CGRP deficiency in small fibre neuropathy may lead to impaired osteogenesis and delayed fracture healing, and also enhance RANKL-mediated osteoclastic activity leading to CN. The link between nerve and bone in CN requires further studies. Nevertheless, the role of neuropathy as a trigger of CN bone destruction is universal.

Inflammation as a Further Driver of Increased Osteoclastic Activity in CN

This extensive osteoclastic activity in CN can only partially be attributed to the enhanced activation of RANKL. Normally, the upregulation of RANKL would lead to systemic bone loss, but in CN, bone loss is limited to the neuropathic affected foot [12, 16]. Furthermore, there is a greater reduction of bone mineral density of the Charcot foot compared with the non-Charcot foot [12] and peripheral osteopenia is not always associated with a reduction of bone mineral density of the axial skeleton [16]. This suggests that factors limited to the affected Charcot foot may be fundamental and the role of inflammation is pivotal.

The Charcot foot classically presents as a red hot swollen foot. This extensive foot inflammation often is not associated with a significant rise of systemic inflammatory markers [37]. C-reactive protein and white blood cell count are often within the normal reference range or mildly elevated [37]. Despite the reported discordance between local and systemic markers, the role of inflammation in the pathogenesis of CN is well recognised and proinflammatory cytokines could be crucial [13]. Data from clinical observation studies of cohorts of Charcot patients reported raised serum concentrations of the proinflammatory cytokines TNF-α and interleukin 6 (IL-6) in the acute active stage of the disease followed by a significant fall at the time of clinical resolution [38, 39]. Serum concentrations of TNF-α and IL-6 correlate with the bone resorption marker C-terminal telopeptide of type 1 collagen [38]. A further study in CN has also shown that the concentration of the pro-inflammatory cytokines in the local circulation is higher compared with the systemic circulation [40]. Moreover, immunohistochemistry of surgical specimens from Charcot patients has indicated that bone resorption in CN takes place in inflammatory environment with increased expression of proinflammatory cytokines (IL-1, IL-6 and TNF-α) [41].

Thus, in CN, trauma on the background of neuropathy leads to an exaggerated cytokine response with release of proinflammatory cytokines [13]. In such pathological conditions with excessive activation of the immune system, osteoclastic activity becomes deregulated due to increased production of pro-inflammatory cytokines by activated T-cells. In neuropathy, it is possible that there is a misbalance between the production of pro-osteoclastogenic cytokines (IL-1β, IL-6, IL-8, IL-11, IL-17, and TNF-α) and anti-osteoclastogenic mediators (IL-4, IL-10, IL-13, IL-18, interferon-γ, and interferon-β) [42]. In CN, a strong correlation between the percentage of CD14-positive cells (osteoclast precursors) and the serum levels of TNF-α has been reported [43]. Moreover, blood monocytes from patients with acute CN spontaneously produced detectable amounts of TNF-α, IL-1β, IL-6 but not IL-4 and IL-10 [39]. When stimulated with lipopolysaccharide, monocytes from Charcot patients had enhanced production of TNF-α, IL-1β, IL-6 but less IL-4 and IL-10 compared with monocytes from diabetic control and healthy control subjects [39]. Overall, these observations indicate a potential link between inflammation and pathological bone resorption in CN [38, 43].

Advances in cellular biology have underpinned the link between inflammation and osteoclast activation. Proinflammatory cytokines can target osteoclasts directly or indirectly by modulating the RANKL/OPG signalling pathway. As an osteoclastogenic mediator, TNF-α induces expression of RANKL in osteoblastic cells, but it can also act directly on osteoclastic precursors (monocytes) to potentiate RANKL-induced osteoclastogenesis and thereby activity [44]. Moreover, experimental work has demonstrated synergism between TNF-α and RANKL in their action on osteoclastic precursors [45–47]. For its osteoclastogenic activity, TNF-α requires permissive levels of RANKL [45]. The role of TNF-α as a modulator of osteoclastic activity in rheumatoid arthritis [48], psoriatic arthritis [49], and also in other forms of inflammatory osteolysis [50] is well established. A further osteoclastogenic mediator, which could be important in CN is IL-6, as it not only enhances RANKL and OPG expression but also can directly stimulate osteoclast differentiation [42, 51]. In addition to trauma, bone fracture itself triggers a coordinated healing cytokine response with induction of proinflammatory cytokines, including IL-1 and TNF-α [52]. RANKL is also increased in fracture healing [53].

The role of TNF-α as an osteoclastogenic mediator has been investigated by traditional osteoclast culture techniques [54]. The addition of high concentration of neutralising antibody to TNF-α decreased the resorbing activity of M-CSF + RANKL-treated osteoclasts derived from Charcot patients. This was evident by a significant reduction of the area of resorption on bovine bone discs on the surface, as assessed by image analysis (Fig. 2a, b). In addition, surface profilometry revealed that the aberrant erosion profile, pit morphology and pit distribution in M-CSF + RANKL-treated cultures in Charcot patients were reversed after the addition of anti-TNF-α (Fig. 2c, d). These findings confirm the role of TNF-α as a promoter of the observed enhanced osteoclast function in M-CSF + RANKL-treated cultures from acute CN patients [54].

These observations suggest that in inflammatory environment, Charcot osteoclasts exhibit enhanced resorbing activity and maintain a continuous resorptive mode, which is not interrupted by osteoclast migration [55]. It is possible that TNF-α modulates the resorption cycle in CN. During the process of bone resorption, osteoclasts solubilise bone mineral followed by the degradation of demineralised organic matrix and in control conditions, the relative rate of collagenolysis is slower than the rate of demineralization [56]. Experimental in vitro studies have shown that agents that can upregulate cathepsin K expression prolong the resorption cycle, and resorption events more frequently present as trenches (continuous resorption) [56]. In contrast, the inhibition of cathepsin K accelerates the resorption cycle, leading to faster accumulation of collagen. This results in resorption events more frequently presenting as shallower and smaller pits (intermittent resorption). Both RANKL and TNF-α stimulate the osteoclasts to produce cathepsin K, which is the major protease responsible for the degradation of collagen [57]. In CN, it is possible that TNF-α via enhanced cathepsin K expression may lead to imbalance between the relative rate of collagenolysis and demineralization and this requires further studies [54].

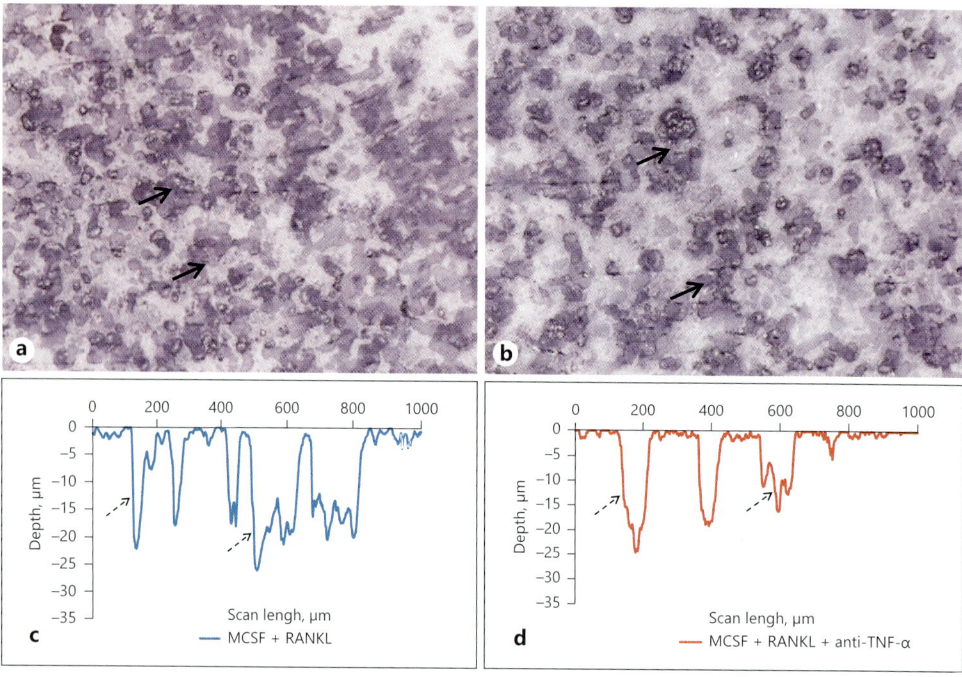

Fig. 2. Resorption on bovine bone discs by newly formed osteoclast generated from monocytes from a Charcot patient. Light microscopy: typical appearance of resorption pits after toluidine blue staining in M-CSF + RANKL-treated culture (**a**) and M-CSF + RANKL + anti-TNF-α-treated culture (**b**). The arrows denote some of the resorption pits. Surface profilometry: typical appearance of erosion profile of resorbed bovine bone discs in M-CSF + RANKL-treated culture (**c**) and M-CSF + RANKL + anti-TNF-α-treated culture (**d**). Dashed arrows denote the below surface profile of pits after surface profilometry (**c, d**).

Summary

Significant progress has been made in our understanding of the pathogenesis of CN in diabetes. Present imaging techniques have significantly contributed to improved recognition of the earliest pathological lesion of CN in diabetes. In addition, advances in cellular biology have elucidated the pathways to pathological bone destruction in CN. Trauma to the neuropathic diabetic foot leads to early osteolysis and uncontrolled inflammation [13]. Bone (micro)fracture is the harbinger of CN [58]. It leads to changes in the bone matrix, which becomes a site of targeted remodelling with increased numbers of apoptotic osteocytes (bone matrix cells) and rapid degradation by activated osteoclasts [24, 59]. Furthermore, bone fracture triggers a coordinated healing cytokine response with the induction of pro-inflammatory cytokines, including TNF-α [52]. In the affected Charcot foot, the inflammatory response to trauma and the associated enhanced cytokine release leads to an upregulation of receptors and adhesion molecules in the endothelium. Indeed, cytokine-activated endothelium recruits osteoclast precursors [60] and promotes the activation of RANK by RANKL,

Petrova

leading to enhanced RANKL-induced migration of osteoclast precursors to the affected Charcot foot. Thus, TNF-α-primed osteoclastic precursors in the presence of increased local expression of RANKL differentiate into highly aggressive osteoclasts with extensive resorbing activity characterised by increased survival, reduced apoptosis and migration [8]. This increased osteoclastic activity may be due to cathepsin K upregulation, which requires further studies. Overall, these observations shed light on the pathogenesis of this devastating condition and may provide a scientific basis for future therapies of this devastating condition in diabetes.

References

1 Petrova NL, Edmonds ME: Charcot neuro-osteoarthropathy-current standards. Diabetes Metab Res Rev 2008;24(suppl 1):S58–S61.

2 Shibuya N, La Fontaine J, Frania SJ: Alcohol-induced neuroarthropathy in the foot: a case series and review of literature. J Foot Ankle Surg 2008;47:118–124.

3 Arapostathi C, Tentolouris N, Jude EB: Charcot foot associated with chronic alcohol abuse. BMJ Case Rep 2013;pii:bcr2012008263.

4 Young N, Neiderer K, Martin B, Jolley D, Dancho JF: HIV neuropathy induced Charcot neuroarthropathy: a case discussion. Foot (Edinb) 2012;22:112–116.

5 Sohn MW, Stuck RM, Pinzur M, Lee TA, Budiman-Mak E: Lower-extremity amputation risk after charcot arthropathy and diabetic foot ulcer. Diabetes Care 2010;33:98–100.

6 Rogers LC, Frykberg RG, Armstrong DG, Boulton AJ, Edmonds M, Van GH, et al: The Charcot foot in diabetes. Diabetes Care 2011;34:2123–2129.

7 Petrova NL, Edmonds ME: Acute Charcot neuro-osteoarthropathy. Diabetes Metab Res Rev 2015;32(suppl 1):281–286.

8 Petrova NL: Studies in the Pathogenesis of Charcotosteoarthropathy. PhD Thesis, King's College London, 2015.

9 Lee L, Blume PA, Sumpio B: Charcot joint disease in diabetes mellitus. Ann Vasc Surg 2003;17:571–580.

10 Brower AC, Allman RM: Pathogenesis of the neurotrophic joint: neurotraumatic vs. neurovascular. Radiology 1981;139:349–354.

11 Chantelau E, Onvlee GJ: Charcot foot in diabetes: farewell to the neurotrophic theory. Horm Metab Res 2006;38:361–367.

12 Petrova NL, Foster AV, Edmonds ME: Calcaneal bone mineral density in patients with Charcot neuropathic osteoarthropathy: differences between type 1 and type 2 diabetes. Diabet Med 2005;22:756–761.

13 Jeffcoate WJ, Game F, Cavanagh PR: The role of proinflammatory cytokines in the cause of neuropathic osteoarthropathy (acute Charcot foot) in diabetes. Lancet 2005;366:2058–2061.

14 Gough A, Abraha H, Li F, Purewal TS, Foster AV, Watkins PJ, et al: Measurement of markers of osteoclast and osteoblast activity in patients with acute and chronic diabetic Charcot neuroarthropathy. Diabet Med 1997;14:527–531.

15 Piaggesi A, Rizzo L, Golia F, Costi D, Baccetti F, Ciaccio S, et al: Biochemical and ultrasound tests for early diagnosis of active neuro-osteoarthropathy (NOA) of the diabetic foot. Diabetes Res Clin Pract 2002;58:1–9.

16 Jirkovská A, Kasalický P, Boucek P, Hosová J, Skibová J: Calcaneal ultrasonometry in patients with Charcot osteoarthropathy and its relationship with densitometry in the lumbar spine and femoral neck and with markers of bone turnover. Diabet Med 2001;18:495–500.

17 Teitelbaum SL: Bone resorption by osteoclasts. Science 2000;289:1504–1508.

18 Boyle WJ, Simonet WS, Lacey DL: Osteoclast differentiation and activation. Nature 2003;423:337–342.

19 Fujikawa Y, Quinn JM, Sabokbar A, McGee JO, Athanasou NA: The human osteoclast precursor circulates in the monocyte fraction. Endocrinology 1996;137:4058–4060.

20 Husheem M, Nyman JK, Vääräniemi J, Vaananen HK, Hentunen TA: Characterization of circulating human osteoclast progenitors: development of in vitro resorption assay. Calcif Tissue Int 2005;76:222–230.

21 Boyce BF, Xing L: Functions of RANKL/RANK/OPG in bone modeling and remodeling. Arch Biochem Biophys 2008;473:139–146.

22 Kostenuik PJ: Osteoprotegerin and RANKL regulate bone resorption, density, geometry and strength. Curr Opin Pharmacol 2005;5:618–625.

23 Yasuda H, Shima N, Nakagawa N, Yamaguchi K, Kinosaki M, Mochizuki S, et al: Osteoclast differentiation factor is a ligand for osteoprotegerin/osteoclastogenesis-inhibitory factor and is identical to TRANCE/RANKL. Proc Natl Acad Sci U S A 1998; 95:3597–3602.

24 Henriksen K, Bollerslev J, Everts V, Karsdal MA: Osteoclast activity and subtypes as a function of physiology and pathology – implications for future treatments of osteoporosis. Endocr Rev 2011;32:31–63.

25 Teitelbaum SL: Osteoclasts: what do they do and how do they do it? Am J Pathol 2007;170:427–435.

26 Susa M, Luong-Nguyen NH, Cappellen D, Zamurovic N, Gamse R: Human primary osteoclasts: in vitro generation and applications as pharmacological and clinical assay. J Transl Med 2004;2:6.

27 Marino S, Logan JG, Mellis D, Capulli M: Generation and culture of osteoclasts. Bonekey Rep 2014;3:570.

28 Sabokbar A, Athanasou NS: Generating human osteoclasts from peripheral blood. Methods Mol Med 2003;80:101–111.

29 Mabilleau G, Petrova NL, Edmonds ME, Sabokbar A: Increased osteoclastic activity in acute Charcot's osteoarthropathy: the role of receptor activator of nuclear factor-kappaB ligand. Diabetologia 2008;51: 1035–1040.

30 Petrova NL, Petrov PK, Edmonds ME, Shanahan CM: Novel use of a Dektak 150 surface profiler unmasks differences in resorption pit profiles between control and Charcot patient osteoclasts. Calcif Tissue Int 2014;94:403–411; erratum in Calcif Tissue Int 2014;94:412–413.

31 Jeffcoate W: Vascular calcification and osteolysis in diabetic neuropathy-is RANK-L the missing link? Diabetologia 2004;47:1488–1492.

32 Pittenger G, Vinik A: Nerve growth factor and diabetic neuropathy. Exp Diabesity Res 2003;4:271–285.

33 Bjurholm A, Kreicbergs A, Schultzberg M, Lerner UH: Neuroendocrine regulation of cyclic AMP formation in osteoblastic cell lines (UMR-106-01, ROS 17/2.8, MC3T3-E1, and Saos-2) and primary bone cells. J Bone Miner Res 1992;7:1011–1019.

34 Bernard GW, Shih C: The osteogenic stimulating effect of neuroactive calcitonin gene-related peptide. Peptides 1990;11:625–632.

35 Santavirta S, Konttinen YT, Nordström D, Mäkelä A, Sorsa T, Hukkanen M, et al: Immunologic studies of nonunited fractures. Acta Orthop Scand 1992;63: 579–586.

36 Wang L, Shi X, Zhao R, Halloran BP, Clark DJ, Jacobs CR, et al: Calcitonin-gene-related peptide stimulates stromal cell osteogenic differentiation and inhibits RANKL induced NF-kappaB activation, osteoclastogenesis and bone resorption. Bone 2010; 46:1369–1379.

37 Petrova NL, Moniz C, Elias DA, Buxton-Thomas M, Bates M, Edmonds ME: Is there a systemic inflammatory response in the acute Charcot foot? Diabetes Care 2007;30:997–998.

38 Petrova NL, Dew TK, Musto RL, Sherwood RA, Bates M, Moniz CF, et al: Inflammatory and bone turnover markers in a cross-sectional and prospective study of acute Charcot osteoarthropathy. Diabet Med 2015;32:267–273.

39 Uccioli L, Sinistro A, Almerighi C, Ciaprini C, Cavazza A, Giurato L, et al: Proinflammatory modulation of the surface and cytokine phenotype of monocytes in patients with acute Charcot foot. Diabetes Care 2010;33:350–355.

40 Divyateja H, Shu KS, Pearson RG, Scammell BE, Game FL, Jeffcoate WJ: Local and systemic concentrations of pro-inflammatory cytokines, osteoprotegerin, sRANKL and bone turnover markers in acute Charcot foot and in controls. Diabetologia 2011; 54:S11–S12.

41 Baumhauer JF, O'Keefe RJ, Schon LC, Pinzur MS: Cytokine-induced osteoclastic bone resorption in charcot arthropathy: an immunohistochemical study. Foot Ankle Int 2006;27:797–800.

42 Zupan J, Jeras M, Marc J: Osteoimmunology and the influence of pro-inflammatory cytokines on osteoclasts. Biochem Med (Zagreb) 2013;23:43–63.

43 Mabilleau G, Petrova N, Edmonds ME, Sabokbar A: Number of circulating CD14-positive cells and the serum levels of TNF-α are raised in acute charcot foot. Diabetes Care 2011;34:e33.

44 Lam J, Abu-Amer Y, Nelson CA, Fremont DH, Ross FP, Teitelbaum SL: Tumour necrosis factor superfamily cytokines and the pathogenesis of inflammatory osteolysis. Ann Rheum Dis 2002;61(suppl 2): ii82–ii83.

45 Lam J, Takeshita S, Barker JE, Kanagawa O, Ross FP, Teitelbaum SL: TNF-alpha induces osteoclastogenesis by direct stimulation of macrophages exposed to permissive levels of RANK ligand. J Clin Invest 2000; 106:1481–1488.

46 Kobayashi K, Takahashi N, Jimi E, Udagawa N, Takami M, Kotake S, et al: Tumor necrosis factor alpha stimulates osteoclast differentiation by a mechanism independent of the ODF/RANKL-RANK interaction. J Exp Med 2000;191:275–286.

47 Fuller K, Murphy C, Kirstein B, Fox SW, Chambers TJ: TNFalpha potently activates osteoclasts, through a direct action independent of and strongly synergistic with RANKL. Endocrinology 2002;143:1108–1118.

48 Romas E: Bone loss in inflammatory arthritis: mechanisms and therapeutic approaches with bisphosphonates. Best Pract Res Clin Rheumatol 2005;19: 1065–1079.

49 Ritchlin CT, Haas-Smith SA, Li P, Hicks DG, Schwarz EM: Mechanisms of TNF-alpha- and RANKL-mediated osteoclastogenesis and bone resorption in psoriatic arthritis. J Clin Invest 2003;111: 821–831.

50 Redlich K, Smolen JS: Inflammatory bone loss: pathogenesis and therapeutic intervention. Nat Rev Drug Discov 2012;11:234–250.

51 Kudo O, Sabokbar A, Pocock A, Itonaga I, Fujikawa Y, Athanasou NA: Interleukin-6 and interleukin-11 support human osteoclast formation by a RANKL-independent mechanism. Bone 2003;32:1–7.

52 Kon T, Cho TJ, Aizawa T, Yamazaki M, Nooh N, Graves D, Gerstenfeld LC, Einhorn TA: Expression of osteoprotegerin, receptor activator of NF-kappaB ligand (osteoprotegerin ligand) and related proinflammatory cytokines during fracture healing. J Bone Miner Res 2001;16:1004–1014.

53 Kon T, Cho TJ, Aizawa T, Yamazaki M, Nooh N, Graves D, et al: Expression of osteoprotegerin, receptor activator of NF-kappaB ligand (osteoprotegerin ligand) and related proinflammatory cytokines during fracture healing. J Bone Miner Res 2001;16: 1004–1014.

54 Petrova NL, Petrov PK, Edmonds ME, Shanahan CM: Inhibition of TNF-α reverses the pathological resorption pit profile of osteoclasts from patients with acute Charcot osteoarthropathy. J Diabetes Res 2015;2015:917945.

55 Søe K, Delaissé JM: Glucocorticoids maintain human osteoclasts in the active mode of their resorption cycle. J Bone Miner Res 2010;25:2184–2192.

56 Søe K, Merrild DM, Delaissé JM: Steering the osteoclast through the demineralization-collagenolysis balance. Bone 2013;56:191–198.

57 Troen BR: The regulation of cathepsin K gene expression. Ann N Y Acad Sci 2006;1068:165–172.

58 Johnson JT: Neuropathic fractures and joint injuries. Pathogenesis and rationale of prevention and treatment. J Bone Joint Surg Am 1967;49:1–30.

59 Heino TJ, Kurata K, Higaki H, Väänänen HK: Evidence for the role of osteocytes in the initiation of targeted remodeling. Technol Health Care 2009;17: 49–56.

60 McGowan NW, Walker EJ, Macpherson H, Ralston SH, Helfrich MH: Cytokine-activated endothelium recruits osteoclast precursors. Endocrinology 2001; 142:1678–1681.

Nina L. Petrova, MD, PhD
Diabetic Foot Clinic
King's College Hospital NHS Foundation Trust
Denmark Hill, London SE5 9RS (UK)
E-Mail nina.petrova@nhs.net

Piaggesi A, Apelqvist J (eds): The Diabetic Foot Syndrome.
Front Diabetes. Basel, Karger, 2018, vol 26, pp 60–69 (DOI: 10.1159/000480046)

Diabetic Peripheral Arteriopathy: A Tale of Two Diseases

Michael E. Edmonds[a] · C. Shanahan[b] · Nina L. Petrova[a]

[a]Diabetic Foot Clinic, King's College Hospital NHS Foundation Trust and Division of Diabetes and Nutritional Sciences, King's College London, and [b]Cardiovascular Division, King's College London, London, UK

Abstract

Peripheral arterial disease is a major risk factor for amputation in patients with diabetes. Its presentation is different from that of the occlusive arterial disease in patients without diabetes. In diabetes, peripheral arterial disease develops at a younger age and women and men are equally affected. The vascular changes have a predominantly distal distribution with the crural vessels being the most severely affected by long occlusions. There is controversy as to whether the presentation of ischaemic foot disease in diabetes can be explained by one disease, namely, atherosclerosis with particular features such as distal arterial involvement or by the occurrence of 2 diseases: a diabetic macroangiopathy, a term for non-atherosclerotic arterial disease, and classical atherosclerosis. The main component of diabetic macroangiopathy is medial arterial calcification of the muscular arteries, which may be accompanied by intimal pathology. This condition has a predilection of disease below the knee. Classic atherosclerosis is noted in the proximal arteries of the diabetic limb, namely, iliac, femoral and popliteal disease. The risk factors for this proximal site disease are hypercholesterolemia and smoking. Further studies are needed to investigate the interaction between macroangiopathy and atherosclerosis in diabetes for improved understanding of the pathogenesis of this severe complication.

Introduction

Peripheral arterial disease is a major risk factor for amputation in patients with diabetes [1]. It has several features that distinguishes it from occlusive arterial disease in the patient without diabetes. Compared with the non-diabetic patient, peripheral arterial disease develops at a younger age, and women are equally affected as men. The vascular changes in diabetic patients are more diffuse and located distally being most severe in the crural vessels [2, 3]. There is a high prevalence of long occlusions in the tibial arteries, which occur more frequently than stenosis [4, 5].

Various clinical and pathological studies have compared arteries in the legs of diabetic patients with those in non-diabetic subjects. A combined clinical and pathological study of large and small arteries in diabetic and non-diabetic patients has shown that the diabetic patient has the same incidence of occlusion in the femoral-popliteal system but a higher incidence of occlusion below the knee [6]. In a further study, casts were made of the vascular lumen of 20 successive extremities amputated for gangrene [7] half of whom were diabetic patients. These subjects had predominant occlusion of the calf vessels and less occlusion in the foot vessels compared with non-diabetic patients. There is controversy as to whether the arteries below the ankle are spared from occlusive disease in diabetes. In amputated legs of diabetic patients, occlusive disease was more severe in arteries above the ankle compared with non-diabetic patients, but no difference was demonstrated in the arteries of the ankle and foot [8]. However, when Ferraresi et al. [9] analyzed the obstructive disease distribution in a series of 1,624 patients with critical limb ischaemia and Rutherford grades 5 and 6, foot arterial disease was present in >70% of patients.

It is not known whether the presentation of ischaemic foot disease in diabetes can be explained by one disease, namely, atherosclerosis, with particular features peculiar to diabetes such as distal arterial involvement or, by the occurrence of 2 separate diseases, first, diabetic macroangiopathy, a term for non-atherosclerotic arterial disease in diabetes, and second, classical atherosclerosis. For the sake of clarity, this paper will first describe the features of diabetic macroangiopathy and second, those of atherosclerosis in ischaemic diabetic patients. It will not consider arteriolar disease.

Diabetic Macroangiopathy

The first notion of a diabetic macroangiopathy was mentioned by Lundbaeck [10]. The main component of diabetic macroangiopathy is medial arterial disease of the muscular arteries, which may be accompanied by intimal pathology. This condition has a predilection of disease below the knee. The medial arterial disease is classically medial arterial calcification although accumulation of laminin, fibronectin and type IV collagen with hyaluronic acid has been described [11]. Diffuse fibrosis of the medial wall has also been reported [12].

Medial Arterial Calcification

Medial arterial calcification is easily detected on radiograph by its classical pipe stem or tramline calcification. Bowen et al. [13] was the first to describe the calcification of the arteries in diabetes in 1924 and related its severity to the duration of diabetes. In 1928, Morrison and Bogan [14] observed that the frequency of calcification in his patients depended also on the duration of diabetes. Ferrier and Ferner [15], in 1964, in a formal study of medial calcification, described it as a characteristic finding in long-term diabetes. Amputation studies have demonstrated that diabetic patients are likely to have more medial calcification in the arteries than non-diabetic patients [8].

Prognosis of Medial Arterial Calcification
Medial wall calcification represents a strong independent predictor of future cardiovascular events and all-cause mortality [16, 17]. There are several studies that link medial calcification with mortality and other complications of diabetes. Everhart initially demonstrated that risk factors for arterial calcification were impaired sensation to vibration, duration of diabetes and high plasma glucose [18]. Interestingly, the risk factors in non-diabetic patients were age, male gender and high serum cholesterol. He then went on to show that diabetic patients with medial calcification had a 1.5-fold mortality rate (95% CI 1.0–2.1), a 5.5-fold rate of amputation (95% CI 2.1–14.1), a 2.4-fold rate of proteinuria (95% CI 1.3–4.5), a 1.7-fold rate of retinopathy (95% CI 0.98–2.8) and a 1.6-fold rate of coronary artery disease (95% CI 0.48–5.4). A further study of 1,059 patients with type 2 diabetes assessed the predicted value of medial calcification in relation to 7-year cardiovascular mortality, coronary heart disease events, stroke and lower extremity amputation. Medial calcification was a strong independent predictor of total (risk factor adjusted odds ratio and 95% CI 1.6; 1.2–2.2), cardiovascular (1.6; 1.1–2.2), and coronary heart disease (1.5; 1.0–2.2) mortality, and also a significant predictor of future coronary heart disease events (fatal or non-fatal myocardial infarction), stroke and amputation. This relationship was observed regardless of glycaemic control and known duration of diabetes [19].

Pathology
In a comparison of lower limb arteries in the legs and feet of 10 diabetic patients with 10 non-diabetic subjects, Ferrier [20] found a higher incidence of advanced medial calcification in the metatarsal arteries of diabetic patients associated with significant metatarsal artery obstruction. Occlusion of the metatarsal arteries was present in 60% of diabetics and 21% of non-diabetics and occlusion was noted in 19% of diabetics and 10% of non-diabetics in the digital arteries. Meema et al. [21] has suggested the possibility that 2 different types of medial calcifications may exist. The first is a benign type, of gradual onset, with thin medial calcifications and no compromise of the lumen. This condition does not result in ischaemia. In contrast, the second type is a rapidly progressive form, in which considerable medial calcification may displace the internal elastica towards the lumen, resulting in luminal narrowing.

Physiological Effects of Calcification
Medial arterial calcification may have several major haemodynamic consequences. It is initially associated with increased blood flow. In a Doppler study of the diabetic neuropathic leg, the arteries were rigid and calcified and blood flow was

increased [22]. In a quantitative angiographic study of the large arteries in the legs of 47 insulin-dependent diabetics, representing a uniform cross section of diabetes duration and the young to middle age range, patients with medial arterial calcification showed no significant decrease of cross-sectional area in any arterial region compared to patients without calcification [23]. Gilbey et al. [24] has shown that in autonomic neuropathy with extensive calcification, the blood flow was high in the hallux as assessed by venous plethysmography and transcutaneous oxygen in the resting supine foot.

Christensen [25] studied the physiology of medial calcification and measured the maximal peak flow, using xenon 133, which was reduced in patients with calcification compared with patients without calcification. In patients with calcification, increasing duration of diabetes was related to decreasing peak flow. Chantelau et al. [26] measured the effect of medial calcification on oxygen supply to exercising diabetic feet. Transcutaneous oxygen decreased with exercise in feet with peripheral vascular disease, regardless of the presence or absence of calcification, and transcutaneous oxygen increased with exercise in feet with calcification but without peripheral vascular disease and also in diabetic control subjects. Neubauer et al. [27] reported in diabetic patients a uniform narrowing of the superficial femoral arteries associated with rugosities, stiffness, medial calcification, norepinephrine depletion and reduced blood flow capacity.

Pathogenesis

Medial arterial calcification occurs independently of atherosclerosis and is strongly associated with aging, chronic kidney disease and diabetes mellitus. Initially, medial calcification was thought to be related to the duration of diabetes, but it has been shown that calcification is a specific complication strongly associated with neuropathy [28]. In 2 large series of cases with Charcot neuroarthropathy, medial calcification was found in 90% [29] and 78% [30] respectively. In a further study of 54 neuropathic patients with foot ulceration compared with 40 neuropathic patients without ulceration, 43 non-neuropathic controls and 50 control subjects, medial arterial calcification was significantly more extensive in the neuropathic patients with foot ulceration. Medial calcification correlated with vibration ($r = 0.35$, $p < 0.01$), duration of diabetes ($r = 0.32$, $p < 0.01$) and serum creatinine ($r = 0.41$, $p < 0.01$) [31]. Furthermore, Forst et al. [32] reported a strong association between medal arterial calcification and diminished heart rate variation and diminished sweat response and Gentile et al. [33] showed linear calcification in 37 out of 41 patients with autonomic neuropathy, which was absent in controls without autonomic neuropathy ($p < 0.001$). Medial arterial calcification has been described in familial amyloid neuropathy and after lumbar sympathectomy. Medial calcification was noted in both feet in 93% of patients who had undergone bilateral lumbar sympathectomy [34]. After unilateral sympathectomy, the incidence of calcified arteries was higher in the affected limb compared with that of the contralateral limb, 89 vs. 18% ($p < $

0.01). Twenty patients with no evidence of previous calcification underwent unilateral sympathectomy, and 13 of these subsequently developed calcification. Seven underwent bilateral sympathectomy and calcification was subsequently seen in 7 out of 7.

Unilateral sympathectomy in animals leads to excess deposition of cholesterol on the operated side [35] and the occurrence of cholesterol sclerosis in the rabbit's aorta was hastened by the removal of the coeliac ganglion [36]. Furthermore, in animal models, denervation of smooth muscle leads to striking pathological changes, including atrophy of muscle fibres with foci of degeneration [37]. Thus, calcification may be related to an underlying autonomic denervation, which may be important in its pathogenesis [38].

Arterial calcification is initiated within the senescent atrophic smooth muscle [39]. Also, long-term administration of calcitonin impeded the formation of calcareous deposits in an experimental model of atherosclerosis in rabbits and reduced the extent of the atherosclerotic process [40].

Medial arterial calcification is an active process involving the deposition of hydroxyapatite crystals along concentric elastin fibres, directly abutting vascular smooth muscle cells. It occurs in the absence of inflammatory cells. Differentiation of vascular smooth muscle cells into osteoblast-like cells is considered to be a mechanism of vascular calcification [41]. Normally, a balance exists between the promoters and inhibitors of calcification [42]. Immunohistochemisty and in situ hybridization techniques have shown that calcified vessels from diabetic patients showed diminished expression of matrix Gla-protein and osteonectin, which are key inhibitors of vascular calcification. Conversely, there was increased expression of osteopontin, alkaline phosphatase, bone sialoprotein, bone Gla protein and collagen II – indicators of osteo/chondrogenesis [41].

Familial aggregation of medial arterial calcification has been noted in the Pima Indians raising the issue of potential genetic factors. To assess whether such familial aggregation was independent of diabetes, members of 1,256 Pima Indian nuclear families with 3,339 offspring were examined radiologically for medial calcification of the feet. Multiple logistic regression analyses were used to compare the presence of the disorder in a parent with the presence of calcification in an offspring and to determine whether familial aggregation of calcification was independent of parental diabetes. Parental calcification confirmed an increased risk of medial calcification in offspring, independent of parental age and disease and independent of offspring age and diabetes. These findings suggest that the factors responsible for the familial clustering of medial calcification may be different from those with diabetes [43].

Impact of Medial Arterial Calcification
Arterial Stiffening
In addition to having a pathological, structural component in the form of medial calcification, macroangiopathy has physiological consequences such as increased

arterial stiffness, which is associated with an increase in pulse wave velocity and increase in pulse pressure. There is a dampening of the "cushioning" effect of the arteries that results in a diminished ability of the arteries to smooth out the pulsatile flow occurring with intermittent ventricular ejection [44]. The principal consequence of arterial stiffening is increased systolic pressure, resulting in elevated cardiac afterload and left ventricular hypertrophy. There is also a decrease in diastolic pressure and impaired coronary perfusion. An impairment of endothelium-dependent relaxation has been described in association with medial arterial calcification using aortic strips from rats with arteriosclerosis [45]. Endothelium-dependent relaxation to acetyl choline was impaired in proportion to the degree of calcification.

Medial Arterial Calcification and Peripheral Arterial Disease
The relationship between medical calcification and the development of clinically important peripheral arterial disease is not fully worked out. Chantelau et al. [46] reported an association of below-knee atherosclerosis to medial arterial calcification. In 42 diabetic patients, subjected to arteriography for peripheral vascular disease, forefoot radiographs were obtained for the assessment of medial calcification. The distribution of the number of partial and total arterial stenoses per leg was assessed according to the co-existence of calcification. A total of 242 partial and complete stenoses were found in 35 legs with medial calcification and 28 without calcification. Legs with medial calcification had more than twice as many stenoses located in the lower leg: 2.6 (95% CI 2.3–2.8) stenoses below knee as compared to 1.3 (95% CI 1.0–1.07) stenoses in the upper leg ($p < 0.05$). Legs with no medial calcification showed stenoses equally distributed above and below the knee.

Medial arterial calcification prevents the compensatory remodelling in response to atherosclerotic lesions and may in this way accelerate the progression of the disease [47]. Furthermore, extensive medial calcification with secondary invasion of the intima increases the risk of thromboembolic events.

Intimal Disease
Diabetic macroangiopathy may have an intimal component that is described as intimal hyperplasia, neointima, hypertrophy and fibroplasia. However, the development in the intima is not simply hyperplasia, as it includes smooth muscle cells, which may have migrated from the media or adventitia, or have been deposited from circulating progenitor cells.

Although intimal thickening has been described in arteriolosclerosis, it also occurs in larger arteries where it is usually labelled as adaptive intimal thickening or diffuse intimal thickening [48]. Recent histology of peripheral arteries has indicated that intimal hyperplasia can lead to significant stenosis and occasional occlusion or thrombus and this is noted in the absence of plaque [49]. Studies of amputated specimens have demonstrated intimal thickening, which has been labelled as atherosclerotic [8, 50].

Occlusion may occur due to concentric intimal thickening or thrombus. It is possible that the occlusive intimal thickening also includes old organized thrombus [49]. The link between intimal thickening and medial calcification is not fully understood, as often the degree of intimal thickening does not relate to the extent of medial calcification [49].

Atherosclerosis

Classic atherosclerosis is noted in the proximal arteries of the diabetic limb and manifests as iliac, femoral and popliteal disease. The risk factors for this proximal site disease are hypercholesterolemia and smoking [51]. Diabetic patients have classic atherosclerotic lesions in the femoral popliteal region at the same frequency as in non-diabetes [6]. The occlusion is often multisegmental and there is poor collateral development. The atherosclerotic disease appears 10 years earlier than in patients without diabetes. It proceeds faster with a high incidence of multiple occlusions [52]. The outlook for survival is less favourable than for non-diabetic patients as associated disease in the coronary and cerebral circulations is more common in diabetes compared with non-diabetes.

Pathology

The development of diabetes-related atherosclerosis is associated with the same pathological course as atherosclerosis in non-diabetic patients [53]. Some authorities state that there is no histological or histochemical evidence to define a specific type of diabetic macroangiopathy [54]. The lesions of atherosclerosis do contain varying amounts and types of lipids, connective tissues, inflammatory cells, and a variety of extracellular components including matrix proteins and enzymes and calcium deposits [55, 56]. However, atherosclerosis in diabetes is associated with excessive intimal calcification in association with macrophages, lipids and the proliferation of vascular smooth muscle cells as a result of proinflammatory cytokine production by activated macrophages. Calcification of advanced atherosclerotic plaques occurs adjacent to lipid and cholesterol depositions and these plaques have necrotic cores. This leads to complex plaque formation, which is vulnerable to rupture and superimposed thrombosis. Heavily calcified plaques do not enhance plaque vulnerability, which seems more associated with a large lipid pool, thin fibrous cap, microcalcifications and excessive local inflammation [57, 58].

Intimal calcification is thought to result from modified lipid accumulation, proinflammatory cytokines, and apoptosis within the plaque that induce osteogenic cell differentiation [59]. Osteogenic differentiation with bone deposition is seldom observed in intimal calcification, although it is often seen in medial arterial calcification [60].

Clinical Presentation

Classic atherosclerosis can occur as a segmental occlusion in aortoiliac region when it presents as intermittent claudication of the buttocks or in the femoro-popliteal region when it is associated with claudication of the calf [61]. In a more advanced stage of atherosclerosis, multiple segmental occlusions can occur. Multiple aortoiliac occlusions result in severe and disabling claudication. Often, multiple occlusions occur in aortoiliac plus superficial femoral arteries, which lead not only to claudication but also to rest pain and necrosis.

Atherosclerosis can be non-segmental specifically in the femoro-popliteal region with occlusion of the superficial femoral artery, and blood flow to the leg is from the deep femoral artery. Intermittent claudication, rest pain and gangrene can occur.

Also, atherosclerosis may be diffuse. It is seen in elderly patients above 70 years old or in diabetic patients in their fifth and sixth decades. There is generalized narrowing of all arteries of the lower limb accompanied by occlusions in the advanced stage. Symptoms are claudication and in advanced cases rest pain and necrosis.

"Diabetic" atherosclerosis is also described. It presents at an early stage, often in the second or third decade. There is specific involvement of the popliteal, leg and foot arteries with progression to the superficial artery. This probably represents diabetic macroangiopathy.

Conclusion

It is controversial whether the presentation of ischaemic foot disease in diabetes can be explained by one disease, namely, atherosclerosis with particular features peculiar to diabetes such as distal arterial involvement or by the occurrence of 2 diseases, namely, diabetic macroangiopathy and classical atherosclerosis. However, the reader may notice some overlap between these conditions as the detailed nature of peripheral arterial occlusive disease in diabetes has not been fully defined.

Of course, in a diabetic patient, particularly a patient who develops arterial disease in later life, both diseases may co-exist.

References

1 Peripheral arterial disease in people with diabetes: American Diabetes Association. Diabetes Care 2003; 26:3333–3341.
2 Faglia E, Favales F, Quarantiello A, et al: Angiographic evaluation of peripheral arterial occlusive disease and its role as a prognostic determinant for major amputation in diabetic subjects with foot ulcers. Diabetes Care 1998;21:625–630.
3 Jude EB, Oyibo SO, Chalmers N, Boulton AJ: Peripheral arterial disease in diabetic and nondiabetic patients: a comparison of severity and outcome. Diabetes Care 2001;24:1433–1437.
4 Graziani L, Silvestro A, Bertone V, Manara E, Andreini R, Sigala A, Mingardi R, De Giglio R: Vascular involvement in diabetic subjects with ischemic foot ulcer: a new morphologic categorization of disease severity. Eur J Vasc Endovasc Surg. 2007;33:453–460.

5   Faglia E: Characteristics of peripheral arterial disease and its relevance to the diabetic population. Int J Low Extrem Wounds 2011;10:152–166.

6   Strandness DE Jr et al: Combined clinical and pathologic study of diabetic and nondiabetic peripheral arterial disease. Diabetes 1964;13:366–372.

7   Conrad MC: Large and small artery occlusion in diabetics and nondiabetics with severe vascular disease. Circulation 1967;36:83–918.

8   Mozes G, Keresztury G, Kadar A, Magyar J, Sipos B, Dzsinich S, Gloviczki P: Atherosclerosis in amputated legs of patients with and without diabetes mellitus. Int Angiol 1998;17:282–286.

9   Ferraresi R, Palena L, Mauri G, Manzi M: Interventional treatment of the below the nkle peripheral artery disease; in Lanzer P (ed): PanVascular Medicine, ed 2. Heidelberg, Springer-Verlag, 2014, pp 3205–3226.

10 Lundbaeck K: Diabetic angiopathy. A new concept of pathogenesis. MMW Munch Med Wochenschr 1977;119:647–654.

11 Andresen JL, Rasmussen LM, Ledet T: Diabetic macroangiopathy and atherosclerosis. Diabetes 1996;45:S91–S94.

12 Capron L: Pharmacologic approaches to the treatment of atherosclerotic arterial obstruction. J Cardiovasc Pharmacol 1995;25(suppl 2):S40–S43.

13 Bowen BD, Koenig EC, Viele A: A study of the lower extremities in diabetes as compared with non-diabetic states from the standpoint of x-ray findings with particular reference to the relationship of arteriosclerosis and diabetes. Bulletin Buffalo Gen Hosp 1924;2:35–41.

14 Morrison LB, Bogan IK: Calcification of the vessels in diabetes. JAMA 1929;92:1424–1426.

15 Ferrier TM, Ferner TM: Radiologically demonstrable arterial calcification in diabetes mellitus. Australas Anns Med 1964;13:222–228.

16 Edmonds M: Medial arterial calcification and diabetes mellitus. 2000;Zeitschrift für Kardiologie 2000;89(suppl 2):S101–S104.

17 David Smith C, Gavin Bilmen J, Iqbal S, Robey S, Pereira M: Medial artery calcification as an indicator of diabetic peripheral vascular disease. Foot Ankle Int 2008;29:185–190.

18 Everhart JE, Pettitt DJ, Knowler WC, Rose FA, Bennett PH: Medial arterial calcification and its association with mortality and complications of diabetes. Diabetologia 1988;31:16–33.

19 Lehto S, Niskanen L, Suhonen M, Ronnemaa T, Laakso M: Medial artery calcification. A neglected harbinger of cardio vascular complications in non insulin dependent diabetes mellitus. Arterioscler Thromb Vasc Biol 1996;16:978–983.

20 Ferrier TM: Comparative study of arterial disease in amputated lower limbs from diabetics and non-diabetics. Med J Aust 1967;1:5–11.

21 Meema HE, Oreopoulos DG, Rapoport A: Serum magnesium level and arterial calcification in end-stage renal disease. Kidney Int 1987;32:388–394.

22 Neubauer B, Gundersen HJ: Calcification, narrowing and rugosities of the leg arteries in diabetic patients. Acta Radiol Diagn 1983;24:401–413.

23 Edmonds ME, Roberts VC, Watkins PJ: Blood flow in the diabetic neuropathic foot. Diabetologia 1982;22:9–15.

24 Gilbey SG, Walters H, Edmonds ME et al: Vascular calcification, autonomic neuropathy, and peripheral flow in patients with diabetic nephropathy. Diabetic Med 1989;6:37–42.

25 Christensen NJ: Muslce blood flow, measured by zenon 133 and vascular calcification in diabetic. Acta Med Scan 1968;183:449–454.

26 Chantelau E, Ma XY, Herrnberger S, Dohmen C, Trappe P, Baba T: Effect of medial arterial calcification on O2 supply to exercising diabetic feet. Diabetes 1990;39:513–516.

27 Neubauer B, Christensen NJ, Christensen T, Gundersen HJ, Jørgensen J: Diabetic macroangiopathy. Medial calcifications, narrowing, rugosities, stiffness, norepinephrine depletion and reduced blood flow capacity in the leg arteries. Acta Med Scand suppl 1984;687:37–45.

28 Edmonds ME, Morrison N, Laws JW, Watkins PJ: Medial arterial calcification and diabetic neuropathy. Br Med J 1982;284:321–323.

29 Sinha S, Munichoodappa CS, Kozak GP: Neuro-arthropathy (Charcot joints) in diabetes mellitus (clinical study of 101 cases). Medicine (Baltimore) 1972;51:191–210.

30 Clouse ME, Gramm HF, Legg M, Flood T: Diabetic osteoarthropathy. Am J Roentgenol Radium Ther Nucl Med 1974;121:22–34.

31 Young MJ, Adams JE, Anderson GF, Boulton AJ, Cavanagh PR: Medial arterial calcification in the feet of diabetic patients and matched non-diabetic control subjects. Diabetologia 1993;36:615–621.

32 Forst T, Pfützner A, Kann P, Lobmann RR, Schäfer H, Beyer J: Association between diabetic-autonomic-C-fibre-neuropathy and medial wall calcification and the significance in the outcome of trophic foot lesions. Experimental and Clinical Endocrinology and Diabetes 1995;103; 94–98.

33 Gentile S, Bizzarro A, Marmo R, de Bellis A, Orlando C: Medial arterial calcification and diabetic neuropathy. Acta Diabetol Lat 1990;27:243–253.

34 Goebel FD, Füessl HS: Mönckeberg's sclerosis after sympathetic denervation in diabetic and non diabetic subjects. Diabetologia 1983;24:347–350.

35 Harrison CV: The effect of sympathectomy on the development of experimental arterial disease. J Pathol 1938;616:353–360.

36 Danisch F: Die sympathischen Ganglien in ihrer Bedeutung für die Cholesterinsklerose des Kaninchens. Beitr Path Anat 1928;79:333–398.

37 Kerper HA, Collier WD: Pathological changes in arteries following partial denervation. Proc Soc Exp Biol Med 1926;24:493–494.

38 Petrova NL, Shanahan CM: Neuropathy and the vascular-bone axis in diabetes: lessons from Charcot osteoarthropathy. Osteoporos Int 2014;25:1197–1207.

39 Morgan AJ: Mineralized deposits in the thoracic aorta of aged rats: ultrastructural and electron probe x-ray microanalysis study. Exp Gerontol 1980;15:563–573.

40 Robert AM, Miskulin M, Godeau G, Tixier JM, Milhaud G: Action of calcitonin on the atherosclerotic modifications of brain microvessels induced in rabbits by cholesterol feeding. Exp Mol Pathol 1982;37:67–73.

41 Shanahan CM, Cary NR, Salisbury JR, Proudfoot D, Weissberg PL, Edmonds ME: Medial localization of mineralization-regulating proteins in association with Mönckeberg's sclerosis: evidence for smooth muscle cell-mediated vascular calcification. Circulation 1999;100:2168–2176.

42 Ho CY, Shanahan CM: Medial Arterial Calcification: An Overlooked Player in Peripheral Arterial Disease. Arterioscler Thromb Vasc Biol 2016;36:1475–1482.

43 Narayan KM, Pettitt DJ, Hanson RL et al: Familial aggregation of medial arterial calcification in Pima Indians with and without diabetes. Diabetes Care 1996;19:968–971.

44 London GM, Guérin AP: Influence of arterial pulse and reflected waves on blood pressure and cardiac function. Am Heart J 1999;138:220–224.

45 Kitagawa S, Yamaguchi Y, Kunitomo M, Amaizame N, Fujiwara M: Impairment of endothelium-dependent relaxation in aorta from rats with arteriosclerosis induced by excess vitamin D and a high-cholesterol diet. Jpn J Pharmacol 1992;59:339–347.

46 Chantclau E, Lee KM, Jungblut R: Association of below-knee atherosclerosis to medial arterial calcification in diabetes mellitus. Diabetes Res Clin Pract 1995;29:169–172.

47 Glagov S, Weisenberg E, Zarins CK, Stankunavicius R, Kolettis GJ: Compensatory enlargement of human atherosclerotic coronary arteries. N Engl J Med 1987;28:316:1371–1375.

48 Fishbein GA, Fishbein MC: Arteriosclerosis: rethinking the current classification. Arch Pathol Lab Med 2009;133:1309–1316.

49 O'Neill WC, Han KH, Schneider TM, Hennigar RA: Prevalence of nonatheromatous lesions in peripheral arterial disease. Arterioscler Thromb Vasc Biol 2015;35:439–447.

50 Soor GS, Vukin I, Leong SW, Oreopoulos G, Butany J: Peripheral vascular disease: who gets it and why? A histomorphological analysis of 261 arterial segments from 58 cases. Pathology 2008;40:385–391.

51 Janka HU, Standl E, Mehnert H: Peripheral vascular disease in diabetes mellitus and its relation to cardiovascular risk factors: screening with the doppler ultrasonic technique. Diabetes Care 1980;3:207–213.

52 Haimovici H: Patterns of arteriosclerotic lesions of the lower extremity. Arch Surg 1967;95:918–933.

53 Siracuse JJ, Chaikof EL: The Pathogenesis of Diabetic Atherosclerosis. G.V. Shrikhande and J.F. McKinsey (eds.), Diabetes and Peripheral Vascular Disease: Diagnosis and Management, Contemporary Diabetes, Springer 2012 pp13–26.

54 Birrer M: Macroangiopathy in diabetes mellitus. Vasa 2001;30:168–174.

55 Stary HC, Blankenhorn DH, Chandler AB, et al: A definition of the intima of human arteries and of its atherosclerosis-prone regions: a report from the Committee on Vascular Lesions of the Council on Arteriosclerosis, American Heart Association. Arterioscler Thromb 1992;12:120–134.

56 Virmani R, Kolodgie FD, Burke AP, Farb A, Schwartz SM: Lessons from sudden coronary death: a comprehensive morphological classification scheme for atherosclerotic lesions. Arterioscler Thromb Vasc Biol 2000;20:1262–1275.

57 Huang H, Virmani R, Younis H et al: The impact of calcification on the biomechanical stability of atherosclerotic plaques. Circulation 2001;103:1051–1056.

58 Kono K, Fujii H, Nakai K, Goto S, Shite J, Hirata K, Fukagawa M, Nishi S: Composition and plaque patterns of coronary culprit lesions and clinical characteristics of patients with chronic kidney disease. Kidney Int 2012;82:344–351.

59 Rocha-Singh KJ, Zeller T, Jaff MR: Peripheral arterial calcification: prevalence, mechanism, detection, and clinical implications. Catheter Cardiovasc Interv 2014;83:E212–E220.

60 Amann K: Media Calcification and Intima Calcification Are Distinct Entities in Chronic Kidney Disease. Clin J Am Soc Nephrol 2008;3:1599–1605.

61 De Wolf VG, Bevan EG: Arteriosclerosis obliterans in the lower extremities: correlation of clinical and angiographic findings. Cardiovasc Clin 1971;3:65–92.

Michael E. Edmonds, MD
Diabetic Foot Clinic
King's College Hospital NHS Foundation Trust
Denmark Hill, London SE5 9RS (UK)
E-Mail michael.edmonds@nhs.net

Piaggesi A, Apelqvist J (eds): The Diabetic Foot Syndrome.
Front Diabetes. Basel, Karger, 2018, vol 26, pp 70–82 (DOI: 10.1159/000480043)

Does Microangiopathy Contribute to the Pathogenesis of the Diabetic Foot Syndrome?

Alberto Coppelli · Lorenza Abbruzzese · Chiara Goretti · Elisabetta Iacopi · Nicola Riitano · Alberto Piaggesi

Diabetic Foot Section, Department of Medicine, University of Pisa, Pisa, Italy

Abstract

Chronic diabetic complications, both micro and macrovascular, have become a serious issue worldwide, and the dramatic rise in the number of patients with diabetes has exacerbated the problem. Hyperglycemia represents the pathologic hallmark of diabetes mellitus and induces vascular damages probably through a common pathway represented by increased intracellular oxidative stress. Among diabetic chronic complications, the pathology related to diabetic foot plays a major role and is the most common reason for hospitalization in diabetic patients. Nearly all components of the lower extremity are involved in the pathological process: skin, subcutaneous cellular tissue, muscles, bones, joints, vessels, nerves. Despite the role of microangiopathic complications in diabetic patients (retinopathy, nephropathy and neuropathy affect most both type 1 and type 2 diabetic patients), the relevance of small vessels damage in the pathogenesis and clinical history of diabetic foot syndrome remains elusive and is still debated. For several years, microangiopathy has not been considered an important pathogenic factor in the development of a diabetic foot ulcer. However, several functional and structural microvascular changes can be detected at the microvascular level in diabetic patients, which might increase the vulnerability of the skin or which can contribute to impaired wound healing. In this review, we highlighted some most exploited pathways involved in the pathogenesis of microangiopathy. We also emphasized the emerging role of microangiopathy in skin ulceration and impaired wound-healing process in diabetic patients.

Introduction

Diabetes mellitus is a very complex and multifactorial metabolic disease characterized by a chronic state of elevated blood glucose; its prevalence is increasing to epidemic proportions throughout the world [1]. In the first half of the last century, Elliot P. Joslin, the father of the modern diabetology, wrote: "The era of coma has given way to the era of complications". Diabetic patients no longer die from acute conditions due to hyperglicemia: it is the chronic complications of the disease that predominate [2]. The high rate of morbidity and mortality in diabetes is reported to be related to the development of micro- (eye, kidney and nerve) and macrovascular (heart and brain) complications [3]. Diabetes, indeed, confers a substantial burden of macrovascular disease, with the risk of any cardiovascular event two- to fourfold greater when compared with non-diabetic subjects [4]. It has been recently reported that the proportion of deaths attributable to diabetes is estimated to be near 12%: diabetes represents the third cause of mortality after cardiovascular and cancer diseases in the United States [5]. Among diabetic chronic complications, pathology related to diabetic foot plays a major role and is the most common reason for hospitalization admission in diabetic patients. Given the increasing prevalence of diabetes predisposing factors, the burden of diabetic foot ulcer is expected to increase in the future; consequently, costs related to diabetic foot ulcer care are estimated to be greater than USD 1 billion annually [6]. Nearly all components of the lower extremity are involved: skin, subcutaneous cellular tissue, muscles, bones, joints, vessels, nerves [7]. Despite the importance of diabetic microangiopathy in health status, the pathogenesis of small vessels damage remains elusive and its relevance in the pathogenesis and clinical history of diabetic foot syndrome is still debated [8, 9].

Physiological Theories of the Pathogenesis of Microangiopathy

In physiological conditions, microvessels are the basic functional unit of the cardio-vascular system comprising of arterioles, capillaries and venules. They differ from macrovessels in both their architecture and cellular components. In contrast to macrovessels supplying blood to organs, microvessels play important roles in transport and exchange of nutrients and waste products of metabolism, tissue defense and repair, maintenance of tissue fluid economy, blood pressure and proper nutrient delivery. All of these processes may be affected by diabetes [8]. Microvascular abnormalities specific to diabetes are represented by microangiopathyc complications of the retina, kidneys and the peripheral nervous system [10, 11]. All these tissues have in common the insulin-dependent intracellular accumulation of glucose. Hyperglyce-mia represents the pathologic hallmark of diabetes mellitus and induces vascular damages probably through a common pathway represented by increased intracellular oxidative stress that links 4 major mechanisms: the polyol pathway, the advanced glycation end products (AGEs) formation, the protein kinase C-diacylglycerol and the hexosamine pathways [12]. Endothelial dysfunction plays a major role in the pathogenesis of the diabetic microangiopathy and anticipates the appearance of the microvascular lesions [13]. Hyperglicemia-induced overproduction of reactive oxygen species as a result of altered glucose metabolism is implicated in the early stages of diabetic atherosclerosis, mediated via the effects of reduced bioavailability of nitric oxide on various pathways including those affecting smooth muscle cell migration and monocyte activation, adhesion and migration, expression of soluble adhesion molecules and the production of vasoconstrictor prostanoids and endhotelin, which increase vascular permeability [14, 15]. In endothelium, high glucose-stimulated reactive oxygen species overproduction plays a crucial role in endothelial cell senescences, which is an early sign of vascular complications in diabetes [16]. According to the "hemodynamic hypothesis," first reported in 1983 by Parving et al. [17], in the early stages of diabetes, there is an increase of the blood flow and capillary permeability; the resulting endothelium injury leads to sclerosis and microvascular hyalinosis. The elasticity of the vessel walls is reduced and an increase in vascular endothelium permeability is also found [18]. The production of AGEs further amplifies this process by activating the proinflammatory pathway resulting in oxidative tissue damages [19–21]. It was found that AGEs formation occurs on extra- and intracellular proteins leading to protein cross-linking, structural and functional changes [21]. At the microvasculature level, increased permeability leads to the expression of vascular endothelial growth factor, a key angiogenic factor in the development of microvascular damage; furthermore, increased endothelium permeability leads to oedema and to a reduction in the supply of nutrients to tissues [18]. With sclerosis and arteriolar hyalinosis, the thickening of the basal membrane is an important feature of these cellular alterations and is an important characteristic of diabetes microangiopathy [18, 22]. These abnormalities are directly related to the capillary pressure and are emphasized on the foot level due to orthostatic position [23]. Furthermore, patients with diabetes has a characteristic dyslipidemia characterized by high tryglicerides levels, low high-density lipoprotein and small, dense low-density lipoprotein [24]. Modified low-density lipoprotein retained in the arterial intima recruits monocyte-derived macrophages that differentiate into foam cells; cytokines and chemokines released by macrophage foam cells support the inflammation process [25]. These molecular defects determine the endothelial dysfuntion, proliferation of plaque macrophages and proliferation of smooth muscle cells that are major source of extracellular matrix, leading to atherosclerotic plaque formation [19]. Neointimal microvessels may also contribute to the delivery of inflammatory mediators and cholesterol to the site of atheroma, suggesting a role in plaque instability. Additionally, rheological mechanisms (increased blood viscosity, reduced red blood cell deformability, increased platelet aggregation) may contribute to microangiopathy development [26]. Vascular abnormalities associated with diabetes include physiological and structural changes in microvessels. In Figure 1, we summarized the main functional and structural abnormalities detected in diabetes microangiopathy.

These vascular changes are detected at the retina, kidneys, skin and peripheral nervous system level, leading to the development of diabetic microangiopathy [27]. Microvascular complications affect a majority of patients with diabetes; they usually affect people with longstanding or uncontrolled disease but can also be present at diagnosis or in those not yet diagnosed as diabetic. The concept according to

Coppelli · Abbruzzese · Goretti · Iacopi · Riitano · Piaggesi

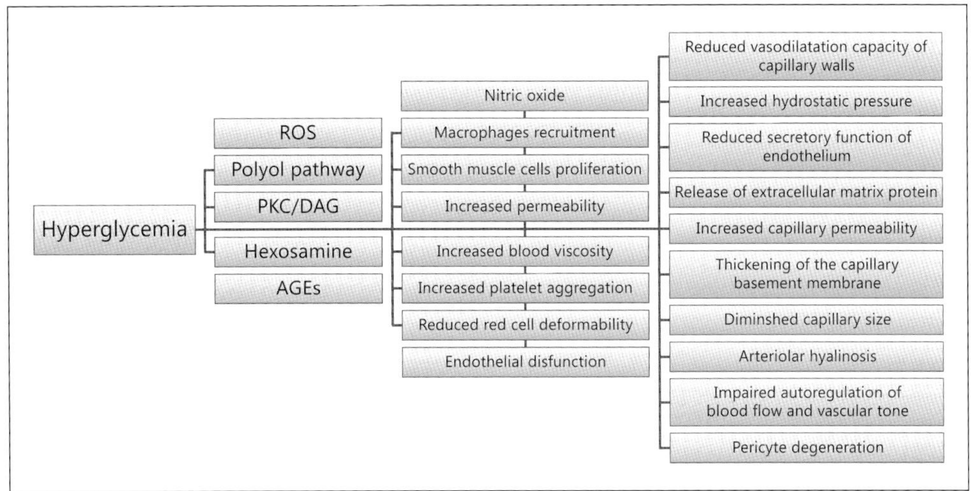

Fig. 1. Main functional and structural microvascular changes in diabetes.

which microcirculation is involved in the pathogenesis of several chronic complications, went through multiple changes over the recent years. Regarding the temporal evolution of the microangiopathy, it is helpful to consider various stages of development: an initial functional stage that is reversible with normalization of blood glucose levels, followed by a period of structural adaptation and remodelling of small vessels that ultimately lead to microvascular failure [8]. The microangiopathy can have a general character and each organ can be affected to a different degree. In certain organs, reparative mechanisms occur, which encompass the clinical presentation of diabetic complications (e.g., retinal neovascularization). In 1950, Friedenwald [28], in discussing the nature of the retinal and glomerular vascular lesions, remarked that it seemed strange that such lesions were limited only to the eyes and kidneys, and he believed that "other organs have as yet not been adequately explored to disclose the full extent of this vascular disease." The term "small vessel disease" was first reported by Goldenberg et al. [29] in 1959. He collected the paraffin blocks of 152 amputation specimens (60% obtained in diabetic patients) at Jewish Hospital in St. Louis (Missouri) and studied large and small vessels primarily for evidence of endothelial proliferation, alterations of elastic structure, and changes in polysaccharide-containing components. He observed that lesions of small arteries in diabetic patients were characterized by endothelial proliferation and deposition of a PAS-positive material in a reticulated pattern. These lesions were found in the vasa vasorum and peri-advential vessels of cognate system arteries, as well as small arteries and arterioles of nerves, muscles and skin, and he postulated that the lesions were closely related to diabetes. In recent years, much attention has been focused on the presence and management of microvascular complications in people with diabetes [30] and a linear relationship between the duration of disease and microvascular complications has been well established [31]. Impairment of the peripheral microcirculation in people with diabetes is often underdiagnosed until complications in the lower limbs such as foot ulcers and/or infections become evident [32]. Although the effects of a chronic state of hyperglycemia on microcirculation have long been recognized, the role of microangiopathy in development of diabetic foot ulcers remains debated. It has been postulated that the alterations of diabetic foot microcirculation play an important role in foot ulceration and in the poor healing of wounds [29, 33].

What Happens at the Skin Level

The skin is composed of 2 layers: epidermis and dermis. The epidermis contains keratin and has no blood supply (nutrition provided by the capillary layer of the dermis); the dermis consists of papillary and reticular layers of collagen and elastic fibers. It consists of a microvascular network that provides tissues with nutrients and eliminates waste products [34]. The skin blood flow is under the regulation of several humoral and neural factors: central neural reflex (from long descending autonomic fibers); reflex arcs through the spinal cord and the integrity of the endothelium [35]. Cutaneous manifestations reach about 30% of diabetic patients. Some dermatoses represent a direct result of metabolic changes such as hyperglicemia and hyperlipidemia. Other skin diseases may result from progressive damage due to vascular, neurological or immune system damage [36]. Microangiopathy of the skin has been described [8]. In physiological conditions, the capillary loops in the epidermis are responsible for the nutritive blood flow of the skin, which is much less than the blood flow in the deeper subpapillary non-nutritive vessels like arteriovenous anastomosis [37]. AGEs collect in the skin dermis and cause skin ageing [38]. Peripheral sympathetic denervation due to autonomic neuropathy can open arteriovenous anastomoses causing an increase in non-nutritive blood flow bypassing the more superficial localized nutritional capillaries [37, 39]. According to the "hemodynamic hypothesis," the capillary blood flow and capillary blood pressure are increased [8]. Furthermore, the capillary permeability like the trans-capillary escape rate of albumin is enhanced [39]. These abnormalities could contribute to the increased swelling rate of the foot during dependency, which in its turn could lead to tissue oedema, hampering diffusion of oxygen and nutrients. These alterations seem to be functional and most likely are caused by chronic hyperglicemia and subsequent metabolic disturbances. The importance of hyperglycemia as central causative factor in vascular abnormalities in diabetic patients is emphasized by the positive effects of long-term glucose normalization on microcirculation of the skin [39, 40]. With time, alterations secondary to chronic hyperglycemia can lead to basement membrane thickening and capillary hyalinosis, contributing to an impaired autoregulation with a subsequent rise of capillary pressure and a decreased vasodilatory reserve; these alterations can lead to reduced

Table 1. Most important molecular mechanisms related to neuronal injury

Glucose-mediated injury [19–21]	Plays a major role through the advanced glycation end products production that tends to decrease the biological function of proteins and initiates an inflammatory signalling cascade that further increases neuronal injury.
Endothelial disfunction [13–15]	Is an early complication of diabetes. Related to excessive reactive oxygen species production and reduction in nitric oxide bioavailability, which impair endothelium-dependent vasodilatation.
Dyslipidemia [24, 25]	Free fatty acids cause lypotoxicity mediated through permeabilization of lysosomal membrane leading to oxidative stress and mitochondrion-activated injury. Furthermore, macrophages are stimulated to release inflammatory cytokines that produce peripheral nerve inflammation.
Insulin resistance [12, 16]	Although neurons do not depend on insulin signalling for glucose utilization, growing body of evidence suggests that insulin resistance contributes to neuronal injury. Insulin resistance acts in particular by accumulating free fatty acids that can lead to cellular inflammation and endoplasmic reticulum stress at peripheral neurons level.
Others mechanisms [16]	Sorbitol accumulation; 12/15 lipoxygenase activation; oxysterols accumulation.

perfusion of the skin, in particular, in situations which require increased blood supply (infections; physical exercise) [33]. The impairment of normal microcirculation may lead to a gradual loss of cutaneous trophism, discromia, and later ulcer.

What Happens at the Nerve Level
The term diabetic neuropathy encompasses several clinically distinct forms of neuropathy, which may occur singly or in combination. Diabetic symmetric polyneuropathy is the most frequent and specific disorder, affecting approximately 50% of patients over the course of their disease and is characterized pathologically as an axonopathy with distal predominance [41]. There is a close connection between the abnormalities of the microcirculation and the diabetic neuropathy, so that this chronic complication is traditionally counted among microvascular complications. Several authors have clearly demonstrated a close correlation between glycaemic control and development of neuropathy [42, 43]. Although the precise nature of the injury to the peripheral nerves from hyperglycemia is not yet certain, the mechanisms of hyperglycemia-induced polyol pathway, injury from AGEs, and enhanced oxidative stress have been implicated in its pathogenesis [44]. Several molecular mechanisms have been postulated and have received different degrees of acceptance (Table 1).

These molecular alterations lead to a profound hemodynamics change with the opening of arterio-venous shunts, abnormal adjustment of the blood flow, an impaired vasodilatory response to various noxious stimuli, and an inflammatory response to the injury. The abnormal adjustment of the microvascular hemodynamics can lead to the thickening of the basal membrane of small vessels and capillary hyalinosis, contributing to an impaired autoregulation with a rise of capillary pressure and a decreased vasodilatory reserve [44]. These alterations can cause diminished skin perfusion. Indeed, in the absence of peripheral neuropathy, total resting skin microcirculation in the diabetic is comparable to that of the nondiabetic foot. In the presence of peripheral neuropathy, however, capillary blood flow is reduced compared to healthy controls [45]. There is a close connection between microvascular abnormalities due to chronic hyperglicemia and the development of neuropathy [46, 47], and the improvements observed in the clinical course of diabetic complications show that long-term glucose normalization improves microvascular complications in diabetic recipients of pancreas transplantation as previously described [48]. Typical symptoms of diabetic neuropathy are pain, numbness, tingling, weakness and difficulties with balance due to proprioceptive loss. Advanced peripheral neuropathy may cause serious complications, such as diabetic foot ulcers or gangrene, and Charcot neuroarthropathy, all of which worsen the quality of life of diabetic patients [49]. Patients with sensory loss appear to have up to a sevenfold increased risk of developing foot ulcers, compared with non-neuropathic diabetic patients [50, 51]. There is scarcity of descriptive information on the morphological changes accompanying the diabetic foot. Popescu et al. [23] performed histopatological examination of tissue fragments obtained in diabetic patients with foot ulcers. The examination showed specific microscopic changes at various levels: at the dermis level, the presence of inflammatory infiltrate (mainly mononuclear cells and polymorphonuclear neutrophils) was shown, while on the microcirculation level the endothelial cells were shown to have a flat smooth inflated aspect. Nervous elements showed degeneration sustained by decreasing in Schwann cells. Sangiorgi et al. [52] reported data on the three-dimensional microvascular architecture constituting the toes of a diabetic patient (lower limb amputation due to extensive necrotic process of soft tissues). He focused the attention mostly on the superficial papillary and sub-papillary vascular networks and in particular on the capillaries entering the dermal papillae. He documented the impairment of the capillary architecture in different cutaneous regions; in particular, a distal capillary impairment was detected. Fiordaliso et al. [53] in a prospective study that was recently published evaluated the presence of microangiopathy by histological analysis of the capillary ultrastructure using transmission electron microscopy and capillary density and arteriolar morphology in the skin of 60 type 2 diabetic patients with foot ulcers (30 neuropathic and 30 neuroischaemic patients). Hystological analysis of the capillary ultrastructure highlighted the presence of an increase in basement membrane thickness and reduced capillary density, both in neuroischaemic and neuropathic diabetic patients. Arteriolar occlusions were also frequently detected in ischaemic patients, indicating the presence of occlusive microvascular disease (hyperplasia of smooth muscle cells in the tunica media was the main detected alteration), despite LoGerfo and Coffman [54] in the late 1980s denied the existence of arteriolar occlusive disease. Kagaya et al. [55] recently reported that the

                                        Coppelli · Abbruzzese · Goretti · Iacopi · Riitano · Piaggesi distribution of ischaemic and non-ischaemic areas in feet of patients with critical limb ischaemia, evaluated by tissue oxygen saturation foot-mapping, is complex, suggesting that microvascular blood flow plays a major role in peripheral tissue perfusion. Collateral microvessels, which strictly connect adjacent angiosomes (three-dimensional units of tissues – skin, subcutaneous tissue, fascia, muscle, bone – fed by a source artery and drained by a specific vein) can be damaged, particularly in patients with diabetes, due to microvascular complications. We recently reported data about positive effects of direct revascularization according to the angiosome model on several outcomes such as healing rate, limb salvage and mortality rate in diabetic patients with critical limb ischaemia [56]. A possible explication of these positive results is that the restoration of good blood flow to the ischaemic area through its specific source artery may have a major effect on diabetic patients, in which microvascular blood flow to the tissue with ulcer is greatly reduced. In our patients, indeed, we observed a high prevalence of diabetic microvascular complications: 78% had some degree of retinopathy and 70% had peripheral neuropathy [56].

It has been recently reported that diabetic patients with proliferative retinopathy has a significantly higher proportion of peripheral arterial disease and proliferative diabetic retinopathy is a stronger independent correlation factor for peripheral arterial disease than a diabetes duration of 10 years [57]. Tomita et al. [58] recently investigated the association between diabetic foot ulcer and microangiopathic complications and concluded that diabetic microangiopathy is an independent predictor of incident diabetic foot ulcer: diabetic patients with retinopathy and nephropathy (albumin excretion rate >20 µg/min during a 24-h urine sample collection) have a significantly increased risk to develop foot ulcers. Moss et al. [59] reported that severe retinopathy was a strong risk factor for major amputation in diabetic patients. Combination of macrovascular and microvascular chronic complications leads to great tissue loss that can impair the wound-healing process and increase the risk of major amputation.

Methods for Studying Microcirculation

Transcutaneous oxygen pressure ($TcPO_2$) measurement [60] has been an integral part of the non-invasive assessment of microcirculatory blood flow since the 1970s. It quantifies the oxygen molecules that are transferred out through the skin, using the basic electrodes of conventional blood gas machine. Oxygen is capable of diffusing throughout the body and the skin and is an indirect measure of the amount of oxygen that is delivered from the blood in the total process of skin microcirculation. When peripheral perfusion is reduced, $TcPO_2$ loses its relationship with the arterial tensions and becomes blood-flow dependent, thus providing quantitative evaluation of blood flow. With the patient in the supine position, a patch of skin area is selected for assessment; the area should not overlie bone, inflammation, or superficial veins. Small electrodes consisting of a circular silver-silver chloride anode surrounding a central platinum cathode are than placed on the skin. A second, control electrode is placed infraclavicularly on the skin of the chest. Normal TcPO$_2$ levels are approximately 60 mm Hg, while levels of 20 mm Hg or less strongly suggest that revascularisation will be required.

Capillaroscopy is one of the most sensitive methods for estimating the nutritional status of skin tissue at microscopic level in vivo. Basic light microscopy can be used to study skin capillaries in vivo. Skin capillaries in an area with a reduced microcirculation change in structure, and it is possible to evaluate the morphology and blood flow of the skin by microscopic studies of these capillary changes. Capillaroscopy provides a 2-D projection of a 3-D network of capillaries. In combination with television and video and/or computer technology capillaroscopy generates high-contrast images of skin capillaries. More recently, dynamic capillaroscopy with sophisticated computer software programs has been used to measure microvascular dynamics, flow distribution and permeability. The addition of fluorescent dyes to dynamic capillaroscopy enables clinicians to distinguish the microvascular from the interstitial compartments and assess transcapillary diffusion [61, 62].

Photo-plethysmography has been introduced in the past to detect changes in blood volume at skin level. This technique requires a light source and a photodetector. When the light enters the skin it gets reflected and absorbed again before reaching the photodetector: the degree of absorption is dependent on the volume of blood in the tissue. With more widespread utilization of ultrasound methods, the use of plethysmography has declined substantially [63].

Laser Doppler Flowmetry and Imaging [64]

The principle is dependent on detecting a phase change in the frequency of laser light incident on the microcirculation. This technique is a non-invasive continuous measurement of the local microcirculatory blood perfusion based on the effect of light on moving red blood cells in a restricted volume of tissue. The magnitude and frequency of change in wavelength can be converted into a measurement technique representing the relative perfusion, rather than absolute values. The technique was developed to produce imaging. Laser Doppler imaging can provide similar data by scanning the entire foot and ankle after the induction of ischaemia using a cuff inflated to suprasystolic pressure at the calf and measuring changes because of reactive hyperaemia after cuff deflation. Laser Doppler imaging has been used to identify poor perfusion in lower extremity ulcers; however, these techniques are vulnerable to motion artefact, ambient temperature changes and inter-operator variability [65].

Conclusions

Foot ulcers rarely result from a single pathology. Several pathological processes usually contribute, which as a consequence of the diabetic state evolve slowly over time and which seem to interact closely. Almost all components of the lower extremity are involved: skin, subcutaneous tissue, muscle, bones, joints, blood vessels, nerves. For several years, microangiopathy has not been considered an important pathogenic factor in the development of a diabetic foot ulcer. However, several abnormalities can be detected at the microvascular level in diabetic patients, which might increase the vulnerability of the skin or which can contribute to impaired wound healing. In particular, an increase in basement membrane thickness and a reduced number of capillary seem to play a major role. The presence of a microvascular complications of diabetes such as peripheral neuropathy can lead to a loss of protective sensation: insensitivity combined with either extrinsic factors such as walking with ill-fitting shoes ultimately results in foot ulceration due to reduced perception of foot trauma. Furthermore, skin microcirculation alterations further increases the risk to develop foot lesions. Skin microcirculation, indeed, plays a prominent role in the skin viability and cutaneous pathology. Alterations in the microcirculatory function of the diabetic foot include both structural and functional abnormalities. Such alterations, together with the neurologic and vascular complications involved in skin blood flow regulation, further render the diabetic foot at risk of ulceration and can contribute to the poor healing of wounds. We must also not forget that a strong association between the presence of microangiopatic chronic complications such as diabetic retinopathy and/or nephropathy and the occurrence of diabetic foot ulcer it has been well demonstrated. Diabetic retinopathy (the most important cause of blindness in western countries in young people) reduces visual acuity, which is an important risk factor for diabetic foot ulcer. In addition, albuminuria and elevated serum creatinine levels and/or dialysis have been reported as risk factors for diabetic foot ulceration in diabetic people. We can summarize mechanisms through which microangiopathy can contribute to skin ulceration and impaired wound healing in diabetic patients:

1. Diabetic symmetric polyneuropathy through the loss of protective sensation.

2. Skin functional and structural abnormalities, which can increase the risk of foot ulceration and contribute to impaired wound healing.

3. Diabetic retinopathy, through the reduction of visual acuity.

4. Diabetic nephropathy/dialysis, risk factors for diabetic foot ulceration.

5. Combination of macrovascular and microvascular complications can lead to great tissue loss, eventually increasing the risk of major amputation.

References

1 Kharroubi AT, Darwish HM: Diabetes mellitus: the epidemic of the century. World J Diabetes 2015;6: 850–867.
2 Chaturvedi N: The burden of diabetes and its complications: trends and implications for intervention. Diabetes Res Clin Pract 2007;76(suppl 1):S3–S12.
3 Zhang PY: Cardiovascular disease in diabetes. Eur Rev Med Pharmacol Sci 2014;18:2205–2214.
4 Shah B, Rockman CB, Guo Y, et al: Diabetes and vascular disease in different arterial territories. Diabetes care 2014;37:1636–1642.
5 Stokes A, Preston SH: Deaths attributable to diabetes in the United States: comparison of data sources and estimation approaches. PLoS One 2017;12:e0170219.

6 Hicks CW, Selvarajah S, Mathioudakis N, Sherman RE, Hines KF, Black JH 3rd, Abularrage CJ: Burden of infected diabetic foot ulcers on hospital admissions and costs. Ann Vasc Surg 2016;33:149–158.

7 Schaper NC, Nabuurs-Franssen MH: The diabetic foot: pathogenesis and clinical evaluation. Semin Vasc Med 2002;2:221–228.

8 Tooke JE: Microvascular function in human diabetes. A physiological perspective. Diabetes 1995;44: 721–726.

9 Flynn MD, Tooke JE: Aetiology of diabetic foot ulceration: a role for the microcirculation? Diabet Med 1992;9:320–329.

10 The Diabetes Control and Complications Trial Research Group, Nathan DM, Genuth S, Lachin J, Cleary P, Crofford O, Davis M, Rand L, Siebert C: The effect of intensive diabetes of treatment on the development and progression of long-term complications in insulin-dependent diabetes mellitus. N Eng J Med 1993;329:977–986.

11 UK Prospective Diabetes Study (UKPDS) Group: Intensive blood-glucose control with sulphonylureas or insulin compared with conventional treatment and risk of complications in patients with type 2 diabetes (UKPDS 33). Lancet 1998;352:837–853.

12 Madonna R, De Caterina R: Cellular and molecular mechanisms of vascular injury in diabetes–part I: pathways of vascular disease in diabetes. Vascul Pharmacol 2011;54:68–74.

13 Leung WK, Gao L, Siu PM, Lai CW: Diabetic nephropathy and endothelial dysfunction: current and future therapies, and emerging of vascular imaging for preclinical renal-kinetic study. Life Sci 2016;166: 121–130.

14 Veves A, Akbari CM, Primavera J, Donaghue VM, Zacharoulis D, Chrzan JS, DeGirolami U, LoGerfo FW, Freeman R: Endothelial dysfunction and the expression of endothelial nitric oxide synthetase in diabetic neuropathy, vascular disease, and foot ulceration. Diabetes 1998;47:457–463.

15 Karunakaran U, Park KG: A systematic review of oxidative stress and safety of antioxidants in diabetes: focus on islets and their defense. Diabetes Metab J 2013;37:106–112.

16 Hammes HP: Pathophysiological mechanisms of diabetic angiopathy. J Diabetes Complications 2003; 17(2 suppl):16–19.

17 Parving HH, Viberti GC, Keen H, Christiansen JS, Lassen NA: Hemodynamic factors in the genesis of diabetic microangiopathy. Metabolism 1983;32: 943–949.

18 Chao CY, Cheing GL: Microvascular dysfunction in diabetic foot disease and ulceration. Diabetes Metab Res Rev 2009;25:604–614.

19 Duran-Jimenez B, Dobler D, Moffatt S, Rabbani N, Streuli CH, Thornalley PJ, Tomlinson DR, Gardiner NJ: Advanced glycation end products in extracellular matrix proteins contribute to the failure of sensory nerve regeneration in diabetes. Diabetes 2009;58: 2893–2903.

20 Vincent AM, Callaghan BC, Smith AL, Feldman EL: Diabetic neuropathy: cellular mechanisms as therapeutic targets. Nat Rev Neurol 2011;7:573–583.

21 Nowotny K, Jung T, Höhn A, Weber D, Grune T: Advanced glycation end products and oxidative stress in type 2 diabetes mellitus. Biomolecules 2015; 5:194–222.

22 Chittenden SJ, Shami SK: Microvascular investigations in diabetes mellitus. Postgrad Med J 1993;69: 419–428.

23 Popescu RM, Cotuţiu C, Graur M, Căruntu ID: Vascular and nerve lesions of the diabetic foot–a morphological study. Rom J Morphol Embryol 2010;51: 483–488.

24 Vincent AM, Hinder LM, Pop-Busui R, Feldman EL: Hyperlipidemia: a new therapeutic target for diabetic neuropathy. J Peripher Nerv Syst 2009;14:257–267.

25 Vincent AM, Hayes JM, McLean LL, Vivekanandan-Giri A, Pennathur S, Feldman EL: Dyslipidemia-induced neuropathy in mice: the role of oxLDL/LOX-1. Diabetes 2009;58:2376–2385.

26 Coppola L, Cerciello T, Boviatsi P, Pastore A, Coppola A, Antonio G, Mastrolorenzo L, Marfella R, Gombos G: Effect of postprandial hyperglycaemia on blood viscosity in aged patients suffering from type 2 diabetes as compared with healthy volunteers. Blood Coagul Fibrinolysis 2007;18:745–50.

27 Khalil H: Diabetes microvascular complications – a clinical update. Diabetes Metab Syndr 2016;pii :S1871-4021(16)30264-8.

28 Friedenwald JS: Diabetic retinopathy. Am J Ophthalmol 1950;33:1187–1199.

29 Goldenberg S, Alex M, Joshi RA, Blumenthal HT: Nonatheromatous peripheral vascular disease of the lower extremity in diabetes mellitus. Diabetes 1959; 8:261–273.

30 Valencia WM, Florez H: How to prevent the microvascular complications of type 2 diabetes beyond glucose control. BMJ 2017;356:j6505.

31 Chawla A, Chawla R, Bhasin GK, Soota K: Profile of adolescent diabetics in North Indian population. J Clin Diabetol 2014;1:1–3.

32 Schramm JC, Dinh T, Veves A: Microvascular changes in the diabetic foot. Int J Low Extrem Wounds 2006;5:149–159.

33 Dinh T, Veves A: Microcirculation of the diabetic foot. Curr Pharm Des 2005;11:2301–2309.

34 Hagisawa S, Shimada T: Skin morphology and its mechanical properties associated with loading. Pressure Ulcer Research: Current and Future Perspectives. Springer-Verlag. Berlin. Germany 2005.

35 Henriksen O: Sympathetic reflex control of blood flow in human peripheral tissues. Acta Physiol Scand Suppl 1991;603:33–39.

36 Murphy-Chutorian B, Han G, Cohen SR: Dermatologic manifestations of diabetes mellitus: a review. Endocrinol Metab Clin North Am 2013;42:869–898.

37 Netten PM, Wollersheim H, Thien T, Lutterman JA: Skin microcirculation of the foot in diabetic neuropathy. Clin Sci (Lond) 1996;91:559–565.

38 Makrantonaki E, Jiang D, Hossini AM, Nikolakis G, Wlaschek M, Scharffetter-Kochanek K, Zouboulis CC: Diabetes mellitus and the skin. Rev Endocr Metab Disord 2016;17:269–282.

39 Eberl N, Piehlmeier W, Dachauer S, König A, Land W, Landgraf R: Blood flow in the skin of type 1 diabetic patients before and after combined pancreas/kidney transplantation. Diabetes Metab Res Rev 2005;21:525–532.

40 Abendroth D, Schmand J, Landgraf R, Illner WD, Land W: Diabetic microangiopathy in type 1 (insulin-dependent) diabetic patients after successful pancreatic and kidney or solitary kidney transplantation. Diabetologia 1991;34(suppl 1):S131–S134.

41 Pop-Busui R, Boulton AJ, Feldman EL, Bril V, Freeman R, Malik RA, Sosenko JM, Ziegler D: Diabetic Neuropathy: a Position Statement by the American Diabetes Association. Diabetes Care 2017;40:136–154.

42 Dyck PJ, Davies JL, Wilson DM, Service FJ, Melton LJ 3rd, O'Brien PC: Risk factors for severity of diabetic polyneuropathy: intensive longitudinal assessment of the Rochester Diabetic Neuropathy Study cohort. Diabetes Care 1999;22:1479–1486.

43 Morales A: A better future for children with type 1 diabetes: review of the conclusions from the diabetes control and complications trial and the epidemiology of diabetes interventions and complications study. J Ark Med Soc 2009;106:90–93.

44 Vincent AM, Callaghan BC, Smith AL, Feldman EL: Diabetic neuropathy: cellular mechanisms as therapeutic targets. Nat Rev Neurol 2011;7:573–583.

45 Jörneskog G, Brismar K, Fagrell B: Skin capillary circulation severely impaired in toes of patients with IDDM, with and without late diabetic complications. Diabetologia 1995;38:474–480.

46 Hile C. Veves A: Diabetic neuropathy and microcirculation. Curr Diab Rep 2003;3:446–451.

47 Flynn MD, Tooke JE: Diabetic neuropathy and the microcirculation. Diabet Med 1995;12:298–301.

48 Boggi U, Vistoli F, Amorese G, Giannarelli R, Coppelli A, Mariotti R, Rondinini L, Barsotti M, Piaggesi A, Tedeschi A, Signori S, De Lio N, Occhipinti M, Mangione E, Cantarovich D, Del Prato S, Mosca F, Marchetti P: Results of pancreas transplantation alone with special attention to native kidney function and proteinuria in type 1 diabetes patients. Rev Diabet Stud 2011;8:259–67.

49 Veves A, Backonja M, Malik RA: Painful diabetic neuropathy: epidemiology, natural history, early diagnosis, and treatment options. Pain Med 2008;9: 660–674.

50 Jude EB, Boulton AJ: Peripheral neuropathy. Clin Podiatr Med Surg 1999;16:81–96.

51 Dinh TL, Veves A: A review of the mechanisms implicated in the pathogenesis of the diabetic foot. Int J Low Extrem Wounds 2005;4:154–159.

52 Sangiorgi S, Manelli A, Reguzzoni M, Ronga M, Protasoni M, Dell'Orbo C: The cutaneous microvascular architecture of human diabetic toe studied by corrosion casting and scanning electron microscopy analysis. Anat Rec (Hoboken) 2010;293:1639–1645.

53 Fiordaliso F, Clerici G, Maggioni S, Caminiti M, Bisighini C, Novelli D, Minnella D, Corbelli A, Morisi R, De Iaco A, Faglia E: Prospective study on microangiopathy in type 2 diabetic foot ulcer. Diabetologia 2016;59:1542–1548.

54 LoGerfo FW, Coffman JD: Current concepts. Vascular and microvascular disease of the foot in diabetes. Implications for foot care. N Engl J Med 1984;311: 1615–1619.

55 Kagaya Y, Ohura N, Suga H, Eto H, Takushima A, Harii K: "Real angiosome" assessment from peripheral tissue perfusion using tissue oxygen saturation foot-mapping in patients with critical limb ischemia. Eur J Vasc Endovasc Surg 2014;47:433–441.

56 Coppelli A, Iacopi E, Bargellini I, Goretti C, Cicorelli A, Lunardi A, Cioni R, Del Prato S, Piaggesi A: Direct revascularization based on the angiosome model reduces risk of major amputations and increases life expectancy in diabetic patients with critical limb ischemia and diabetic foot ulcerations. Diabetes. June 2015;64(suppl 1):139OR.

57 Chen YW, Wang YY, Zhao D, Yu CG, Xin Z, Cao X, Shi J, Yang GR, Yuan MX, Yang JK: High prevalence of lower extremity peripheral artery disease in type 2 diabetes patients with proliferative diabetic retinopathy. PLoS One 2015;10:e0122022.

58 Tomita M, Kabeya Y, Okisugi M, Katsuki T, Oikawa Y, Atsumi Y, Matsuoka K, Shimada A: Diabetic microangiopathy is an independent predictor of incident diabetic foot ulcer. J Diabetes Res 2016;2016: 5938540.

59 Moss SE, Klein R, Klein BE: The 14-year incidence of lower-extremity amputations in a diabetic population. The Wisconsin Epidemiologic Study of Diabetic Retinopathy. Diabetes Care 1999;22:951–959.

60 Brownrigg JR, Hinchliffe RJ, Apelqvist J, Boyko EJ, Fitridge R, Mills JL, Reekers J, Shearman CP, Zierler RE, Schaper NC; International Working Group on the Diabetic Foot: Performance of prognostic markers in the prediction of wound healing or amputation among patients with foot ulcers in diabetes: a systematic review. Diabetes Metab Res Rev 2016; 32(suppl 1):128–135.

61 Abularrage CJ, Sidawy AN, Aidinian G, Singh N, Weiswasser JM, Arora S: Evaluation of the microcirculation in vascular disease. J Vasc Surg 2005;42: 574–581.

62 Shore AC: Capillaroscopy and the measurement of capillary pressure. Br J Clin Pharmacol 2000;50:501– 513.

63 Allen J, Frame JR, Murray A: Microvascular blood flow and skin temperature changes in the fingers following a deep nspiratory gasp. Physiol Meas 2002;23: 365–373.

64 Andersen CA: Noninvasive assessment of lower extremity hemodynamics in individuals with diabetes mellitus. J Vasc Surg 2010;52(3 suppl):76S–80S.

65 Mathieu D, Mani R: A review of the clinical significance of tissue hypoxia measurements in lower extremity wound management. Int J Low Extrem Wounds 2007;6:273–283.

Alberto Coppelli, MD
Diabetic Foot Section
Department of Medicine, University of Pisa
Via Paradisa 2, IT–56124 Pisa (Italy)
E-Mail albcoppy@yahoo.it

Piaggesi A, Apelqvist J (eds): The Diabetic Foot Syndrome.
Front Diabetes. Basel, Karger, 2018, vol 26, pp 83–96 (DOI: 10.1159/000480054)

The Organization of Care for the Diabetic Foot Syndrome: A Time-Dependent Network

Alberto Piaggesi · Lorenza Abbruzzese · Alberto Coppelli ·
Elisabetta Iacopi · Nicola Riitano · Chiara Goretti

Diabetic Foot Section, Department of Medicine, University of Pisa, Italy

Abstract

The diabetic foot (DF) is a progressive and destructive complication of diabetes mellitus. It has a multifaceted pathogenesis and a complex clinical course, with different phases and patterns, so much so that it is befitting to define it more as the "DF syndrome." The problems of the management of this disease are not only related to the complexity of the interventions and their integration into a strategy, which addresses the different questions that arise in the different phases of the pathology, but also inherent to the organization of care that should overcome the criticalities of a chronic, worsening and poorly symptomatic illness. Delayed referral of the early pathology to multidisciplinary care, the lack of adequate treatment of urgencies and emergencies and the lack of a dedicated follow-up are the chief aspects of this problem. The implementation of a time-dependent network with the characteristics indicated by the international guidelines is the only way to address the aforementioned problem with successful outcomes as the recent European experiences demonstrated. Only by combining the adequate organizational structure with the multidisciplinary team approach in a time-dependent dedicated network can we have the possibility of successfully managing a pathology that is bound to increase fourfold in the next 10 years. This initiative will however absorb a majority of the resources dedicated to diabetes care throughout the world. This paper focuses on the different critical aspects that should be addressed when the structure of a complex therapeutic strategy for the DF syndrome has to be developed, the challenges that are to be faced and possible solutions to overcome them.

The Diabetic Foot Syndrome

The so-called diabetic foot (DF) is actually a syndrome that affects the lower limbs of diabetic patients, which develops gradually and continuously right from the onset of the disease, throughout the lifespan of the patients, characterized by a progressive involvement of both the nervous and the vascular structures within the limb. This

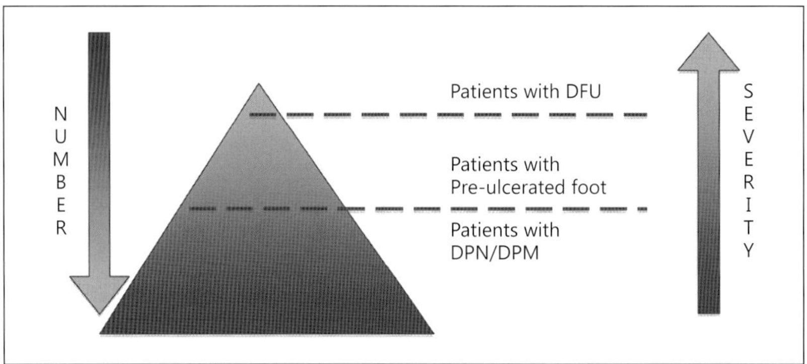

Fig. 1. The pyramid of the DF syndrome. The progression of the disease increases the severity of the pathology over time, while the number of patients decreases. The patients at the top of the pyramid (10–15%) are those who consume the majority (≈85%) of the resources.

in turn determines a morphological and functional deterioration at the level of the foot, which may evolve in different forms of local pathologies, all progressing towards end-stage conditions culminating in lower extremity amputations (LEAs) or death.

The pathogenesis of the pathology is related to the macro- and micro-angiopathic modifications that happen due to the chronic derangement of glycaemic controls and follows the progressions of the metabolic disease and it is influenced by the level of metabolic control of the patients in the long-term, being more frequent and more severe in patients characterized by a worse metabolic control and with a long duration of diabetes [1–3].

It is difficult to establish the prevalence of the DF syndrome, since it changes depending on the basis on which we set our measurements: if we look at the prevalence from the the nervous and vascular involvement of the limb perspective (i.e., diabetic peripheral neuropathy [DPN] and diabetic peripheral macroangiopathy [DPM]), we will find a prevalence of 40–60% for DPN and of 20–50% for DPM depending upon the series and with a large overlapping of neuro-ischaemic conditions [4–8]. The pre-ulcerative conditions at the level of the foot that create a high ulcerative risk are as frequent as 20–40% and the prevalence of the active pathology may range from 1% in the case of the acute Charcot foot to almost 7% for the ulcerated DF, with an annual incidence of 2% in the diabetic population [9–14].

So we can depict a pathology that has a great impact over the general diabetic population and which worsens to more severe phases in a significant number of patients, according to a pyramidal model in which we may identify 3 different areas: a base, where there is a large number of patients with DPN and DPM, an intermediate level where a number of patients who develop pre-ulcerative foot pathology are grouped, and a summit, where a limited but still significant number of patients progress towards DF ulcers (DFUs) and active Charcot foot (Fig. 1).

Piaggesi · Abbruzzese · Coppelli · Iacopi · Riitano · Goretti

The progression of the pathology is largely unpredictable, and the passages from one condition to the other are difficult to detect because of the scarce or even absent symptoms due to the presence of DPN; it is not infrequent that patients are diagnosed of having type 2 diabetes because of a DF-related condition [15].

Usually the DF syndrome in the DPN/DPM stage develops in years, without any evident symptom, but with signs that can be easily detected if adequately searched by expert caregivers.

The pre-ulcerative stage represents the vast majority of the cases of the symptomless evolution of the previous condition, with foot problems that can – or cannot – be perceived by the patients, like corns, calluses, deformities, cold sensation, swelling, toes and foot deformities, discoloration and cyanosis, loss of skin hair and anhydrosis [16].

The transition towards the DFU state can be dramatic for its rapid progression and poorly symptomatic both at the same time, thus creating a true emergency for the ultimate risk of loosing a limb, or even the patient, in just a few hours [17].

The Dramas of the Delayed Referral

The long duration of the first stages during which limb ischaemia and insensitivity develop, thereby exposing the foot, which is deformed by motor neuropathy, to injuries that suddenly evolve into real dramas together with the virtual absence of any symptom can explain the delay that happens when patients are referred to specialized care [18, 19].

Delay is the most important cause of negative outcomes in the management of the critical conditions that characterize the ulcerated phase; by avoiding delays and providing timely treatment, recurrences can be prevented and the issue of patients at high risk progressing fast from the pre-ulcerative phase to the ulcerative one can be addressed effectively [20, 21].

In the EURODIALE study, which followed 1,232 patients in 14 highly specialized clinics in 10 different European countries for 1 year, the prevalence of delayed referral in some of the centres reached an impressive rate of 55%; it was identified as one of the most significant determinants for LEAs and considered the most important risk factor from a caregiver point of view [22].

Time is an issue in DF management; it is not only crucial from a therapeutic point of view, since timely interventions do make a difference in the fast-evolving acute phases of the disease, but also of paramount importance in primary and secondary prevention, where the possibilities of success are higher and the costs are lower [23].

In these phases, both in primary prevention, where patients have DPN/DPM but not yet any complication at the level of the foot, and in secondary prevention, where patients have a pathologic condition at the foot, time is considered to be an important

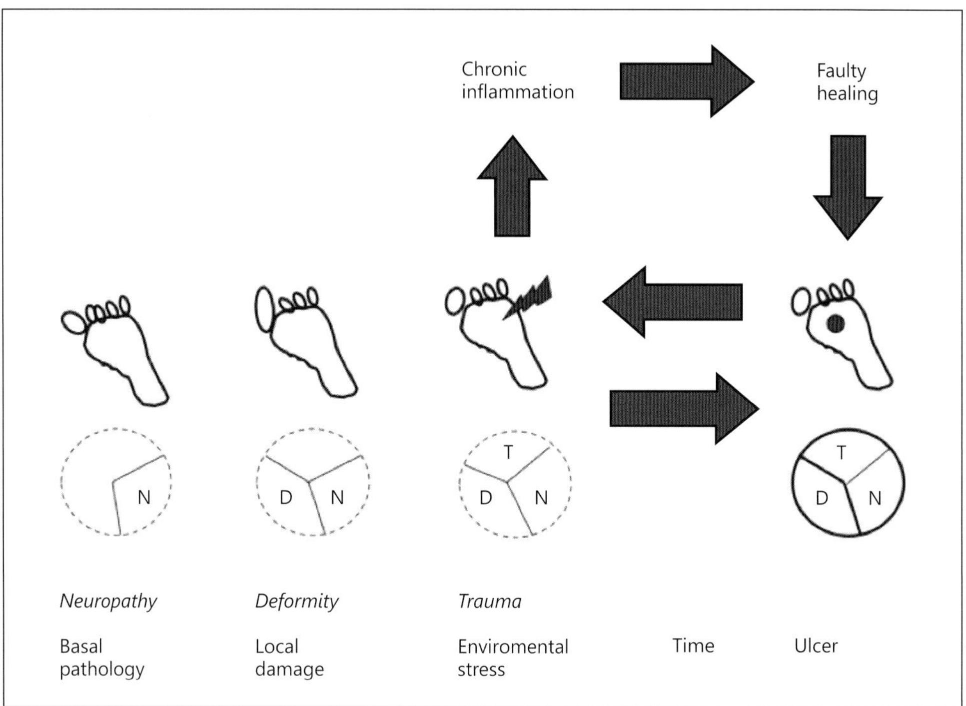

Fig. 2. The progression of the DF syndrome: from chronic complications in the limb the pathology progress to structural deformities in the foot which, under the influence of a trauma produce an ulcer which does not heal and that trigger a vicious cycle that impede to the situation to improve. To effectively intervene in this pathway at any level means stop/reduce the progression toward the major amputation or death.

parameter required to correct the factors that make the pathology progress or recur, since it takes years for DPN/DPM to induce foot pathologic changes and months for the DFUs to recur (Fig. 2) [24].

In this phase, the intensive treatment of diabetes with the target of restoring a near-normoglycemic condition for the longest time possible is crucial for delaying the onset and slowing down the progression of the chronic complications (including DPN and DPM) of diabetes mellitus (DM).

The Diabetes Control and Complications Trial for type 1 DM and the UK Prospective Diabetes Study for type 2 diabetes demonstrated in large cohorts of patients how the achievement and maintenance of near-normal glycaemic levels are able to prevent or reduce the progression of micro-and macro-vascular complications of DM, and in the case of micro-angiopathic complications, also to reverse the progression of the early forms of the disease [25, 26].

The follow-up of patients for a long elapse of time helped in establishing how for each 1% of reduction of glycated haemoglobin A1c, which is a medium-term indicator of the metabolic control, the risk of developing chronic complications decreased

Piaggesi · Abbruzzese · Coppelli · Iacopi · Riitano · Goretti

by 21%, with an estimated cost lesser than 30,000 USD per patient, while the average costs related to amputations were estimated as 15,000 USD in the year of amputation and 4,200 USD per year during the lifetime of the patient [27, 28].

It has been demonstrated how interventions in these early phases when delivered at appropriate times are able to reduce the incidence of DFUs in DF patients by means of education, preventative podiatric care and early treatment [29, 30].

Again, the delayed referral of progressing cases to specialized care, related to poor symptomatology of the cases for the presence of DPN, is the more important cause for the progression of the disease from the early preventable and treatable phases to the more severe and dramatic ones. In a large study involving more than 17,000 patients in one year, Gavan et al. [31] showed that delaying the referring of cases for more than 1 month from the diagnosis state to specialist care would increase significantly the risk of DFUs, gangrene and amputations; a delay longer than 2 years doubled the OR for all the 3 conditions. The pro-active screening, widely applied to the population at risk actually represents the most effective tool for contrasting the delayed referral.

The Pro-Active Screening

Since the very beginning of the establishment of diabetology as a specialty, conducting an active search to recognize the presence of complications was one of the most important clinical activities of the specialists, who aimed to prevent, detect and treat as early as possible the chronic complications of the disease.

Elliot P. Joslin, the father of modern diabetology, was a strenuous promoter of the pro-active screening of lower limb complications and established a dedicated program for this purpose in his Boston diabetic clinic [32].

Since then, the pro-active screening for DF has been promoted by many different institutions, scientific societies and organizations, which produced guidelines, procedures and instructions on how to organize and carry on such an activity on the diabetic population.

Formosa et al. [33], in a recent review, described 10 different DF screening guidelines, published between 2011 and 2015, and pointed out how between them there was a great variability in methods and grading systems, making it difficult to compare them with each other.

Both the American Diabetes Association and the International Working Group on Diabetic Foot (IWGDF) have independently released guidelines on the screening procedures for DF and their recommendations are quite similar, suggesting that both DPN- and DPM-related items, together with the foot aspects should be investigated at least yearly in at-risk diabetic patients [34, 35].

The problems start when the implementation of such guidelines, both at the technical and organizational level, is considered. van Acker et al. [36], in a recent review on the actual implementation of DF guidelines in 5 European countries, concluded that "implementation of the guidelines and set-up of multidisciplinary clinics for holistic management of the DF disorders varies across Europe and remains suboptimal."

The reasons for this far-from-optimal level of implementation of a highly effective form of prevention and early treatment are mainly related to the barriers that the local organization of care at the level of GPs and community services create to the pro-active screening of DF. In a recent review, van Houtum [37] pointed out how such barriers at the basal level, made by the lack of sensitivity of the doctors and the other care professionals towards the pathology, and by the organization of the health care systems, actually prevent the possibility for the DF patients to access the multidisciplinary care that they need, and argued for implementing strategies to overcome this problem.

At present, little has been done in this direction; the initiatives aimed in promoting the implementation of guidelines have been targeted so far mainly, if not exclusively, on the organization of the specialized, multi-disciplinary clinics, with sporadic experiences at the basal level with generally unsatisfactory outcomes [38–40].

Urgencies and Emergencies

Another significant problem is represented by the urgencies and emergencies that frequently complicate the clinical course of DF [41].

Events like unnoticed trauma, which may trigger the active phase of a Charcot neuroarthropathy, or an infection complicating an ischaemic ulceration, may turn a chronic disease into a dramatically acute condition fast-progressing towards progressive and irreversible destruction of the foot, even putting at risk the life of the patients.

The frequent underestimation of the severity and progressiveness of the actual conditions of the patients is due to the lack of symptoms to identify the presence of neuropathy, which affects the same districts where peripheral arteriopathy is progressing at the same level of severity of ischemia: while non-diabetic patients unavoidably mention worsening pain, diabetic patients do not [42].

Pain is reduced or even absent, and inflammatory signs, which are mediated by neural reflexes, are reduced, both at local and systemic levels: it is not infrequent to find an active Charcot patient walking painless and with little or no swelling, or a severely infected patient with a leukocyte count within the normal range [43].

This is something that confuses both the patients and the doctors; they both strongly rely on pain and inflammation for evaluating the severity of the clinical picture, and it is the most dangerous condition because it delays the administration of medical care, which is very much needed and which should be delivered on time in order to be effective [44].

DF is a subtle disease and patients, and especially doctors, should be trained not to underestimate any possible sign – even if it is weak or unexpected – and be well

Table 1. Emergencies in DF; action needed, people responsible and time frame

Emergency	Intervention needed	People responsible	Time frame
Active Charcot	Offloading	Diabetologist	Immediate
Necrotising Fascitis	Fasciotomy	Surgeon/anesthesiologist	Immediate
Abscess/Phlegmon	Drainage	Diabetologist	Within 12 h
Wet Gangrene	Amputation	Diabetologist/surgeon Anaesthesiologist	Within 24 h
Critical Limb Ischemia[1]	Revascularization	Endovascular specialist Vascular surgeon	Within 24 h
Pre-critical limb ischemia[2]	Revascularization	Endovascular specialist Vascular surgeon	Within 48 h

[1] Rest pain, progressing necrosis; [2] no rest pain, stable lesions.

prepared in their mind such that the worse should be presumed until the contrary gets proven.

Once detected, the critical condition should be handled with a timely action in order to prevent the progression of the harm that the condition may bring to the patient not only to the foot, since sepsis is a frequent and a death-precipitating event in DF patients [45].

Although in the majority of guidelines it is indicated that 24 h is the time frame in which DF emergencies (critical ischaemia, deep infection, active Charcot) should be addressed, there is actually a hierarchy of interventions that should be time dependant; according to the pathology and its grade of progression, interventions that have to be made in a time range from immediate to 48 hrs of delay are summarized in Table 1.

Time Is Tissue

To effectively manage the emergencies, the time-dependency aspect of the interventions is of paramount importance, because as the cardiologists say by referring to the management of the acute myocardial infarction (AMI), "time is tissue."

Actually, in all the situations that drive the progression of the DF pathology, there is a turning point, which is the divide between reversibility and non-reversibility and that is also the criterion by which an emergent solution is defined: the onset of necrobiosis for ischaemia, the deep tissues involvement for infection and the active phase of neuro-arthropathy beyond stage zero, all indicate that the pathology has reached the point of non-reversibility and that is the time to act, since any delay will translate to a destruction of the foot, which will be proportional to the length of the delay. In an elegant retrospective study on patients with infection and ischaemia at the level of the foot, Faglia et al. [46] demonstrated how a prompt surgical intervention was associated with a significant reduction in the number and the level of foot amputations, and how any day of delay was associated with a 61% increase in the risk of a higher level amputation.

"Time is limb" and the emergencies in DF patients should be considered and managed in the same way that AMI is treated because the dynamics are quite the same, with the possible concomitance of infection, which it was if, in a patient with an acute myocardial infarction, a pancarditis would intervene complicating the scenario.

The same resources that contributed to save lives in patients with acute myocardial ischaemia – quickly referring to the specialized unit, coordinated multi-disciplinary approach, prompt revascularization, strict monitoring of the general conditions of the patients – all of them, with the adjunct of timely surgical debridement, should be set in place in the third-level specialized centres to save the limbs (and lives) of the DF patients [47].

It takes a paradigm shift and a cultural change in the mentality of the caregivers who are committed to the care of DF to consider this a critical pathology until the contrary has been proven.

DF Patients Are Forever: The Follow-Up

Due to the progressive nature of the underlying pathologies, the acute phase of DF is bound to recur and this is totally unavoidable. The risk of recurrence is 60 times higher compared to the risk of a first lesion, and more than 60% of the patients will experience a recurrence within one year; more than healing, we should think in terms of time free from ulcers, in the case of recurring DF patients, to be more close to the reality of the pathology [48, 49].

These considerations, together with the little or even absent symptomatology, which characterize the neuropathic DF patient, have highlighted the importance of a close follow-up to intercept as soon as possible the episodes of recurrence, which are usually more severe and limb- and life-threatening than the first ones.

Both vascular and neurologic aspects should be evaluated in this context: the surveillance of revascularized patients should be pursued with non-invasive means like duplex-scanning to map the vessels of the lower limbs and $TcPO_2$ to explore the functional status at the level of the foot in terms of oxygen delivery.

Neuropathy and the consequent deformities that create pressure imbalances and concentrations, which will eventually progress to a new DFU, should be monitored with clinical inspection, searching for the presence of pre-ulcerative lesions such as hyperkeratosis, skin breaks, anhydrosis and bony prominences.

Foot temperature has been demonstrated to be a good proxy for the early inflammatory changes that precede the appearance of a DFU and it should be measured frequently, eventually with the direct involvement of the patient [50].

In any case, whatever strategy will be chosen, the timing is again crucial and a time schedule for the different situations from which the patients come is shown in Table 2.

Table 2. A follow-up schedule for recurrent DF patients

Condition	Follow-up	Responsible	Time frame
Previous active Charcot	Clinical/imaging/ skin temperature	Diabetologist/radiologist	Every 3 months
Minor amputation	Clinical/duplex scanning/ pressure evaluation	Diabetologist/podologist	Every 6 months
Major amputation	Duplex scanning of contra-lateral limb/control of the stump for prosthesis	Diabetologist/ vascular surgeon	Every 6 months
Previous revascularization	Duplex scanning of both limbs/TcPO$_2$/Clinical	Diabetologist/ vascular surgeon	Every 3 months
Previous DFU – neuropathic	Clinical/pressure measurements	Diabetologist/podologist	Every 6 months
Previous DFU – ischemic	Duplex scanning of both limbs/TcPO$_2$/clinical	Diabetologist/ vascular surgeon	Every 3 months

Times are only indicative and they should be customized according to the history of each patient.

The Network for DF

All the previous considerations converge on a time-related issue, which is the management of DF in each stage of its progression: only the timely delivery of appropriate care can be effective in arresting the progression of the disease in the early phases, can successfully treat the acute manifestation and can prevent amputations.

From this perspective it is not only "what" but also "when" and "who" that make the difference between an effective intervention and a failure, with potential negative consequences for the patient and a waste of resources; we should think in terms of time/effectiveness, when DF care is the issue.

In other words, what is needed is an organizational model that may connect the pathology with the adequate care at each step of its progression.

Since more than 20 years, the IWGDF promoted a organizational model based on the multi-disciplinary approach and on a 3-level hierarchy according to the grade of complexity of the disease: the more complex and severe the pathology, the higher the level; in Table 3, a synthetic description of the characteristics of such a model is reported.

According to this model, each level should take care only of the cases compatible with the resources and expertise that are available at that level, and timely refer the more complex cases to the centres at the higher level and the less complex cases to the lower levels, to optimize the clinical pathways and the resource allocation.

The matching of clinical pictures to the level of management is shown in Table 4 using the Texas University Score for DF wounds as a paradigm.

Table 3. The three-level organizative model for DF care*

Level	Location	Personnel	Facilities	Activities
First level	Community	GP, nurse	Equipped medical studies	Screening, therapy of the risk factors, prevention
Second level	Hospital	Diabetologist, nurse, podologist/podiatrist	DF clinic	Management of acute non-ischaemic conditions, offloading, treatment of mild-to moderate infections, clinical follow-up, urgent referral for acute infections
Third level	Teaching hospital	Multidisciplinary team including at least a DF specialist and a vascular interventional specialist, coordinated by a diabetologist	DF unit, with dedicated beds and access to revascularization and DF surgery	All the activities of the DF clinic plus management of ischaemia and severe infections, with the possibility to admit patients, revascularization and surgical management. Urgent referral for critical limb ischaemia and emergent foot surgery

* Each level corresponds to a pattern, including location activities and characteristics to which the centres should refer in order to fit into the model.

Table 4. The Texas University score for the classification of the DF ulcers

	0	I	II	III
A	No open lesion	Superficial ulcer	Ulcer dep to fascia, tendon or joint	Ulcer penetrating joint or bone
B	+ infection	+ infection	+ infection	+ infection
C	+ ischaemia	+ ischaemia	+ ischaemia	+ ischaemia
D	+ ischaemia and infection	+ ischaemia and infection	+ ischaemia and infection	+ ischaemia and infection

For each stage, a code in color has been associated according to the relative level of management. ☐ First level; ▨ second level; ◼ third level.

The objective of this organization is to create a network committed to the management of the DF and intercommunicating in order to promptly refer the case to the adequate level of care according to its severity, reducing the delayed referral, tackling urgencies and emergencies and intercepting early cases, thereby preventing their evolution towards more complex clinical forms.

Both [51] Germany and Belgium [39] recently implemented a national program on the IWGDF model for DF, and the results in terms of reduction in amputations were encouraging [52, 53].

Carinci et al. [54], in a review of national data obtained from 26 different countries members of the Organization for the Economic Cooperation and Development, confirmed how in 10 years the rates of LEAs reduced significantly among diabetic patients and how the reduction was significantly more important in those countries that had a public health service based on general taxation, compared to the ones that had an insurance-based system.

Since 2003, the Health Authority of Tuscany, one of the 20 administrative regions of Italy, whose health service is public, based on taxation and providing universal coverage, promoted the IWGDF model by means of a specific legislation, which had been adjourned in 2016, and which endorsed the 3-level multidisciplinary model [55, 56].

The positive effects of this approach have been confirmed by the constant trend of reduction in the rate of major amputations from 2001 to 2010, which reached an impressive value of – 30.7% at the national level, with Tuscany showing the best results both for amputations and revascularizations.

Despite these generally satisfactory figures, a closer analysis of the data at a regional level showed a huge variability within the region, with areas that were far from optimal and areas that showed performances among the best in Italy [57].

This was the main drive for the implementation of a novel approach to DF, which directly involved the GPs, committed to actively screening the DF in their population of diabetic patients, and to promptly refer them to the second level in case of any sign of the pathology.

This "second step" of the organization of care at the regional level was paralleled by an adjournment of the legislation on DF, as we said, which defined the criteria of referral of the cases, the increase in the number of third-level centres from 1 to 3, the creation of a fast track for emergent cases, and more in general the definition of the protocols for the prompt referral of the cases to the different levels of the network, according to the principles of the multi-disciplinary "community of practice" oriented on the cases.

Although it is too early to evaluate whether this paradigm shift would produce the expected results in terms of further reduction in amputation and in the homogenization of the outcome throughout the region, the first effects can be traced to the increasing number of cases referred to our third-level centres (+32% in the first 3 months of 2017) from the first- and second-level centres of our area.

Conclusions

Due to its progressiveness, aggressiveness and scarce clinical evidence, the DF syndrome, poses a number of problems to the specialists committed to its management.

Timely interception of the disease in its early manifestations to reduce the progression towards worse clinical forms, prompt management of urgencies and emergencies to avoid the irreversible tissue damage due to a delay in the treatment and a close follow-up to prevent the recurrences are the pillars on which an adequate management strategy of such a complex pathology should be founded.

Beyond the clinical and technical aspects of care, there are organizational and political issues that need to be addressed to successfully implement an adequate therapeutic program; the organization of a dedicated network, which works on an integrated program to actively screen, timely treat and systematically follow-up the DF patients is what is needed to improve the quality of the treatment of this dramatic complication of diabetes.

The recent experiences in some European countries and regions confirm the goodness of this approach, which brought the clinicians and the public health policymakers together in a joint effort to set up appropriate strategies to prevent limb amputations and save the lives of our patients.

References

1 Brownlee M: The pathobiology of diabetic complications: a unifying mechanism. Diabetes 2005;54: 1615–1625.
2 Salvotelli L, Stoico V, Perrone F, Cacciatori V, Negri C, Brangani C, Pichiri I, Targher G, Bonora E, Zoppini G: Prevalence of neuropathy in type 2 diabetic patients and its association with other diabetes complications: The Verona Diabetic Foot Screening Program. J Diabetes Complications 2015;29:1066–1070.
3 Dekker RG 2nd, Qin C, Ho BS, Kadakia AR: The effect of cumulative glycemic burden on the incidence of diabetic foot disease. J Orthop Surg Res 2016;11: 143.
4 Tesfaye S, Vileikyte L, Rayman G, et al: Painful diabetic peripheral neuropathy: consensus recommendations on diagnosis, assessment and management. Diabetes Metab Res Rev 2011;27:629–638.
5 Juster-Switlyk K, Smith AG: Updates in diabetic peripheral neuropathy. F1000Res 2016;5.
6 Faglia E, Caravaggi C, Marchetti R, Mingardi R, Morabito A, Piaggesi A, Uccioli L, Ceriello A; SCAR (SCreening for ARteriopathy) Study Group: Screening for peripheral arterial disease by means of the ankle-brachial index in newly diagnosed Type 2 diabetic patients. Diabet Med 2005;22:1310–1314.
7 Beks PJ, Mackaay AJ, de Neeling JN, de Vries H, Bouter LM, Heine RJ: Peripheral arterial disease in relation to glycaemic level in an elderly Caucasian population: the Hoorn study. Diabetologia 1995;38: 86–96.
8 Selvin E1, Marinopoulos S, Berkenblit G, Rami T, Brancati FL, Powe NR, Golden SH: Meta-analysis: glycosylated hemoglobin and cardiovascular disease in diabetes mellitus. Ann Intern Med 2004;141:421–431.
9 Bekler HI, Ertav A: Preclinical symptoms of the diabetic foot. J Am Podiatr Med Assoc 2009;99:114–112.
10 Tang UH, Zügner R, Lisovskaja V, Karlsson J, Hagberg K, Tranberg R: Foot deformities, function in the lower extremities, and plantar pressure in patients with diabetes at high risk to develop foot ulcers. Diabet Foot Ankle 2015;6:27593.
11 Formosa C, Gatt A, Chockalingam N: The importance of clinical biomechanical assessment of foot deformity and joint mobility in people living with type-2 diabetes within a primary care setting. Prim Care Diabetes 2013;7:45–50.
12 Trieb K: The Charcot foot: pathophysiology, diagnosis and classification. Bone Joint J 2016;98-B:1155–1159.
13 Zhang P, Lu J, Jing Y, Tang S, Zhu D, Bi Y: Global epidemiology of diabetic foot ulceration: a systematic review and meta-analysis †. Ann Med 2017;49: 106–116.
14 Abbott CA, Carrington AL, Ashe H, et al: The North-West Diabetes Foot Care Study: incidence of, and risk factors for, new diabetic foot ulceration in a community-based patient cohort. Diabet Med 2002; 19:377–384.

15 Gavan NA, Veresiu IA, Vinik EJ, Vinik AI, Florea B, Bondor CI: Delay between onset of symptoms and seeking physician intervention increases risk of diabetic foot complications: results of a cross-sectional population-based survey. J Diabetes Res 2016;2016: 1567405.

16 Schaper NC, Van Netten JJ, Apelqvist J, Lipsky BA, Bakker K; International Working Group on the Diabetic Foot: Prevention and management of foot problems in diabetes: a Summary Guidance for Daily Practice 2015, based on the IWGDF Guidance Documents. Diabetes Metab Res Rev 2016;32(suppl 1):7–15.

17 Skrepnek GH, Mills JL Sr, Armstrong DG: A Diabetic Emergency One Million Feet Long: Disparities and Burdens of Illness among Diabetic Foot Ulcer Cases within Emergency Departments in the United States, 2006-2010. PLoS One 2015;10:e0134914.

18 Mills JL, Beckett WC, Taylor SM: The diabetic foot: consequences of delayed treatment and referral. South Med J 1991;84:970–974.

19 Chantelau E: The perils of procrastination: effects of early vs. delayed detection and treatment of incipient Charcot fracture. Diabet Med 2005;22:1707–1712.

20 Mantey I, Foster AV, Spencer S, Edmonds ME: Why do foot ulcers recur in diabetic patients? Diabet Med 1999;16:245–249.

21 Prompers L, Huijberts M, Apelqvist J, Jude E, Piaggesi A, Bakker K, Edmonds M, Holstein P, Jirkovska A, Mauricio D, Ragnarson Tennvall G, Reike H, Spraul M, Uccioli L, Urbancic V, Van Acker K, van Baal J, van Merode F, Schaper N: High prevalence of ischaemia, infection and serious comorbidity in patients with diabetic foot disease in Europe. Baseline results from the Eurodiale study. Diabetologia 2007; 50:18–25.

22 Schaper NC: Lessons from Eurodiale. Diabetes Metab Res Rev 2012;28(suppl 1):21–26.

23 Ortegon MM, Redekop WK, Niessen LW: Cost-effectiveness of prevention and treatment of the diabetic foot: a Markov analysis. Diabetes Care 2004;27: 901–907.

24 Edmonds M: A natural history and framework for managing diabetic foot ulcers. Br J Nurs 2008;17:S20, S22, S24–S29.

25 Klein R: Hyperglycemia and microvascular and macrovascular disease in diabetes. Diabetes Care 1995; 18:258–268.

26 Stratton IM, Adler AI, Neil HA, Matthews DR, Manley SE, Cull CA, Hadden D, Turner RC, Holman RR: Association of glycaemia with macrovascular and microvascular complications of type 2 diabetes (UKPDS 35): prospective observational study. BMJ 2000; 321:405–412.

27 Lifetime benefits and costs of intensive therapy as practiced in the diabetes control and complications trial. The Diabetes Control and Complications Trial Research Group. JAMA 1996;276:1409–1415.

28 Alva ML, Gray A, Mihaylova B, Leal J, Holman RR: The impact of diabetes-related complications on healthcare costs: new results from the UKPDS (UKPDS 84). Diabet Med 2015;32:459–466.

29 Ren M, Yang C, Lin DZ, Xiao HS, Mai LF, Guo YC, Yan L: Effect of intensive nursing education on the prevention of diabetic foot ulceration among patients with high-risk diabetic foot: a follow-up analysis. Diabetes Technol Ther 2014;16:576–581.

30 Hoogeveen RC, Dorresteijn JA, Kriegsman DM, Valk GD: Complex interventions for preventing diabetic foot ulceration. Cochrane Database Syst Rev 2015;8:CD007610.

31 Gavan NA, Veresiu IA, Vinik EJ, Vinik AI, Florea B, Bondor CI: Delay between onset of symptoms and seeking physician intervention increases risk of diabetic foot complications: results of a cross-sectional population-based survey. J Diabetes Res 2016;2016: 1567405.

32 Sanders LJ, Robbins JM, Edmonds ME: History of the team approach to amputation prevention: pioneers and milestones. J Am Podiatr Med Assoc 2010; 100:317–334.

33 Formosa C, Gatt A, Chockalingam N: A critical evaluation of existing diabetic foot screening guidelines. Rev Diabet Stud 2016;13:158–186.

34 Boulton AJ, Armstrong DG, Albert SF, Frykberg RG, Hellman R, Kirkman MS, Lavery LA, LeMaster JW, Mills JL Sr, Mueller MJ, Sheehan P, Wukich DK: Comprehensive foot examination and risk assessment. A report of the Task Force of the Foot Care Interest Group of the American Diabetes Association, with endorsement by the American Association of Clinical Endocrinologists Diabetes Care 2008;31: 1679–1685.

35 Schaper NC, Van Netten JJ, Apelqvist J, Lipsky BA, Bakker K; International Working Group on the Diabetic Foot (IWGDF): Prevention and management of foot problems in diabetes: a Summary Guidance for Daily Practice 2015, based on the IWGDF guidance documents. Diabetes Res Clin Pract 2017;124:84–92.

36 van Acker K, Léger P, Hartemann A, Chawla A, Siddiqui MK: Burden of diabetic foot disorders, guidelines for management and disparities in implementation in Europe: a systematic literature review. Diabetes Metab Res Rev 2014;30:635–645.

37 van Houtum WH: Barriers to implementing foot care. Diabetes Metab Res Rev 2012;28(suppl 1):112–115.

38 Internal Clinical Guidelines Team: Diabetic Foot Problems: Prevention and Management. London, National Institute for Health and Care Excellence (UK), 2015.

39 Morbach S, Kersken J, Lobmann R, Nobels F, Doggen K, Van Acker K: The German and Belgian accreditation models for diabetic foot services. Diabetes Metab Res Rev 2016;32(suppl 1):318–325.

40 Schoen DE, Gausia K, Glance DG, Thompson SC: Improving rural and remote practitioners' knowledge of the diabetic foot: findings from an educational intervention. J Foot Ankle Res 2016;9:26.

41 Skrepnek GH, Mills JL Sr, Armstrong DG: A Diabetic Emergency One Million Feet Long: Disparities and Burdens of Illness among Diabetic Foot Ulcer Cases within Emergency Departments in the United States, 2006–2010. PLoS One 2015;10:e0134914.

42 Noronen K, Saarinen E, Albäck A, Venermo M: Analysis of the Elective Treatment Process for Critical Limb Ischaemia with Tissue Loss: Diabetic Patients Require Rapid Revascularisation. Eur J Vasc Endovasc Surg 2017;53:206–213.

43 Remington AC, Hernandez-Boussard T, Warstadt NM, Finnegan MA, Shaffer R, Kwong JZ, Curtin C: Analyzing treatment aggressiveness and identifying high-risk patients in diabetic foot ulcer return to care. Wound Repair Regen 2016;24:731–736.

44 Iacopi E, Coppelli A, Goretti C, Piaggesi A: Necrotizing Fasciitis and The Diabetic Foot. Int J Low Extrem Wounds 2015;14:316–327.

45 Brennan MB, Hess TM, Bartle B, Cooper JM, Kang J, Huang ES, Smith M, Sohn MW, Crnich C. Diabetic foot ulcer severity predicts mortality among veterans with type 2 diabetes. J Diabetes Complications 2017; 31:556–561.

46 Faglia E, Clerici G, Caminiti M, Quarantiello A, Gino M, Morabito A: The role of early surgical debridement and revascularization in patients with diabetes and deep foot space abscess: retrospective review of 106 patients with diabetes. J Foot Ankle Surg 2006;45:220–226.

47 Piaggesi A, Coppelli A, Goretti C, Iacopi E, Mattaliano C: Do you want to organize a multidisciplinary diabetic foot clinic? We can help. Int J Low Extrem Wounds 2014;13:363–370.

48 Edmonds M: A natural history and framework for managing diabetic foot ulcers. Br J Nurs 2008;17:S20, S22, S24–S29.

49 Jeffcoate WJ, Chipchase SY, Ince P, Game FL: Assessing the outcome of the management of diabetic foot ulcers using ulcer-related and person-related measures. Diabetes Care 2006;29:1784–1787.

50 Rutkove SB, Chapman KM, Acosta JA, Larrabee JE: Foot temperature in diabetic polyneuropathy: innocent bystander or unrecognized accomplice? Diabet Med 2005;22:231–238.

51 Jeffcoate W, Edmonds M, Rayman G, Shearman C, Stuart L, Turner B; Putting Feet First Implementation Group: Putting feet first – national guidance at last. Diabet Med 2009;26:1081–1082.

52 Ahmad N, Thomas GN, Gill P, Torella F: The prevalence of major lower limb amputation in the diabetic and non-diabetic population of England 2003–2013. Diab Vasc Dis Res 2016;13:348–353.

53 Kröger K, Berg C, Santosa F, Malyar N, Reinecke H: Lower limb amputation in Germany. Dtsch Arztebl Int 2017;114:130–136.

54 Carinci F, Massi Benedetti M, Klazinga NS, Uccioli L: Lower extremity amputation rates in people with diabetes as an indicator of health systems performance. A critical appraisal of the data collection 2000-2011 by the Organization for Economic Cooperation and Development (OECD). Acta Diabetol 2016;53:825–832.

55 Regione Toscana, Delibera Consiglio Regionale 603 del 24 Dicembre 2003. Linee-guida organizzative per la gestione del piede diabetico 2003.

56 Regione Toscana, Delibera Consiglio Regionale 698 del 19 Luglio 2016. Percorso diagnostico terapeutico assistenziale per la persona affetta da piede diabetico. Linee di indirizzo regionali 2016.

57 Lombardo FL, Maggini M, De Bellis A, Seghieri G, Anichini R: Lower extremity amputations in persons with and without diabetes in Italy: 2001–2010. PLoS One 2014;9:e86405.

Alberto Piaggesi, MD
Diabetic Foot Section
Department of Medicine, University of Pisa
Via Paradisa 2, IT–56124 Pisa (Italy)
E-Mail piaggesi@immr.med.unipi.it

Piaggesi · Abbruzzese · Coppelli · Iacopi · Riitano · Goretti

Piaggesi A, Apelqvist J (eds): The Diabetic Foot Syndrome.
Front Diabetes. Basel, Karger, 2018, vol 26, pp 97–106 (DOI: 10.1159/000480056)

Offloading the Diabetic Foot: The Evolution of an Integrated Strategy

Sicco A. Bus

Department of Rehabilitation, Academic Medical Center, University of Amsterdam, Amsterdam Movement Sciences, Amsterdam, The Netherlands

Abstract

When there is loss of protective sensation, elevated plantar pressure is a causative factor in the development of plantar foot ulcers in persons with diabetes. Therefore, to prevent and heal these foot ulcers, offloading is an important aspect of treatment. Neuropathic plantar forefoot ulcers can be best offloaded with knee-high devices such as a total contact cast or walker, and healing of the ulcer occurs most effectively when these devices are non-removable, probably because this guarantees that the foot is offloaded with each step the patient takes. There is no adequate evidence for using any removable device or a surgical offloading procedure, even though removable offloading devices are commonly used. This is recommended only when the adherence levels of the patient in wearing the device are good. Regarding the prevention of plantar foot ulcer recurrence in high-risk patients, recent trials show that it is the combination of providing adequate and demonstrated pressure relief using custom-made footwear and a good adherence in wearing this footwear that gives the best clinical outcome; more than half of the recurrent plantar foot ulcers can be prevented using this approach. It has been demonstrated that offloading is an important procedure in ulcer prevention and healing, but it requires an integrated approach through implementing the use of devices that force adherence or it is essential to pump in efforts to increase adherence by using removable modalities to achieve the best outcome for the patient.

Introduction

As a complication of diabetes mellitus, about half of all patients are likely to develop loss of protective sensation in the feet that is secondary to peripheral neuropathy [1]. When there is loss of protective sensation, the repetitive application of elevated plantar foot pressure during ambulation is a causative factor for the development of ulcers on the plantar foot surface [2]. These patients become unaware about high levels of pressure present under their feet, and this can then progress to cause trauma and injury to the foot [3, 4]. These high plantar pressure levels are generally caused by changes in the structure of the foot, such as with deformity, loss of fat pad quality, and limited mobility in the joints of the ankle and foot.

Reducing these high plantar pressures is called "offloading," which is considered one of the cornerstones of treatment for treating plantar foot ulcers in diabetes [3]. The annual incidence of foot ulcers when neuropathy is present is about 7–8%, but after an ulcer has healed, the risk of recurrence is much higher, around 40% in the first 12 months after healing, and 60% at 3 years [4]. This shows the need for continuous attention to the patient's foot health, including the offloading of regions that show high plantar pressures and that are at high ulcer risk.

The following review of the available medical-scientific literature will show that effective offloading of the foot in diabetic patients is important for both the healing and the prevention of foot ulcers. Prevention deals with everything that is done to prevent ulcer recurrence. Recurrence is studied much more frequently than first ulcer development because of the much higher ulcer risk included, which generally requires fewer subjects to show the effect of an intervention. While the aetiological pathway of ulcer development and the role of offloading are quite clear, there is insufficient evidence to support offloading for first ulcer prevention and more investigations are needed in this area [5].

But it will also become apparent that effective offloading alone is not enough to adequately prevent and treat plantar foot ulcers in diabetes. The best offloading modality can be developed, but if it is not worn by the patient, the foot ulcer will not heal or ulcer recurrence will not be prevented. Good adherence to treatment is needed and requires specific attention by clinicians and other involved health care providers and illustrates the evolution of an integrated strategy for offloading the diabetic foot.

Offloading Modalities

Many different casts, walkers, shoes, surgical techniques, and other offloading modalities have been developed and studied over the last 30 years to understand their effect on peak pressure in the high-risk diabetic patient. Very consistently, the total contact cast (TCC) and knee-high (removable) walkers have been shown to most effectively offload the plantar foot surface [6, 7]. Due to the high design of these devices to fit under the knee, in relation to the cone shape of the lower leg, a significant portion of the load on the lower-extremity is exerted on the lower leg instead of the foot [8, 9]. And due to the custom-moulded interface of the device with the foot, pressures on the foot are redistributed from high-risk or ulcer regions to other foot regions. In addition to limiting the ankle joint motion and reducing gait speed with these devices, these mechanisms can lead to a peak pressure reduction at the forefoot by up to 87% compared to a standard control condition [7, 10].

Shoes that extend to the ankle or just above the ankle, such as cast shoes, forefoot offloading shoes and orthopaedic shoes, cannot use this redistribution of load to the lower leg. They are therefore generally less effective in offloading the foot than knee-high devices: ~40–60% relief in peak pressure compared to a standard control condition has been found [11, 12].

Different therapeutic footwear designs, which are mainly used in the prevention of foot ulcers, can effectively offload at-risk foot regions [6]. Among these, a rocker-bottom outsole seems most effective, with up to 52% pressure relief found [13, 14], although one will have to realize that balance and gait stability in these neuropathic patients can be compromised by using significant rigid rocker configurations. A compromise between efficacy and usability may have to be made. Custom-made insoles and the construction elements that constitute these insoles can be effective in relieving peak pressure [15]. Recent studies have provided additional support to the existing knowledge base on the efficacy of using metatarsal pads and bars and medial arch supports in offloading the forefoot of the diabetic neuropathic patient [16, 17], under the condition that they are correctly placed with respect to the metatarsal heads [18]. Additionally, different open and closed cell foam materials that are used as top layer of the insole have been shown to be able to significantly relieve pressure across the entire plantar foot surface, whereas local pressure relief can be achieved by deepening and/or softening insole materials at at-risk locations [17]. Both barefoot and in-shoe plantar pressure measurements have been proven to be useful methods to guide the design of these offloading elements and insoles and to optimize the pressure result where indicated [19, 20].

Many surgical techniques have been shown to effectively relieve forefoot peak pressures in patients with an active foot ulcer. These techniques include Achilles tendon lengthening, metatarsal head resections and liquid silicone injections [21–23]. It should be realized though that these effects may only be temporary, as is the case with liquid silicone injections.

Other modalities that are used to relieve pressure on the foot are callus removal and felted foam materials. The removal of abundant forms of callus, which develop more commonly in the neuropathic than in the non-neuropathic foot, can reduce peak pressures by as much as 30%. How often such callus needs to be removed to create a continuum in offloading is unknown [24, 25]. Felted foam has shown to significantly relieve areas of high pressure, but the effect may last only for short times, requiring many frequent changes in dressing in order for the ulcer to heal.

Clearly, different interventions exhibit a great variation in offloading capacity and this likely influences their efficacy to heal foot ulcers or prevent ulcer recurrence in diabetic patients [7].

Ulcer Healing

The largest available evidence base on the role of offloading is for the treatment of non-ischaemic non-infected neuropathic plantar forefoot ulcers [6]. Surprisingly, the direct association between offloading and healing of a foot ulcer has hardly been studied [26]. The proportion of patients healed in a given time and the time taken to achieve complete healing are the most reported and most relevant clinical outcomes in healing.

Multiple recent and well-conducted meta-analyses and systematic reviews have been conducted on the topic of plantar foot ulcer healing [6, 27–29]. It should be stressed that this concerns the treatment of non-complicated neuropathic forefoot ulcers. Each meta-analysis and systematic review shows that non-removable offloading is more effective than removable offloading in healing these ulcers, both in terms of healing proportions (e.g., at 12 weeks) and time to healing. One randomized controlled trial (RCT) showed similar healing rates between the TCC and a removable walker [30]. The TCC has been considered by many to be the gold standard of treatment. These studies show that non-removable offloading with a knee-high device rather than necessarily only a cast device is now the gold standard in treatment. This provides centres where casting or adequate skills in casting are not available to use evidence-based offloading for treating plantar foot ulcers. Other reasons to use a different device than a TCC may be that they can cause iatrogenic ulcers due to poor casting and are known to reduce activity level and lead to difficulty in sleeping or driving a car. Whether these issues also relate to removable walkers being rendered irremovable has not been reported.

Removable forms of offloading always is associated with the issue that the patient may not be adherent to wearing the device or shoe, thereby reducing the effectiveness of healing the plantar ulcer that requires continuous offloading. A recent study on adherence and ulcer healing confirmed for the first time that adherence plays a pivotal role in the healing of plantar ulcers [31]. But an important study on the use of removable walkers found that patients used their prescribed removable knee-high walker for an average of only 29% of their total daily number of steps [32]. This demonstrates the potential problem of removable devices in managing a situation that is acute with risk of infection. While recognized and recently shown to be a decisive factor in ulcer healing, there is lack of information or knowledge on what the best way is to improve adherence [6, 33]. Until we know how to improve this aspect, patients who lack good adherence are best treated with a non-removable offloading device.

The evidence for using forefoot offloading shoes, cast shoes and custom-made temporary shoes for healing plantar foot ulcer is at the most meagre and based mainly on retrospective studies [34–36]. While such shoes can promote ulcer healing and sometime show healing proportions similar to the TCC, properly conducted and controlled prospective trials are needed to draw definite conclusions.

Surgical interventions such as Achilles tendon lengthening, metatarsal-phalangeal joint arthroplasty, and metatarsal head resection may promote healing, as several controlled studies including some RCTs have shown, but they often seem to have only limited additional value compared to non-surgical treatment, sometimes in the form of only a shorter time to healing. These surgical interventions are generally considered only after non-surgical treatment has failed, which seems to be the appropriate procedure, given the available evidence [6]. Next, more information on the balance between efficacy and safety of surgical procedures is needed before their application can be widely recommended, even as the "last resort" option for previously failed healing with non-surgical modalities. The effect of digital flexor tenotomy in healing apex toe ulcers has been assessed only in several retrospective case series. In a total of 231 treated patients in these 7 studies, 92–100% of ulcers healed in a mean 21–40 days. Therefore, this seems to be a promising technique, but prospective trials are needed to confirm this finding [6].

Prevention of Ulcer Recurrence
For the prevention of foot ulcer recurrence, offloading is generally achieved by the provision of therapeutic footwear that is either fully custom-made according to the patient's foot or has custom-made insoles fitted in a pre-fabricated diabetic shoe. The diabetic shoe often has extra depth in order to accommodate deformities and it has a rigid rocker outsole for pressure reduction. Several RCTs and cohort studies on the prevention of plantar foot ulcer recurrence have been conducted. Until 2013, these studies were mostly clinical trials that showed a beneficial effect of the use of therapeutic footwear compared to the use of standard footwear in preventing ulcer recurrence, while one RCT showed no effect whatsoever [5, 6]. The drawback of these trials was, however, that they lack information about the offloading efficacy of the footwear used in the studies and used a wide range of intervention and control shoes. This complicates the comparison between footwear tested within one study and also the comparison between results from different studies, and may explain some contrasting results in this area [37]. Two more recent RCTs have specifically used plantar pressure measurements in the design and evaluation of custom-made footwear and have provided the opportunity to study the role of pressure relief and optimization in the prevention of plantar foot ulcer recurrence [38, 39]. In one, the analysis of in-shoe plantar pressures while walking was used as a guidance tool for modifying the custom-made shoe of the patient, if needed, when high pressure locations were found. The trial showed that the custom-made footwear could be significantly improved for its pressure-relieving properties using this approach, and it showed an 11% reduction in ulcer recurrence incidence compared to custom-made footwear that did not undergo such improvement in pressure [38]. While this was a non-significant improvement, it can be considered a clinically relevant improvement. Since footwear adherence was measured objectively in these patients using a sensor in the shoe [40], a sub-analysis of the intervention was possible in the group of adherent patients, considering that a good shoe can be effective only if worn by the patient. In this sub-group of adherent patients, those with pressure-improved footwear showed a significant 46% lower ulcer incidence rate of plantar foot ulcer recurrence compared to the adherent patients whose shoes did not undergo pressure improvement. In the other trial, innovative custom-made insoles were designed and manufactured using barefoot plantar pressure and 3D foot shape data as input to a computer-assisted design and manufacturing algorithm.

According to a proof-of-principle study, these innovative insoles were found to be more effective in reducing peak pressure at the metatarsal heads than traditionally manufactured custom-made insoles [41]. In the trial, both types of insoles were worn in an off-the-shelf extra-depth shoe with a rigid rocker outsole and patients were frequently instructed to always wear these shoes while active. The results of the 15-month follow-up showed a 63% reduction in the recurrence of plantar metatarsal head ulcers using the innovative insoles compared to the use of standard-of-care insoles [39]. These 2 trials demonstrate that it is the combination of adequate pressure relief and adherence to wearing the footwear that gives the best clinical effect.

We have several indications that a 200 kPa level of in-shoe peak pressure may be a useful target for effective footwear design and manufacturing. That is, it may be a useful target when plantar pressure is measured with a validated and calibrated system that uses pressure sensors that have a surface area of 1 cm^2 (a different sensor surface area will likely result in a different pressure outcome under a given load). One study examined patients who had remained healed after plantar ulceration and found a mean pressure of approximately 200 kPa at the prior ulcer site [42]. Data from the above-mentioned trial showed that when peak pressure was <200 kPa at the previous ulcer location, further adaptation of the footwear did not result in a reduction of peak pressure [20]. And a risk factor analysis of pressure-related plantar foot ulcer recurrence using data from the same trial showed that when peak pressure is <200 kPa and footwear adherence is >80%, the risk of ulcer recurrence reduces by 60% compared to when these conditions are not met [43]. An in-shoe pressure threshold for foot ulceration is likely to be unique to each individual, but we use this 200 kPa value in clinical footwear practice as a helpful target for offloading high-risk patients.

Several surgical interventions such as Achilles tendon lengthening and metatarsal head resection have been show to effectively reduce pressure under the forefoot and may reduce ulcer recurrence rates compared to non-surgical treatment in selected patients who do not seem to respond to non-surgical treatment. Quite interestingly, studies have shown these surgical interventions to be relatively more effective in the prevention of ulcer recurrence than in the healing of foot ulcers for which they are primarily chosen [6]. Overall, the evidence base to support the safe use of surgical procedures for ulcer prevention is still weak, with very few recent controlled studies conducted [6]. Additionally, complications with these procedures such as transfer ulcers and impaired balance during walking have been shown and make some of the procedures less popular for diabetic foot care.

The Evolution of an Integrated Strategy

The evidence on foot ulcer healing shows that neuropathic plantar forefoot ulcers that are not complicated by infection or ischemia, and which represent approximately 25% of foot ulcers treated in specialized clinics [44], can heal in approximately 6–8 weeks when an appropriate offloading device is used. Non-removable offloading is the current "gold standard" treatment. Where offloading devices cannot be made non-removable or where contraindications for using non-removable offloading exist, an integrated approach of using a good offloading device and instructing and motivating the patient to wear this device at all times when the patient is loading the foot, and monitor its use, should be used. Several studies show that non-removable devices for which most evidence exists are underused in clinical practice [45–47]. This gap between evidence/recommendations and clinical practice needs to be bridged, and previously several suggestions have been made on how to do this [48].

Most ulcers, however (one study showing this to be 75% of foot ulcers in specialized foot clinics), are complicated by factors such as infection and/or peripheral vascular disease including ischemia [44, 49]. These ulcers take much longer to heal, some do not heal, but very little data is available on what would be the reasonable time to healing. At minimum, treatment requires an integrated approach in which the infection has to be controlled and the ischaemia has to be resolved, through a revascularization procedure [50]. Due to the neuropathic and often biomechanical origin of these ulcers, offloading should still be considered a cornerstone of treatment in such complex wounds because of the enhanced risk of limb loss in these patients. The most recent guidance document of the International Working Group on the Diabetic Foot on offloading includes several suggestions on the use of offloading in the treatment of more complicated plantar foot ulcers [51].

Measurable and effective pressure reduction should result from all prescribed interventions for offloading the foot to prevent or heal plantar foot ulcers [7]. More clinics and footwear companies are introducing the use of barefoot and in-shoe plantar pressure measurement for this purpose and experience the advantage of having these objective tools to assess offloading efficacy. Given the added value in preventing foot ulcer recurrence in diabetes, these tools are expected to be cost-effective, although this will have to be demonstrated. The use of such tools will transform the offloading field from being a more experienced and trial-and-error based field to being a more scientific and data-driven based field in the future.

Measurable and effective pressure reduction is necessary but not sufficient for healing foot ulcers or preventing recurrence. The behaviour of the patient is also important if the device that the patient wears cannot be made non-removable. Forced adherence to offloading in ulcer treatment should always be given consideration where there is no contraindication. Considerations for preventing ulcer recurrence are somewhat different because applying a non-removable shoe is not an option, and therefore even more important. Ulcer-free survival is poor after a patient has healed from a foot ulcer [4]. Adherence to wearing prescribed footwear has been shown to be low, in particular when patients are at home [33]. And it is the combination of a good pressure-relieving shoe and adequate adherence that gives the best clinical result in prevention of recurrence. Therefore, an integrated approach aimed at biomechanical optimization through good orthotic management and improvement of adherence through a behavioural intervention is required. Effective strategies to do the latter have not yet been reported. The provision of offloading footwear for specific use inside the house, where adherence is lowest, may help [33]. The provision of attractive footwear may help, and an educational intervention such as motivational interviewing to empower the patient in taking responsibility for their own treatment and outcome, may help. Adherence is an important component in clinical outcome and therefore future studies should focus on this subject so that we learn how adherence can be improved upon and when integrated with orthotic care, how it can heal and prevent foot ulcers in diabetic patients.

Conclusions

This overview informs clinicians and other health care professionals working with diabetic foot patients about effective offloading treatment for healing plantar foot ulcers and preventing their recurrence. It clearly demonstrates that it is the combination of having a good offloading device or shoe and good adherence or forced adherence to wearing the device that gives the best clinical outcomes. Therefore, treatment should focus on an integrated approach of good orthotic care and behavioural interventions for the healing and prevention of foot ulcers in diabetes.

References

1 Armstrong DG: Loss of protective sensation: a practical evidence-based definition. J Foot Ankle Surg 1999;38:79–80.
2 Monteiro-Soares M, Boyko EJ, Ribeiro J, Ribeiro I, Dinis-Ribeiro M: Predictive factors for diabetic foot ulceration: a systematic review. Diabetes Metab Res Rev 2012;28:574–600.
3 Wu SC, Crews RT, Armstrong DG: The pivotal role of offloading in the management of neuropathic foot ulceration. Curr Diab Rep 2005;5:423–429.
4 Armstrong DG, Boulton AJM, Bus SA: Diabetic foot ulcers and their recurrence. N Engl J Med 2017;376: 2367–2375.
5 van Netten JJ, Price PE, Lavery LA, et al: Prevention of foot ulcers in the at-risk patient with diabetes: a systematic review. Diabetes Metab Res Rev 2016; 32(suppl 1):84–98.
6 Bus SA, van Deursen RW, Armstrong DG, et al: Footwear and offloading interventions to prevent and heal foot ulcers and reduce plantar pressure in patients with diabetes: a systematic review. Diabetes Metab Res Rev 2016;32(suppl 1):99–118.
7 Cavanagh PR, Bus SA: Off-loading the diabetic foot for ulcer prevention and healing. Plast Reconstr Surg 2011;127(suppl 1):248S–256S.
8 Shaw JE, Hsi WL, Ulbrecht JS, Norkitis A, Becker MB, Cavanagh PR: The mechanism of plantar unloading in total contact casts: implications for design and clinical use. Foot Ankle Int 1997;18:809–817.
9 Begg L, McLaughlin P, Vicaretti M, Fletcher J, Burns J: Total contact cast wall load in patients with a plantar forefoot ulcer and diabetes. J Foot Ankle Res 2016;9:2.
10 Fleischli JG, Lavery LA, Vela SA, Ashry H, Lavery DC: 1997 William J. Stickel Bronze Award. Comparison of strategies for reducing pressure at the site of neuropathic ulcers. J Am Podiatr Med Assoc 1997; 87:466–72.
11 Beuker BJ, van Deursen RW, Price P, Manning EA, van Baal JG, Harding KG: Plantar pressure in offloading devices used in diabetic ulcer treatment. Wound Repair Regen 2005;13:537–542.
12 Bus SA, van Deursen RW, Kanade RV, et al: Plantar pressure relief in the diabetic foot using forefoot offloading shoes. Gait Posture 2009;29:618–622.
13 van Schie C, Ulbrecht JS, Becker MB, Cavanagh PR: Design criteria for rigid rocker shoes. Foot Ankle Int 2000;21:833–844.

14 Praet SF, Louwerens JW: The influence of shoe design on plantar pressures in neuropathic feet. diabetes care 2003;26:441–445.

15 Bus SA, Ulbrecht JS, Cavanagh PR: Pressure relief and load redistribution by custom-made insoles in diabetic patients with neuropathy and foot deformity. Clin Biomech 2004;19:629–638.

16 Guldemond NA, Leffers P, Schaper NC, et al: The effects of insole configurations on forefoot plantar pressure and walking convenience in diabetic patients with neuropathic feet. Clin Biomech 2007;22:81–87.

17 Arts ML, de Haart M, Waaijman R, et al: Data-driven directions for effective footwear provision for the high-risk diabetic foot. Diabet Med 2015;32:790–797.

18 Hastings MK, Mueller MJ, Pilgram TK, Lott DJ, Commean PK, Johnson JE: Effect of metatarsal pad placement on plantar pressure in people with diabetes mellitus and peripheral neuropathy. Foot Ankle Int 2007;28:84–88.

19 Bus SA, Haspels R, Busch-Westbroek TE: Evaluation and optimization of therapeutic footwear for neuropathic diabetic foot patients using in-shoe plantar pressure analysis. Diabetes Care 2011;34:1595–1600.

20 Waaijman R, Arts ML, Haspels R, Busch-Westbroek TE, Nollet F, Bus SA: Pressure-reduction and preservation in custom-made footwear of patients with diabetes and a history of plantar ulceration. DiabetMed 2012;29:1542–1549.

21 van Schie CH, Whalley A, Armstrong DG, Vileikyte L, Boulton AJ: The effect of silicone injections in the diabetic foot on peak plantar pressure and plantar tissue thickness: a 2-year follow-up. Arch Phys Med Rehabil 2002;83:919–923.

22 Maluf KS, Mueller MJ, Strube MJ, Engsberg JR, Johnson JE: Tendon Achilles lengthening for the treatment of neuropathic ulcers causes a temporary reduction in forefoot pressure associated with changes in plantar flexor power rather than ankle motion during gait. J Biomech 2004;37:897–906.

23 Patel VG, Wieman TJ: Effect of metatarsal head resection for diabetic foot ulcers on the dynamic plantar pressure distribution. AmJ Surg 1994;167:297–301.

24 Pitei DL, Foster A, Edmonds M: The effect of regular callus removal on foot pressures. J Foot Ankle Surg 1999;38:251–255.

25 Young MJ, Cavanagh PR, Thomas G, Johnson MM, Murray H, Boulton AJ: The effect of callus removal on dynamic plantar foot pressures in diabetic patients. Diabet Med 1992;9:55–57.

26 Gutekunst DJ, Hastings MK, Bohnert KL, Strube MJ, Sinacore DR: Removable cast walker boots yield greater forefoot off-loading than total contact casts. ClinBiomech(Bristol, Avon) 2011;26:649–654.

27 Lewis J, Lipp A: Pressure-relieving interventions for treating diabetic foot ulcers. Cochrane Database Syst Rev 2013;1:CD002302.

28 Morona JK, Buckley ES, Jones S, Reddin EA, Merlin TL: Comparison of the clinical effectiveness of different off-loading devices for the treatment of neuropathic foot ulcers in patients with diabetes: a systematic review and meta-analysis. Diabetes Metab Res Rev 2013;29:183–193.

29 Elraiyah T, Prutsky G, Domecq JP, et al: A systematic review and meta-analysis of off-loading methods for diabetic foot ulcers. J Vasc Surg 2016;63(2 suppl):59S–68S.e1-2.

30 Faglia E, Caravaggi C, Clerici G, et al: Effectiveness of removable walker cast versus nonremovable fiberglass off-bearing cast in the healing of diabetic plantar foot ulcer: a randomized controlled trial. Diabetes Care 2010;33:1419–1423.

31 Crews RT, Shen BJ, Campbell L, et al: Role and Determinants of Adherence to Off-loading in Diabetic Foot Ulcer Healing: A Prospective Investigation. Diabetes Care 2016;39:1371–1377.

32 Armstrong DG, Lavery LA, Kimbriel HR, Nixon BP, Boulton AJ: Activity patterns of patients with diabetic foot ulceration: patients with active ulceration may not adhere to a standard pressure off-loading regimen. Diabetes Care 2003;26:2595–2597.

33 Waaijman R, Keukenkamp R, de haart M, Polomski WP, Nollet F, Bus SA: Adherence to wearing prescription custom-made footwear in patients with diabetes at high risk for plantar foot ulceration. Diabetes Care 2013;36:1613–1618.

34 Hissink RJ, Manning HA, van Baal JG: The MABAL shoe, an alternative method in contact casting for the treatment of neuropathic diabetic foot ulcers. Foot Ankle Int 2000;21:320–323.

35 Dumont IJ, Lepeut MS, Tsirtsikolou DM, et al: A proof-of-concept study of the effectiveness of a removable device for offloading in patients with neuropathic ulceration of the foot: the Ransart boot. Diabet Med 2009;26:778–782.

36 Van De Weg FB, Van Der Windt DA, Vahl AC: Wound healing: total contact cast vs. custom-made temporary footwear for patients with diabetic foot ulceration. ProsthetOrthotInt 2008;32:3–11.

37 Cavanagh PR, Bus SA: Off-loading the diabetic foot for ulcer prevention and healing. J Am Podiatr Med Assoc 2010;100:360–368.

38 Bus SA, Waaijman R, Arts M, et al: Effect of custom-made footwear on foot ulcer recurrence in diabetes: a multicenter randomized controlled trial. Diabetes Care 2013;36:4109–4116.

39 Ulbrecht JS, Hurley T, Mauger DT, Cavanagh PR: Prevention of Recurrent Foot Ulcers With Plantar Pressure-Based In-Shoe Orthoses: the CareFUL prevention multicenter randomized controlled trial. diabetes care 2014;37:1982–1989.

40 Bus SA, Waaijman R, Nollet F: New monitoring technology to objectively assess adherence to prescribed footwear and assistive devices during ambulatory activity. Arch Phys Med Rehabil 2012;93: 2075–2079.

41 Owings TM, Woerner JL, Frampton JD, Cavanagh PR, Botek G: Custom therapeutic insoles based on both foot shape and plantar pressure measurement provide enhanced pressure relief. Diabetes Care 2008;31:839–844.

42 Owings TM, Apelqvist J, Stenstrom A, et al: Plantar pressures in diabetic patients with foot ulcers which have remained healed. Diabet Med 2009;26:1141–1146.

43 Waaijman R, de Haart M, Arts ML, et al: Risk factors for plantar foot ulcer recurrence in neuropathic diabetic patients. Diabetes Care 2014;37:1697–1705.

44 Prompers L, Huijberts M, Apelqvist J, et al: High prevalence of ischaemia, infection and serious comorbidity in patients with diabetic foot disease in Europe. Baseline results from the Eurodiale study. Diabetologia 2007;50:18–25.

45 Wu SC, Jensen JL, Weber AK, Robinson DE, Armstrong DG: Use of pressure offloading devices in diabetic foot ulcers: do we practice what we preach? Diabetes Care 2008;31:2118–2119.

46 Prompers L, Huijberts M, Apelqvist J, et al: Delivery of care to diabetic patients with foot ulcers in daily practice: results of the Eurodiale Study, a prospective cohort study. Diabet Med 2008;25:700–707.

47 Raspovic A, Landorf KB: A survey of offloading practices for diabetes-related plantar neuropathic foot ulcers. J Foot Ankle Res 2014;7:35.

48 Bus SA: The Role of Pressure Offloading on Diabetic Foot Ulcer Healing and Prevention of Recurrence. Plast Reconstr Surg 2016;138(3 suppl):179S–187S.

49 Cavanagh PR, Lipsky BA, Bradbury AW, Botek G: Treatment for diabetic foot ulcers. Lancet 2005;366: 1725–1735.

50 Nabuurs-Franssen MH, Sleegers R, Huijberts MS, et al: Total contact casting of the diabetic foot in daily practice: a prospective follow-up study. Diabetes Care 2005;28:243–247.

51 Bus SA, Armstrong DG, van Deursen RW, et al: IWGDF guidance on footwear and offloading interventions to prevent and heal foot ulcers in patients with diabetes. Diabetes Metab Res Rev 2016;32(suppl 1): 25–36.

Sicco A. Bus, PhD
Department of Rehabilitation, Room A01-419
Academic Medical Center, University of Amsterdam, Amsterdam Movement Sciences
PO Box 22660, NL–1100 DD Amsterdam (The Netherlands)
E-Mail s.a.bus@amc.uva.nl

Piaggesi A, Apelqvist J (eds): The Diabetic Foot Syndrome.
Front Diabetes. Basel, Karger, 2018, vol 26, pp 107–130 (DOI: 10.1159/000480057)

Surgical Management of the Charcot Foot

Luca Dalla Paola · Giuseppe Scavone · Anna Carone ·
Lucian Vasilache · Giulio Boscarino

Diabetic Foot Unit, Maria Cecilia Hospital, GVM Care and Research, Cotignola, Italy

Abstract

Charcot neuropathic osteoarthropathy is a severe complication of diabetic neuropathy. Even today the disease is difficult to recognize and treat. While in the early stages conservative therapy is extremely efficient and avoids progression into more advanced phases, when there are structural deformities and osteoarticular alterations, surgery often takes on the role of limb salvage therapy. Within this scenario, we take into consideration the physiopathology and anatomical/functional conditions that support the indication for surgery. In this paper, we review the surgical techniques, both in the field of reconstructive and prophylactic surgery aiming at correcting deformity and instability before ulcerative lesions onset, and in the field of emergent surgery once there is a complicated condition due to osteomyelitis in the bone structures.   © 2018 S. Karger AG, Basel

Introduction

Charcot neuropathic osteoarthropathy (CN) involving the foot and/or the ankle is a challenging clinical condition that causes progressive bone deformity and osteoarticular instability, which leads to ulcerations, spread of infection and, consequently, an elevated risk of amputation [1–7]. CN does not only entail a high risk of losing the limb; this condition is also linked to a reduction in the quality of life, high disability and increased risk of mortality [8–15].

Even if J.M. Charcot gave the first detailed description of the clinical aspect of the disease in 1868, CN is a pathological process still difficult to recognize and treat. As diabetes exponentially increases worldwide, all the health professionals need to be aware of its possible limb-threatening progression [16–19].

It is also important to notice how progression – from neuropathy to structural deformity – also involves transitional stages, and during the early phases it becomes possible to efficiently treat the condition, thereby preventing progression. The earlier CN is diagnosed and treated (total off-loading), the lesser the risk to develop deformity and articular instability that can lead to ulceration, osteomyelitis and, thus, amputation.

Fifty years ago, Eichenholtz [20] defined for the first time (in a landmark paper based on clinical examination and radiographic findings) the 3 independent but linear stages of CN: development, coalescent and reconstructive. The system proposed by Eichenholtz was modified by Shibata et al. [21] adding a stage prior to that of development characterized by lack of injury or osteoarticular disorders.

Chantelau has recently proposed a new CN classification based on magnetic resonance imaging (MRI) [22]. Stage A includes the acute or active phase, while stage B refers to the quiescent phase. These are differentiated by the presence or absence of bone marrow oedema on MRI. Each stage presents different numerical gradings (grade 0 is characterized by the absence of cortical fractures; grade 1 by the presence of cortical fractures). The stage influences decisions on treatment, while grading regards functionality, orthotic aid possibilities and prognosis. Each of the 4 categories clinically differs from each other in terms of histopathology and radiological imaging. It is extremely important to recognize the different stages of progression in order to effectively choose a treatment strategy. Indeed, the approach may vary according to the different stages of the natural history of the CN.

It is presently not possible to predict the onset of this complex pathology in diabetic patients with peripheral neuropathy. Yet, it is possible to diagnose early and detect the first clinical signs and symptoms. Recognizing the condition in its early stages, when there is no anatomic alteration yet, would allow the possibily to opt for a conservative approach, avoiding deformity and osteoarticular instability stages that translate into the risk for amputation.

Early diagnosis of CN is based both on patient's history and on clinical data. Any time a neuropathic patient presents a red, hot, swollen foot, we are led to thinking about an acute stage CN. The diagnosis is then confirmed once we get to know the patient's history. The careful and accurate analysis of the medical history will enhance the diagnostic hypothesis and, in particular, will allow the opportunity to make a differential diagnosis as compared to other conditions (e.g., gout, arthritis, algodistrophy, osteomyelitis), which may show similar clinical and instrumental (radiological) findings.

The localization of the undermining anatomical-structural condition is equally important to define and predict the magnitude of the deformity and assess the need for corrective surgery.

In CN, Frykberg and Sanders [4–6] identified 5 patterns of damage in the foot and ankle and associated these different anatomical patterns (Fig. 1).

The location at Lisfranc and at the ankle/subtalar joints are the locations where the most severe structural deformity and instability are found. The pattern V is rare but may be correlated with an avulsion injury or isolated pathologic fracture of the posterior calcaneal tuberosity.

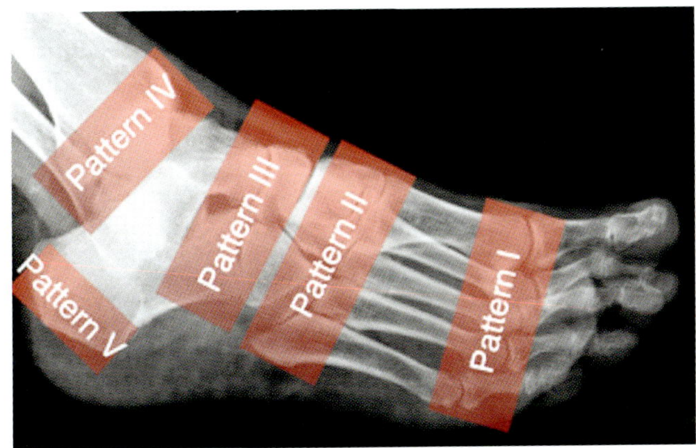

Fig. 1. Frykberg and Sanders anatomical classification of CN.

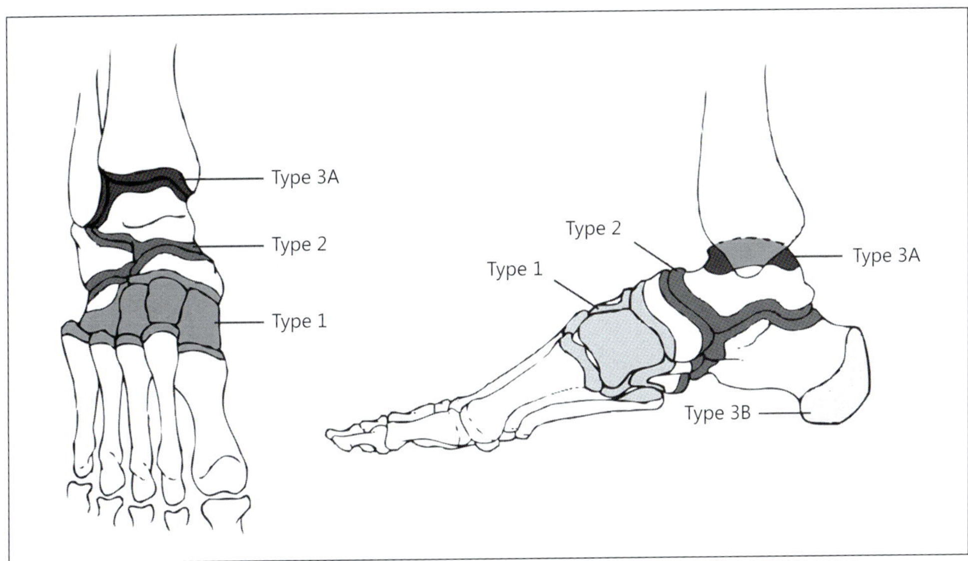

Fig. 2. Brodsky anatomical classification of CN.

Based on the 4 regions most commonly affected by CN, an anatomical classification is described also by Brodsky and Rouse (Fig. 2) [23].

This classification was further differentiated into a supplementary number of classes as of the elevated percentage of involvement of the midfoot and of the medial column [24–26].

Acquired deformities are often complicated by large wounds that develop alongside bone deformities, and the progression of infection to osteomyelitis is frequent, with an increased risk of major amputation (Fig. 3) [12, 19, 23–29].

Bevan and Tomlinson [30] found (studying the radiographic images in weight-bearing conditions) that patients are at low risk of developing ulcerations or infections if their feet are radiographically consistently plantigrade. They observed that the risk

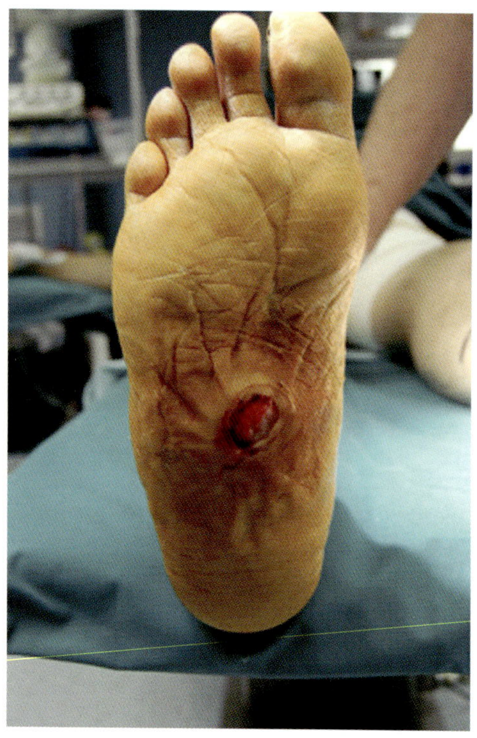

Fig. 3. Charcot foot complicated by plantar ulceration.

of developing a wound was reduced if the axis of the hindfoot was reasonably collinear with the axis of the forefoot.

In CN, the degree of instability and deformity correlates with the risk of developing an ulcer and it must be considered the primary risk factor for amputation [13]. In these terms, the most proximal the deformity and instability is, the highest is the risk of wound onset. In the case of ankle involvement, the surgical approach should be carried out as soon as possible even before the onset of an ulcer [13, 25, 31–35].

The existence of a foot ulcer may require further investigations and treatment, including hospitalization, non-weight-bearing, specific antibiotic regimen and diagnostic imaging such as MRI or bone scans. The presence of a wound becomes the primary indication for surgical treatment of CN because it compromises the limb functionality, causing a high-risk of spreading infection through soft tissue and osteomyelitis [13].

Indications for Surgical Approach

Surgical treatment of Charcot neuroarthropathy is an extremely important chapter of the whole surgical approach to the diabetic foot. Actually, the Charcot foot surgery also embraces all the distinct classes of surgery described in the classification published by Armstrong and Frykberg (Table 1) [36].

Dalla Paola · Scavone · Carone · Vasilache · Boscarino

Table 1. Classes of diabetic foot surgery

Diabetic foot surgery class	Description	Potential risk for high level amputation
Class IV: emergent	Procedure performed to limit progression of acute infection	High
Class III: curative	Procedure performed to assist in healing open wound	Moderate
Class II: prophilactic	Procedure performed to reduce risk of ulceration or reulceration in person with loss of protective sensation but without open wound	Low
Class I: elective	Procedure performed to alleviate pain or limitation of motion in a person without loss of protective sensation	Very low

The ideal and standard surgical approach for CN has not yet reached a consensus due to the lack of robust data supporting any particular approach. All this has not prevented surgeons to surgically treat deformity, articular instability and more or less complex ulceration complicated or not by osteomyelitis.

Surgical procedures are recommended when all conservative treatments fail to prevent ulcerations [17]. These restrictive indications are bound to the perception of a significant risk of not being able to reach a sufficient stabilization or a high percentage of post-surgery complications in patients with multiple comorbidities.

The CN surgery indications are exostosis with high-risk of ulceration despite an optimal orthotic treatment, severe articular instability, pain associated with malalignment and relapsing wounds [37].

In centres specialized in the treatment of the diabetic foot, the percentage of patients with CN undergoing major and/or minor surgery ranges from 14% [18] to 51% [29].

In the literature, the percentage of major amputation ranges in CN population from 3 to 9%. Some authors state that the risk of amputation increases with the progression of the infection, expecially in the more proximal osteomyelitis localizations [38]. Recently, another study underlined that neither the extension of osteomyelitis or its staging according to the Cierny and Mader classification, nor the localization of the deformity and bone infection according to Frykberg and Sanders classification should be considered as negative prognostic factors for amputation [39].

Saltzman et al. [40] report that in their series, the greater demand for amputation is observed in patients who develop midtarsal deformities compared to patients with more proximal deformities. The most important factor for prognosis would have been the presence of recurrent ulcerations (36% of amputations) compared to patients who do not develop ulcerative lesions (6% of amputations).

The 2 main phases of Charcot foot surgery consist of correcting the deformity through prophylactic surgery and of the treatment of ulcerative lesions associated or not to the presence of osteomyelitis in an unstable and deformed foot. The endpoint of prophylactic surgery is to achieve a stable, plantigrade foot with a reduced risk of ulceration. This result allows patients to use rigid rocker sole footwear and custom moulded, multilayer, total contact insoles. Thus, surgical planning entails not only an evaluation of the deformity observed in the radiological exams, but also and most of all, the need to take into consideration the local and overall clinical condition of the patient and his/her risk factors associated to comorbidity. In other words, a severe deformity condition, which is radiologically evident, if it does not entail a high-risk of ulcer with an appropriate orthothic aid, then it will probably not translate into an indication for surgery; on the contrary, in the event of a relapsing ulceration despite the use of appropriate shoes and insoles, it will translate into an indication to surgically correct any kind of deformity. For these reasons, a first attempt with conservative therapy must always be implemented. This point was highlighted by Pinzur [41], who showed that 60% of patients with midfoot CN reached the desired endpoint without the need for surgery.

Failure to properly treat CN with conservative or surgical treatment carries the risk of progression and development of ulcers and a subsequent infection onset and osteomyelitic involvement of bone structures next to the cutaneous lesion.

If an ulceration is present – particularly if complicated by osteomyelitis – surgical approach must be considered salvage treatment, as there is a high risk for amputation [13, 42, 43].

Prophilactic Surgical Treatment

The aim of the prophilactic surgical treatment is to control and correct the alignment of the foot, so as to decrease the risk of ulceration. The prophylactic surgical treatment must be understood with a scale of complexity in which the surgical aggression is directly related to the degree of deformity and instability, as well as its location. Being elective procedures, it is essential that for patients with an indication to this type of treatment, we also consider the comorbidities that can lead to treatment complications. We believe that any patient eligible for elective CN surgery needs a cardiological assessment (including specialized evaluation, electrocardiogram and echocardiography) possibly integrated with a stress test to highlight an inducible ischemic heart disease. Thirty percent of patients with CN show peripheral arterial disease [44]. Thus, all patients with CN who are eligible for surgical treatment need – before surgery – an appropriate vascular assessment, and in the event of critical ischaemia, a percutaneous or surgical revascularization [34, 39].

The appropriate timing for surgery is usually considered at stages II–III according to Eichenholtz classification. In fact, during the acute phase, the risk of failure of

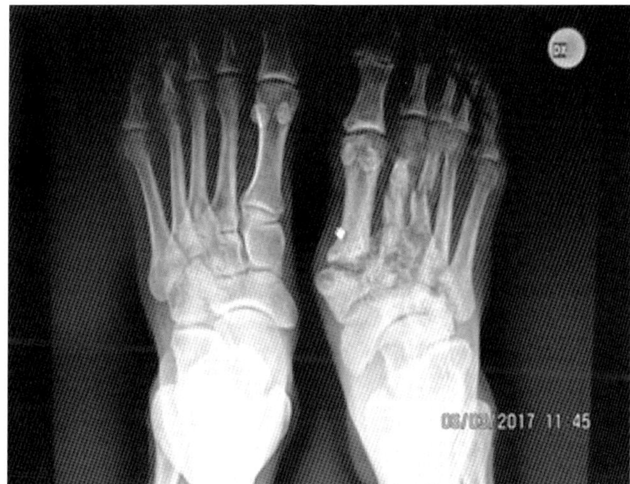

Fig. 4. Midfoot CN.

stabilization in relation to the active inflammatory condition and to the osteoarticular destruction is considered rather high. There are currently no data showing the opportunity to move surgery up to earlier stages of the disease. Indeed, there are only a few papers that report on surgery in the acute phase [45, 46].

Surgical planning must take into account the clinical condition with careful consideration of the exostoses and their location. The patient should be clinically evaluated in the offloading and weightbearing state. The standard radiological study (plain radiographs) will evaluate the deformity that is evident on the sagittal plane, assessing the lateral talar-first metatarsal angle (or Meary's angle), cuboid height, medial column height, calcaneal fifth metatarsal angle, lateral tibiotalar angle and the transverse plane (hindfoot-forefoot angle and AP talar first metatarsal angle) [42].

Surgical options range from simple decompressive exostectomy to more extensive realignment and arthrodesis of the foot and ankle with internal or external fixation. Osseous correction is achieved with exostectomy, osteotomies and/or arthrodesis. Sometimes, in the event of very complex deformities, there is an indication for the combination of the 3 approaches. Once the intraoperative correction is obtained, Kirshner wires and Steinmann pins need to be used for a temporary stabilization.

The midfoot location (class 2–3 using Frykberg and Sanders classification; class 1 using the Brodsky classification) is the most frequent one with 70% of cases (Fig. 4).

Exostectomy is most effectively used when tarso-metatarsal joints are involved [47]. Patients presenting bony prominences without other deformities only need a simple exostectomy (Fig. 5) [48].

This exostectomy technique has been successfully used by different authors in their study on Charcot midfoot deformity [8, 23, 49–51].

If the surgical exostectomy procedure fails to prevent ulceration or recurrence, then more extensive arthrodesis and fusion interventions are needed.

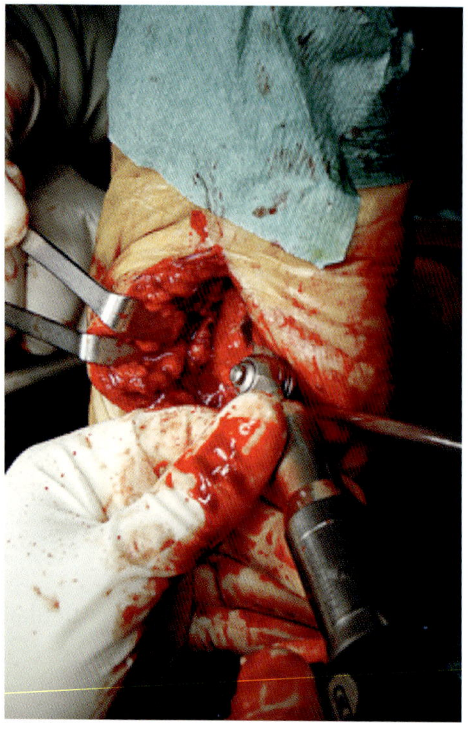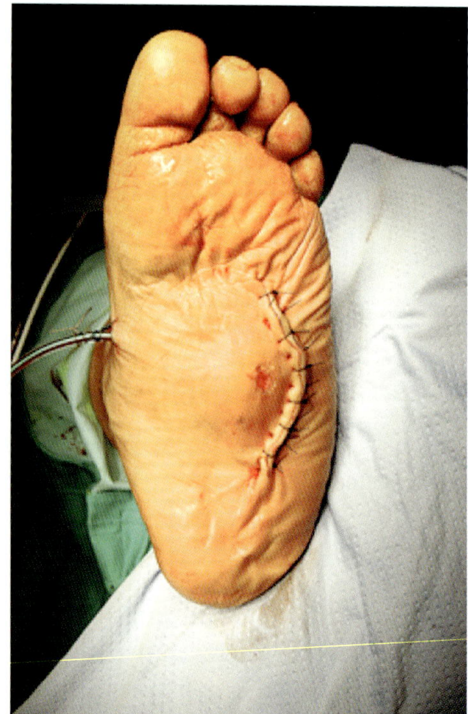

Fig. 5. Midfoot exostectomy.

Translation of medial or lateral metatarsal bones is associated with a shortening of the medial column. The deformity is located in the region of the navicular bone with talus and navicular in plantar flexion, while the cuneiforms are located dorsally with the first metatarsal. Class 2 (using Frykberg and Sanders classification) is very often combined with class 3. The latter shows the cuboid bone in plantar dislocation and prominence. The clinical presentation is configured with a rocker-bottom foot development of a plantar ulceration at the bony prominences. Usually, this type of deformity prevents conservative treatment. In general, it is necessary to reconstruct the medial and lateral column. and in cases of complex deformities, it is also appropriate to associate with the arthrodesis of the subtalar joint.

This complex surgical approach involves a triple arthrodesis (subtalar, calcaneocuboid and talonavicular joints). The first step is the improvement of the calcaneal inclination angle by posterior muscle group lenghtening. Then the subtalar and calcaneocuboid joints are exposed with an incision from the peroneal malleolus to the base of the 5th metatarsal. To access the medial column and the talonavicular joints, an incision may be carried out between the anterior and posterior tibialis tendons.

The deformity at the ankle (class 4 using Frykberg and Sanders classification; class 3A of Brodsky's classification) can involve only the tibio-talar joint, or in complex forms it can also involve the subtalar joint (Fig. 6).

   Dalla Paola · Scavone · Carone · Vasilache · Boscarino

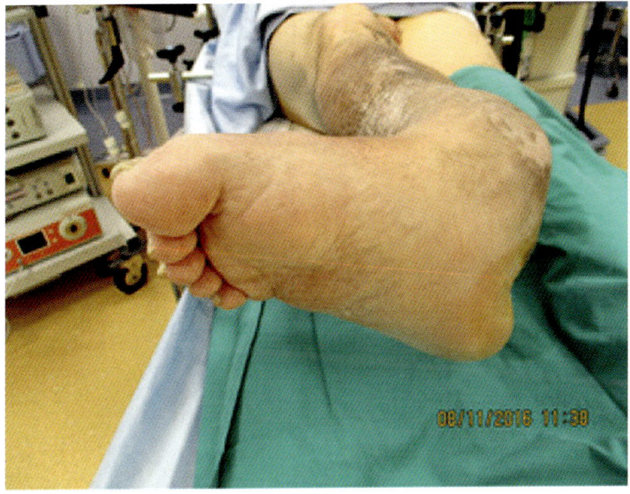

Fig. 6. Ankle deformity in CN.

The ankle arthrodesis or the stabilization of the hindfoot is the treatment of choice for the deformity of the area. The goal of the arthrodesis is the foot realignment on the leg axis to obtain a stable plantigrade position, which is braceable and walkable. The surgical approach involves different ways of access, but the easiest way that allows a straightforward approach to the ankle joint is the transfibular one. During the procedure, it is almost the rule to perform osteotomy to correct alignment of the ankle and hindfoot [52].

If the deformity and the instability only affect the subtalar joint associated with less deformity of the Chopart joints, the triple arthrodesis may be considered to be the procedure of choice.

If the impairment of stability affects the ankle joint with collapse or destruction of the talus, it is necessary to perform an ankle (TTC) or tibiocalcaneal arthrodesis. In the case of complex deformities, we prefer to perform the total removal of the talus and run a tibiocalcaneal fusion (Fig. 7).

To succeed in this procedure, we need to accurately remove the articular cartilage, continuing until the bleeding cancellous bone is reached. Subsequently, it is necessary to prepare the bone surfaces to be opposed and achieve the maximum contact surface. Even the soft tissues must sometimes be cleaned up and thus a stable fixation needs to be done [37, 53].

The calcaneal fracture as provided in class 5 of the Frykberg and Sanders classification and 3B following the Brodsky classification must undergo surgical treatment in case of deformity progression, when there is a dislocation of the posterior portion of the calcaneous in relation to the contraction of the Achilles tendon (Fig. 8). The objective is to correct the deformity and to prevent ulcerative lesions.

A stable pseudarthrosis is an acceptable outcome in patients with CN, since it allows to stabilize and use a prosthetic aid walk [54].

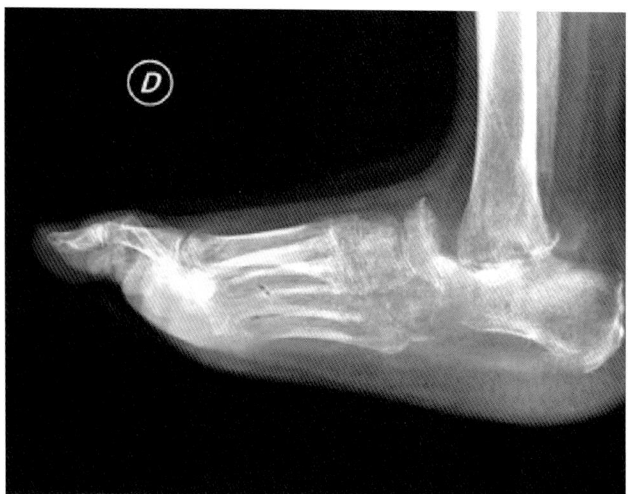

Fig. 7. Tibiocalcaneal arthrodesis with total talectomy.

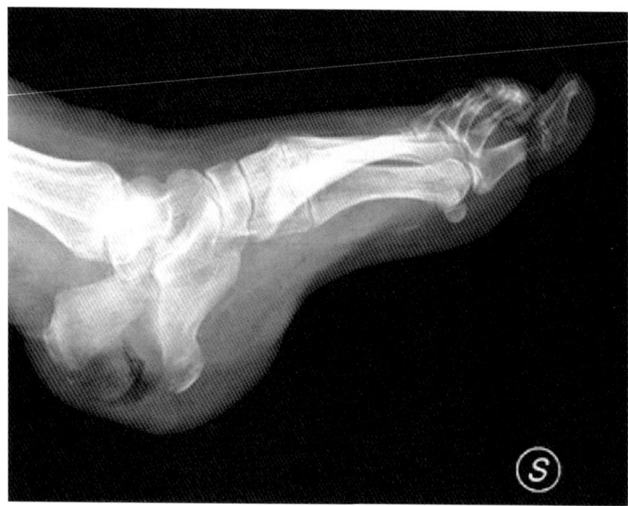

Fig. 8. Calcaneal fracture.

Since ankle equinus is considered an important alteration that contributes to the deformity of the midfoot, most reconstructive interventions provide – as adjuvant treatment – the Achilles tendon or the gastrocnemius muscle lenghtening. Contracture of the Achilles tendon has been analysed and is a factor that leads to midfoot collapse due to lack of adequate foot dorsiflexion.

The lengthening of the gastrocnemius-soleus muscle unit, achieved by percutaneous lengthening of the Achilles tendon or fractional lengthening of the musculotendineous junction, is the primary step in scheduling complex surgery for this disease [28, 55, 56].

Choosing the fixation method (internal/external or hybrid) depends on a complex evaluation that considers the bone quality, soft tissue condition, the presence and

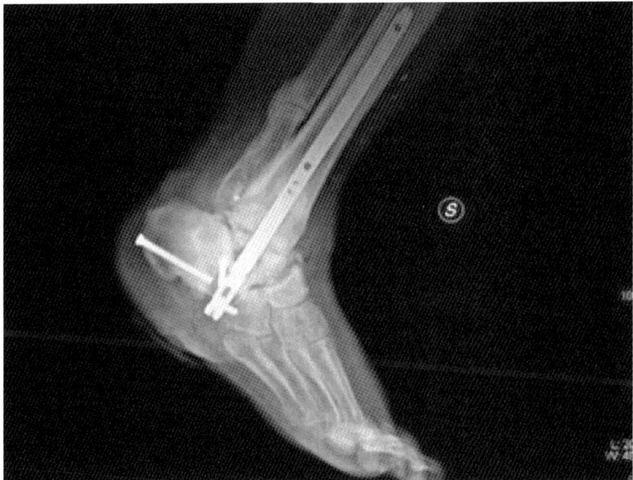

Fig. 9. Dislocation of intramedullary nail.

entity of fracture and/or dislocation, the history of previous surgery, positive osteo-myelitis history, walking ability, comorbidities and degree of obesity.

The internal fixation systems for CN with involvement of the foot or ankle include intramedullary implants (screws, cannulated screws, nails, rods) or extramedullary implants like locking or nonlocking plates or fixed angle plates. Recently, solid or can-nulated intramedullary screws (i.e., midfoot beaming) have been used in CN midfoot fusion. The advantages described are restoration of anatomic alignment and fixation beyond the localization of deformity [57].

The localization of the CN to the ankle corresponds to the earliest indication for surgery. The target is then the fusion of the joints to obtain a plantigrade foot able to handle weightbearing and walk. From different studies, it has been found that the use of the retrograde transcalcaneal nail has shown a fusion rate ranging from 70 to 100% and a limb salvage rate ranging from 75 to 100% [52, 58–61].

Complications are not uncommon when using the intramedullary nail for ankle stabilization. All patients need to be seen at frequent intervals during the follow-up, so that early signs of infection can be identified and treated. If a cast is placed, it must be changed frequently, so the surgical margins can be inspected. Tibial stress fracture can occur with the use of an inadequate length nail. Interlocking screws can loosen (Fig. 9).

External fixation can also be considered for foot and ankle reconstruction. The ex-ternal fixation systems may have different features and their use can diversify into different situations. We may consider several categories of external fixators: static, dynamic or for off-loading stabilization. Several papers have shown varying percent-ages of correction and stabilization using circular frames (Fig. 10) [28, 62–68].

All these studies confirm the possible positive approach of external fixation on dif-ferent pathophysiological aspects of CN through the following factors: decreased bone mineral density, bone loss, osteomyelitis, non-union, peripheral vascular disease and compromised soft tissue coverage of the surgical site. Circular external fixation

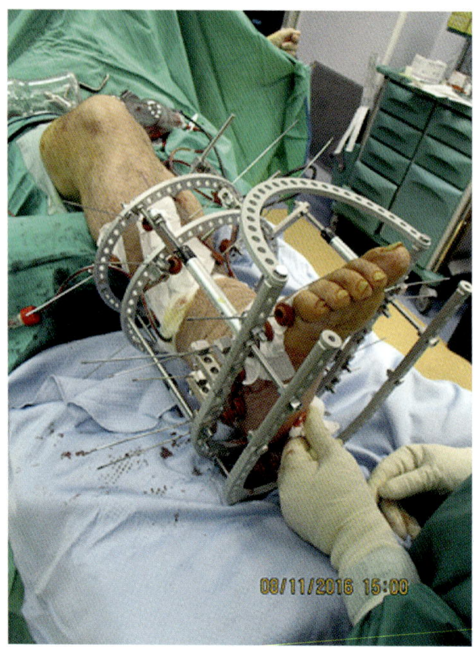

Fig. 10. Circular external fixator.

allows surgeons to perform even complex deformity corrections. In some cases, it is possible to use – through a gradual deformity correction – the original Ilizarov technique, that also considers dynamic external construction.

The use of internal and external fixation techniques depends on the characteristics of the pathology to be treated, the kind of patient and his or her comorbidities. The choice of one or the other may have advantages and disadvantages. Currently, the literature does not show conclusive evidence of which technique is actually superior to the other to approach fusion in the treatment of Charcot neuroarthropathy. Recently, some studies have moved the attention to the potential synergy of the 2 techniques for the treatment of patients with CN and complex deformities [69]. The conditions that allow taking into consideration a hybrid technique are the absence of ulceration or a history of osteomyelitis. The synergy of the 2 techniques allows the possibilty not only to obtain a compression/stabilization of the fusion sites but also to undergo a complete foot and ankle offloading. This aspect should not be overlooked, particularly when it involves a large soft tissue reconstruction [70, 71].

Bone grafts can be considered to fill osseous defects and stimulate bone regeneration. Autologous bone grafts for complete histocompatibility and the cancellation of the risk of disease transmission should be considered gold standard. The most frequently used donor site is the iliac crest [72]. Proximal and distal portions of the tibia, calcaneus and fibula may also be donor sites.

Currently, new composite biocompatible materials based on calcium sulphate and hydroxyapatite are used in these surgical approaches also in case of osteomyelitis localizations [73].

Dalla Paola · Scavone · Carone · Vasilache · Boscarino

Surgery in relation to treatment complexity and comorbidities may present complications such as dehiscence and infection of the surgical site, delayed fusion, loss of fixation and recurrence of deformity. Also, the use of external fixation may have some complications, such as superficial pin site/tract infection, fine wires breakage, deep infections, tibia fracture, vascular damage, if not considered anatomic safe zones [74]. Thus, a really close post-surgery follow-up is essential. It needs to provide for frequent control both in the case of preventive surgery and in the event of curative surgery regarding ulcerations and osteomyelitis localization. Frequent and carefully conducted outpatient follow-up enables the identification of complications and to treat them even while they are in the early stage.

Diagnosis of Osteomyelitis

The possibility of differentiating the picture of osteoarticular disintegration due to CN as compared to osteomyelitis localization becomes critical in planning the therapeutic surgical approach. A careful medical history analysis will help in effectively differentiating CN from osteomyelitis.

The clinical starting point – that is, the oedema and the increase in skin temperature – is the first sign to define the aetiology of the osteoarticular alteration. Such suspicion should then be supported with standard and advanced radiological exams.

If the patient's history was negative for ulcerative lesions, it will probably be possible to exclude osteomyelitis. If the patient presents with ulceration, or if there is a history of previous cutaneous injury, then performing the differential diagnosis and selecting the most appropriate treatment become mandatory. It is even clearer when in addition to the availability of anamnesis and radiological data, blood chemistry data (inflammatory markers, white blood cells count), clinical data (appearance of the lesion, probe-to-bone maneuvre), microbiology and histology data are also available. Additionally, information on the association between the location of the wound and the radiological location of the bone destruction will help in selecting an appropriate treatment plan. For example, a location of the ulcerated lesion in correspondence with a metatarsal head associated to an alteration of the Lisfranc joint that "jumps" the undermining metatarsal bones argues in favour of a condition of osteoarthropathy and not of osteomyelitis.

If instead radiology confirms a continuity of the ulcerated lesion and the bone-destructed location, then there is a high probability of an osteomyelitis condition.

The "gold standard" for detecting osteomyelitis foci (sensitivity 95%, specificity 99%) is represented by surgical percutaneous bone biopsy specimens after an antibiotic-free period of 2 weeks [75, 76].

Butalia et al. published a study in 2008 that confirmed that bone biopsy should be considered the "gold standard" for the diagnosis of osteomyelitis. They highlighted

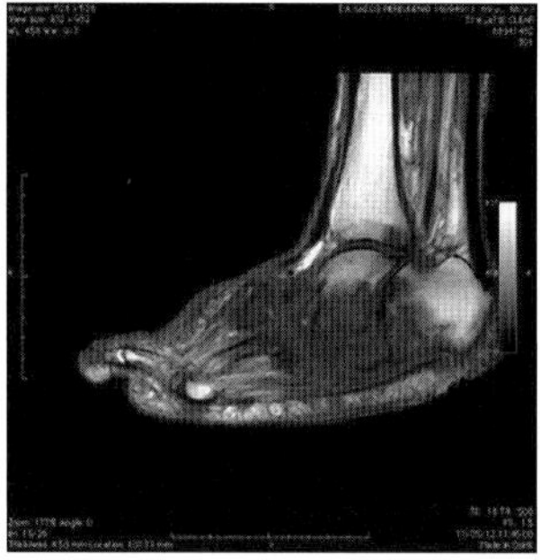

Fig. 11. T1 image.

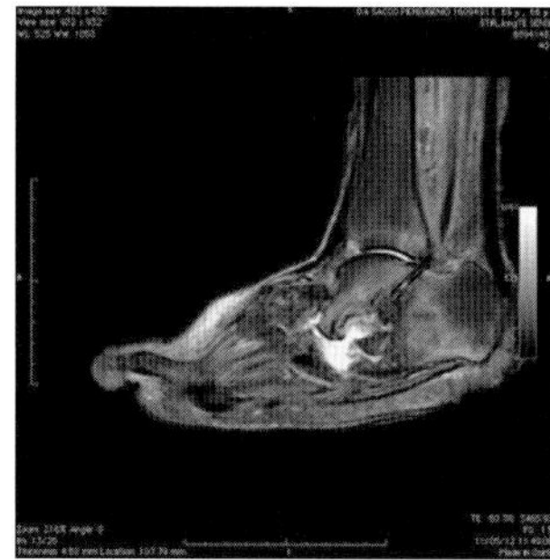

Fig. 12. T2 image.

that the physical examination (examining lesions extending more than 2 cm^2 and performing positive probe-to-bone test), the plain standard radiographs and the laboratory tests (ESR >70 mm/h) can support the correct diagnosis of osteomyelitis in the diabetic foot [77].

From the histological point of view, the chronic infection appears as plasmacells and lymphocytes infiltration, while the acute infection has neutrophils infiltration. Both deep soft tissue and bone must be sent for histopathological analysis because organisms found in soft tissue may not always reveal the organism involved in the underlying osteomyelitis [78]. Ge et al. [79] studied in 2002 the microbiological profile of infected diabetic foot ulcers and discovered that 75% of lesions had multiple pathogens with an average of 2.4 pathogens per lesion.

To support the diagnosis of osteomyelitis, the imaging studies must be interpreted in combination with the clinical examination and the laboratory values.

Although sensitivity and specificity of plain films are modest, imaging techniques using them should be the basic imaging technique to use (easy to obtain and relatively economical in comparison to other imaging modalities). Cortical defects, permeative radiolucencies, destructive alterations and/or periosteal new bone development indicate osteomyelitis [80].

Bone scans with Technetium-99methylene diphosphonate (Tc^{99m}) detect alterations in bone in a more timely fashion when compared to plain film radiographs. An improvement over plain film radiography is the sensitivity for this imaging modality (approaches 90% when using 3- or 4-phase scans) [81].

The specificity is much inferior (<50%) and is subordinate to increased bone turnover in most bone disorders (fractures, post-surgery transformations and non-infected CN).

MRI is useful in patients with surrounding soft tissue infection because it captures both soft tissue and bone (specificity 80–100%, sensitivity 90–100%) and can help in the diagnosis due to altered signal intensity of the affected bone [81].

The T1 image shows decreased signal intensity due to marrow fat in the bone, while the T2 image shows increased signal intensity (Fig. 11, 12).

     Dalla Paola · Scavone · Carone · Vasilache · Boscarino

Although costly, MRI is an irreplaceable tool in surgical planning because it provides for great anatomical detail. Recently, 2 different meta-analyses on the helpfulness of MRI in diagnosing foot osteomyelitis were published [80, 82].

In the diagnosis of foot osteomyelitis, MRI was found to be superior (sensitivity 90%, specificity 83%, overall accuracy 89%) to CT bone scanning, labeled white cell scans and plain radiography.

According to Dinh et al. [80], both CT and positron emission tomography have not been sufficiently tested in diabetic patients to recommend their use for the diagnosis of osteomyelitis.

Surgical Treatment of Charcot Osteoarthropathy Complicated by Osteomyelitis

Surgery must be considered the most effective therapeutic approach to diabetic Charcot foot complicated by wounds and osteomyelitis [28, 48, 55, 56, 83].

To choose a surgical treatment, we must take into consideration not only the osteomyelitic foci – more or less extended – usually involving the area of deformity, but also the infected soft tissue. The treatment of choice needs to address both. Most likely, from the point of view of prognosis for limb salvage, the extent of the soft tissues damage is very important in relation to the size of the infectious involvement of bone structures [39, 84].

From a surgical point of view, all ulcerations should be debrided to obtain drainage of any visible purulence. As well as allowing the surgeon to visualize the wound bed properly, debridement converts a chronic wound to an acute one, aiding in the healing process. Debridement also permits the elimination of devitalized tissue that aids to decrease the bacterial load. The incision lines for drainage of infected tissues should take into account the anatomical aspects of the reconstruction, the biomechanics and the chance to get a plantigrade attitude of the foot at low risk of ulcer recurrence.

When it is planned to surgically treat a patient with osteomyelitis of the foot, there are several key concepts that a clinician must keep in mind. He should resect all infected and necrotic bone to obtain bleeding viable bone. If the infected bone is resected along with all soft tissue involvement, primary closure is an option [85]. If the surgical sites are clinically infected, they should be left open, and multiple debridements could be required [55, 86–88].

When the surgical site appears clean and free from infection, delayed primary closure could be chosen. If primary closure seems not suitable, when bleeding and clinically observable infectious components are under control, the use of negative pressure wound therapy (NPWT) may be suitable. During the previous years, instillation of antiseptic agents associated to NPWT seems to be helpful [89–91]. After a variable period of treatment with NPWT, other techniques for covering exposed cancellous bone, like dermal substitutes or surgical flaps, could be used.

Antibiotic-loaded bone cement can help in filling the empty space left by resection of bone and may be useful in the face of infection. After surgical debridement, culture-guided antibiotic therapy (AT) should be started and continued for 2–6 weeks.

CN Complicated by Forefoot Wounds and Osteomyelitis

The surgical treatment of Charcot foot complicated by forefoot wound and osteomyelitis does not differ from the treatment of complicated neuropathic ulceration. The target should be the drainage of infection from bone and soft tissues, surgical closure of the wound and stabilization of the surgical area.

Ha Van et al. [92] reported on the role of conservative surgery versus non-surgical management of diabetic foot osteomyelitis. One group was treated non-surgically with offloading, AT and wound care. The other group was treated similarly with the addition of surgery (resection of a phalanx or metatarsal bone). The healing rate of the non-surgical group was 57%, with a mean healing time of 15.4 months. The healing rate of conservative surgery was 78% with a mean healing time of 6 months. The number of secondary surgical procedures, which included amputation and revascularisation, was significantly higher in the non-surgical cohort. Also, the duration of AT was longer in the non-surgical group (246 days) than in the surgical one (111 days).

Aragon-Sanchez et al. [93] described in a recent paper their experience in the treatment of patients with diabetic foot osteomyelitis, where a conservative approach (no amputation of any part of the foot) had been taken. Treating surgically within 12 h of admission with prioritization of foot-sparing surgery and avoidance of amputation, they analysed the factors that determine the results of surgical treatment of osteomyelitis of the foot in diabetic patients. They found that the risks of failure in the case of conservative surgery were necrotizing soft tissue infection, the presence of ischaemia and exposed bone. Conservative surgery without local or high-level amputation was successful in almost 50% of the patients.

The use of dermal substitutes and/or skin grafting and NPWT may be necessary for these patients [34]. When deformity involves the forefoot, metatarsal head(s) are a common location of osteomyelitis. Metatarsal head resection may be a common and standardized treatment. If the number of metatarsal head involved is more than one, the surgical approach should be a pan-metatarsal head resection (Fig. 13) [93–98].

CN Complicated by Midfoot Wound and Osteomyelitis

The most common surgical procedure for CN is that of the midfoot. The goals of treatment in the case of Charcot neuroarthropathy with midfoot or ankle deformity and osteomyelitis are the surgical correction of altered anatomy and treatment of os-

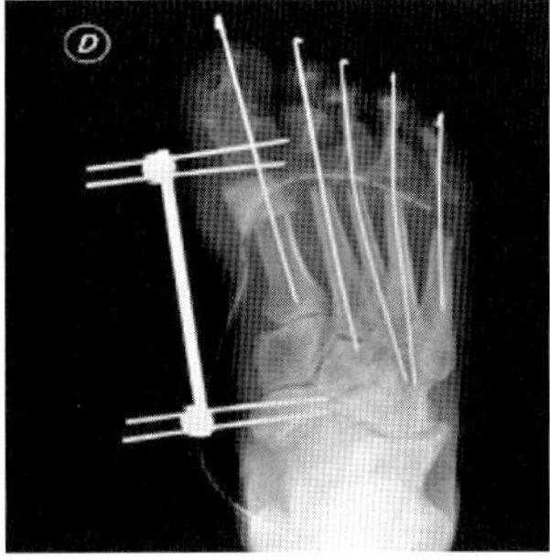

Fig. 13. Panmetatarsal head resection.

teomyelitis foci. The goal is a complete fusion, although pseudoarthrosis can generate a stable lower extremity allowing ambulation and reduced risk of ulceration/re-ulceration. External fixation and arthrodesis versus exostectomy are effective options for surgical reconstruction.

Excision of all tissues (soft tissue and bone) involved in the infection is the first step.

For histopathologic and microbiological assessment, intraoperative bone biopsies should be sent to the laboratory, as the culture isolates should serve as a guide for parenteral AT. Patients with clinically infected wounds should undergo a course of parenteral AT even in the presence of negative cultures.

"Silent" bone infection (patients with a wound at the level of an exostosis that had positive cultures obtained from the resected bone portion) should be treated with targeted AT.

The correction of the deformity is the second step. The goal is to create a plantigrade foot (clinically and radiographically). If there is significant infectious involvement of the soft tissues, it may be postponed after the resolution of the acute infection. Sometimes the first and the second step may be carried out at the same time.

Treatment options range from simple tangential sequestrectomy to more complex surgery such as triple arthrodesis.

The midfoot at the level of Lisfranc joint (pattern II using Sanders and Frykberg classification) is the most frequent location for collapse and joint dislocation.

A simple ostectomy is considered effective in the treatment of the deformity of the medial column complicated by ulcerative lesion. Catanzariti et al achieved a healing rate of 94% of ulcerative lesions of the medial column, but only 34% of the lateral column wounds healed [49]. These low percentages of healing lesions involving the lateral column have been confirmed in other studies [50, 51].

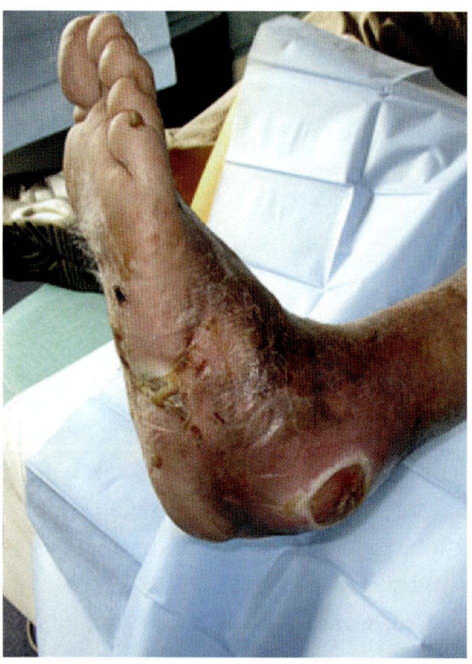

Fig. 14. Ankle CN complicated by lateral ulceration.

CN Complicated by Ankle/Hindfoot Wound and Osteomyelitis

If the bony structures of the hindfoot and/or ankle are also involved (Fig. 14), osteotomy must be executed so as to reunite 2 often conflicting needs, that is, the need to eliminate as much infected bone as possible and the need to preserve sufficient bony structures for fusion.

In case of complete infective talar involvement, in the presence of subluxation or dislocation of the talus, the treatment possibilities range from a simple wedge osteotomy of the heads of the subtalar joint and/or tibio-talar joint (consequently achieving a correction of the ankle varus or valgus deformity) to total talectomy with tibiocalcaneal fusion [34, 99].

The surgeon usually executes a primary intention closure after soft tissue debridement and correction of the deformity. If surgical margins are too tight or if a large debridement is performed, it is possible to plan closure by second intention. Once bleeding is controlled, the use of NPWT with or without instillation of antimicrobial agents is a valid option [34].

After correction of the bony deformity, reconstructive plastic surgery has occasionally been used. Final coverage can be accomplished with the use of dermal substitutes and subsequent skin grafting.

The third step is to warrant the immobilization/stabilization of the foot and ankle using a preconstructed circular external fixator [28, 32–34, 47, 55, 56, 100].

External fixation makes it possible to address at the same time both the component of deformity of the foot and ankle, and the demolitive/reconstructive approach of

Dalla Paola · Scavone · Carone · Vasilache · Boscarino

ulcer and tissue damage. Off-loading circular external fixation provides stabilization and continued access for local wound care [101].

In order to produce solid clinical constructs, the surgeon applies the Ilizarov technique with the use of fine-tensioned K-wires. Using the Ilizarov technique we cannot have any implant at the site of the previous infection or corrective surgery.

This surgical technique enables the stabilization of bone tissue without the use of internal hardware. During the healing period, the external circular frame offers an extremely stable construct without the use of large, encumbering casts.

A study conducted on the largest cohort of patients with Charcot arthropathy and osteomyelitis has been published by Pinzur et al. [17] in 2012. He treated these patients with a single-stage procedure. After surgical eradication of the infected bone, tissue cultures from the resected bone were used to guide parenteral AT. To consent correction of the deformity to a plantigrade situation, sufficient bone was removed. Large smooth percutaneous pins were used for temporary fixation. A 3-level preconstructed static circular external fixator was used to preserve the correction obtained surgically obtained previously. When the wounds could not be closed, they were reapproximated if possible and managed with dressings and wound care. In patients with a deformity in the midfoot, the circular external fixator was kept for 8 weeks and when the ankle was involved, it was kept for a minimum period of 12 weeks. Patients were managed in a weight-bearing total contact cast for 4–6 weeks after removal of the circular external fixator. Patients were transitioned from a commercially available walker to a commercially available therapeutic footwear (depth-inlay shoes and custom accommodative foot orthoses). As result, limb salvage was achieved in 95.7% of the patients and they were able to ambulate in commercially available therapeutic footwear.

Several studies with a similar protocol achieved high limb salvage rates when treating Charcot osteoarthropathy with midfoot or ankle osteomyelitis [17, 28, 32–34].

Patients with Charcot osteoarthropathy often have a series of comorbidities added to osteomyelitis complication. To get the best results, treatments should be carried out in a specialized multidisciplinary setting [102].

Postoperative Care

The postoperative treatment depends on the type of procedure performed, the location of the deformity treated and the type of implant used (internal or external fixation). Off-loading should be considered essential in the early postoperative period. One of the benefits of the external fixation is the even earlier possibility of weight-bearing. If using internal fixation, it is necessary to provide a full offloading and to use a plaster cast for 3–4 months. After the removal of the external fixator or the plaster cast, you should prepare a custom-moulded orthoses and gradually increase weight-bearing. The follow-up should be combined with that of lifelong diabetes.

CN Surgery and Evidence-Based Medicine

When there is an indication for prophylactic surgery for the correction of a significant degree of deformity and instability, the analysis of what has been published in the literature reveals a low degree of evidence, as there are only non-controlled retrospective case series, case reports and expert opinions (level 4 or 5 evidence) [55].

Recently, a meta-analysis done by Schneekloth et al. [103] has shown that the quality of published data on surgical management of CN has improved during the last few years. This conclusion is related to the publication, over the past 5 years, of studies showing better quality evidence. Manuscripts currently comparing different fixation techniques are encouraging as well as publications taking into consideration the cost of salvage reconstructive treatment as compared to amputation surgery. Randomised, prospective multicentre studies addressing this topic are not yet available. The ideal timing for corrective treatment is still to be defined. The goal of treatment – conservative or surgical – is the achievement of a plantigrade and stable foot with low ulcerative risk. If the deformity involves the most proximal anatomical regions (ankle and hindfoot), the surgical treatment need becomes clearer. Despite the development of more sophisticated surgery techniques and dedicated devices associated with a greater selection of patients, approximately 9% of patients with CN undergoing surgery will require the execution of a major amputation.

References

1 Rogers LC, Frykberg RG, Armstrong DG, Boulton AJ, Edmonds M, Van GH, et al: The Charcot foot in diabetes. J Am Podiatr Med Assoc 2011;101:437–446.
2 Armstrong DG, Peters EJ: Charcot's arthropathy of the foot. J Am Podiatr Med Assoc 2002;92:390–394.
3 Frykberg RG, Belczyk R: Epidemiology of the Charcot foot. Clin Podiatr Med Surg 2008;25:17–28, v.
4 Sanders LJ, FR: Diabetic neuropathic osteoarthropathy: the Charcot foot. In: Frykberg R, editor. The high risk foot in diabetes mellitus. New York: Churchill Livingstone; 1991, pp 297–338.
5 Frykberg RG, Sage RA, Wukich DK, Pinzur MS, Schuberth JM: Charcot arthropathy. Foot Ankle Spec 2012;5:262–271.
6 Sanders LJ FR: The Charcot foot (Pied de Charcot); in Bowker J, Pfeifer M (eds): Levin and O'Neal's the Diabetic Foot, ed 7. Philadelphia, Mosby Elsevier, 2008, pp 257–283.
7 Rajbhandari SM, Jenkins RC, Davies C, Tesfaye S: Charcot neuroarthropathy in diabetes mellitus. Diabetologia 2002;45:1085–1096.
8 Myerson MS, Henderson MR, Saxby T, Short KW: Management of midfoot diabetic neuroarthropathy. Foot Ankle Int 1994;15:233–241.
9 Centers for Disease Control and Prevention: National Diabetes Fact Sheet: National Estimates and General Information on Diabetes and Prediabetes in the United States, 2011. Atalanta, US Department of Health and Human Services, 2011.
10 Dhawan V, Spratt KF, Pinzur MS, Baumhauer J, Rudicel S, Saltzman CL: Reliability of AOFAS diabetic foot questionnaire in Charcot arthropathy: stability, internal consistency, and measurable difference. Foot Ankle Int 2005;26:717–731.
11 Pakarinen TK, Laine HJ, Mäenpää H, Mattila P, Lahtela J: Long-term outcome and quality of life in patients with Charcot foot. Foot Ankle Surg 2009;15:187–191.
12 Rogers LC, Frykberg RG, Armstrong DG, Boulton AJ, Edmonds M, Van GH, et al: The Charcot foot in diabetes. Diabetes Care 2011;34:2123–2129.

13 Sohn MW, Stuck RM, Pinzur M, Lee TA, Budiman-Mak E: Lower-extremity amputation risk after Charcot arthropathy and diabetic foot ulcer. Diabetes Care 2010;33:98–100.

14 Gazis A, Pound N, Macfarlane R, Treece K, Game F, Jeffcoate W: Mortality in patients with diabetic neuropathic osteoarthropathy (Charcot foot). Diabet Med 2004;21:1243–1246.

15 Lee L, Blume PA, Sumpio B: Charcot joint disease in diabetes mellitus. Ann Vasc Surg 2003;17:571–580.

16 Wild S, Roglic G, Green A, Sicree R, King H: Global prevalence of diabetes: estimates for the year 2000 and projections for 2030. Diabetes Care 2004;27:1047–1053.

17 Pinzur MS, Sage R, Stuck R, Kaminsky S, Zmuda A: A treatment algorithm for neuropathic (Charcot) midfoot deformity. Foot Ankle 1993;14:189–197.

18 Fabrin J, Larsen K, Holstein PE: Long-term follow-up in diabetic Charcot feet with spontaneous onset. Diabetes Care 2000;23:796–800.

19 Pinzur MS: Current concepts review: Charcot arthropathy of the foot and ankle. Foot Ankle Int 2007;28:952–959.

20 Eichenholtz SN: Charcot Joints. Springfield, Charles C Thomas, pp 3–8.

21 Shibata T, Tada K, Hashizume C: The results of arthrodesis of the ankle for leprotic neuroarthropathy. J Bone Joint Surg Am 1990;72:749–756.

22 Chantelau EA, Grützner G: Is the Eichenholtz classification still valid for the diabetic Charcot foot? Swiss Med Wkly 2014;144:w13948.

23 Brodsky JW, Rouse AM: Exostectomy for symptomatic bony prominences in diabetic Charcot feet. Clin Orthop Relat Res 1993;21–26.

24 Trepman E, Nihal A, Pinzur MS: Current topics review: Charcot neuroarthropathy of the foot and ankle. Foot Ankle Int 2005;26:46–63.

25 Schon LC, Weinfeld SB, Horton GA, Resch S: Radiographic and clinical classification of acquired midtarsus deformities. Foot Ankle Int 1998;19:394–404.

26 Sella EJ, Barrette C: Staging of Charcot neuroarthropathy along the medial column of the foot in the diabetic patient. J Foot Ankle Surg 1999;38:34–40.

27 Frykberg RG, Rogers LC: The aiabetic Charcot foot: a primer on conservative and surgical management. J Diabetic Foot Complications 2009;1.

28 Pinzur MS: Neutral ring fixation for high-risk non-plantigrade Charcot midfoot deformity. Foot Ankle Int 2007;28:961–966.

29 Pinzur MS: Benchmark analysis of diabetic patients with neuropathic (Charcot) foot deformity. Foot Ankle Int 1999;20:564–567.

30 Bevan WP, Tomlinson MP: Radiographic measures as a predictor of ulcer formation in diabetic Charcot midfoot. Foot Ankle Int 2008;29:568–573.

31 Wukich DK, Sung W: Charcot arthropathy of the foot and ankle: modern concepts and management review. J Diabetes Complications 2009;23:409–426.

32 Farber DC, Juliano PJ, Cavanagh PR, Ulbrecht J, Caputo G: Single stage correction with external fixation of the ulcerated foot in individuals with Charcot neuroarthropathy. Foot Ankle Int 2002;23:130–134.

33 Saltzman CL: Salvage of diffuse ankle osteomyelitis by single-stage resection and circumferential frame compression arthrodesis. Iowa Orthop J 2005;25:47–52.

34 Dalla Paola L, Brocco E, Ceccacci T, Ninkovic S, Sorgentone S, Marinescu MG, et al: Limb salvage in Charcot foot and ankle osteomyelitis: combined use single stage/double stage of arthrodesis and external fixation. Foot Ankle Int 2009;30:1065–1070.

35 van der Ven A, Chapman CB, Bowker JH: Charcot neuroarthropathy of the foot and ankle. J Am Acad Orthop Surg 2009;17:562–571.

36 Armstrong DG, Frykberg RG: Classifying diabetic foot surgery: toward a rational definition. Diabet Med 2003;20:329–331.

37 Burns PR, Wukich DK: Surgical reconstruction of the Charcot rearfoot and ankle. Clin Podiatr Med Surg 2008;25:95–120, vii–viii.

38 Rogers LC, Bevilacqua NJ: The diagnosis of Charcot foot. Clin Podiatr Med Surg 2008;25:43–51, vi.

39 Dalla Paola L, Carone A, Baglioni M, Boscarino G, Vasilache L: Extension and grading of osteomyelitis are not related to limb salvage in Charcot neuropathic osteoarthropathy: a cohort prospective study. J Diabetes Complications 2016;30:608–612.

40 Saltzman CL, Hagy ML, Zimmerman B, Estin M, Cooper R: How effective is intensive nonoperative initial treatment of patients with diabetes and Charcot arthropathy of the feet? Clin Orthop Relat Res 2005:185–190.

41 Pinzur M: Surgical versus accommodative treatment for Charcot arthropathy of the midfoot. Foot Ankle Int 2004;25:545–549.

42 Wukich DK, Raspovic KM, Hobizal KB, Rosario B: Radiographic analysis of diabetic midfoot Charcot neuroarthropathy with and without midfoot ulceration. Foot Ankle Int 2014;35:1108–1115.

43 Wukich DK, Sadoskas D, Vaudreuil NJ, Fourman M: Comparison of diabetic Charcot patients with and without foot wounds. Foot Ankle Int 2017;38:140–148.

44 Wukich DK, Raspovic KM, Suder NC: Prevalence of peripheral arterial disease in patients with diabetic Charcot neuroarthropathy. J Foot Ankle Surg 2016;55:727–731.

45 Simon SR, Tejwani SG, Wilson DL, Santner TJ, Denniston NL: Arthrodesis as an early alternative to nonoperative management of Charcot arthropathy of the diabetic foot. J Bone Joint Surg Am 2000;82-A:939–950.

46 Mittlmeier T, Klaue K, Haar P, Beck M: Should one consider primary surgical reconstruction in Charcot arthropathy of the feet? Clin Orthop Relat Res 2010; 468:1002–1011.

47 Shen W, Wukich D: Orthopaedic surgery and the diabetic Charcot foot. Med Clin North Am 2013;97: 873–882.

48 Brodsky JW: The diabetic foot. In: Coughlin MJ, Mann RA, editors. Surgery of the foot and ankle. 7th ed. St. Louis (MO): Mosby 1999, pp 895–969.

49 Catanzariti AR, Mendicino R, Haverstock B: Ostectomy for diabetic neuroarthropathy involving the midfoot. J Foot Ankle Surg 2000;39:291–300.

50 Rosenblum BI, Giurini JM, Miller LB, Chrzan JS, Habershaw GM: Neuropathic ulcerations plantar to the lateral column in patients with Charcot foot deformity: a flexible approach to limb salvage. J Foot Ankle Surg 1997;36:360–363.

51 Laurinaviciene R, Kirketerp-Moeller K, Holstein PE: Exostectomy for chronic midfoot plantar ulcer in Charcot deformity. J Wound Care 2008;17:53–55, 57–58.

52 Siebachmeyer M, Boddu K, Bilal A, Hester TW, Hardwick T, Fox TP, et al: Outcome of one-stage correction of deformities of the ankle and hindfoot and fusion in Charcot neuroarthropathy using a retrograde intramedullary hindfoot arthrodesis nail. Bone Joint J 2015;97-B:76–82.

53 Wukich DK, Raspovic KM, Hobizal KB, Sadoskas D: Surgical management of Charcot neuroarthropathy of the ankle and hindfoot in patients with diabetes. Diabetes Metab Res Rev 2016;32(suppl 1):292–296.

54 Ettinger S, Plaass C, Claassen L, Stukenborg-Colsman C, Yao D, Daniilidis K: Surgical management of Charcot deformity for the foot and ankle-radiologic outcome after internal/external fixation. J Foot Ankle Surg 2016;55:522–528.

55 Lowery NJ, Woods JB, Armstrong DG, Wukich DK: Surgical management of Charcot neuroarthropathy of the foot and ankle: a systematic review. Foot Ankle Int 2012;33:113–121.

56 Pinzur MS: Use of platelet-rich concentrate and bone marrow aspirate in high-risk patients with Charcot arthropathy of the foot. Foot Ankle Int 2009;30:124–127.

57 Lamm BM, Siddiqui NA, Nair AK, LaPorta G: Intramedullary foot fixation for midfoot Charcot neuroarthropathy. J Foot Ankle Surg 2012;51:531–536.

58 Caravaggi C, Cimmino M, Caruso S, Dalla Noce S: Intramedullary compressive nail fixation for the treatment of severe Charcot deformity of the ankle and rear foot. J Foot Ankle Surg 2006;45:20–24.

59 Dalla Paola L, Volpe A, Varotto D, Postorino A, Brocco E, Senesi A, et al: Use of a retrograde nail for ankle arthrodesis in Charcot neuroarthropathy: a limb salvage procedure. Foot Ankle Int 2007;28:967–970.

60 DeVries JG, Berlet GC, Hyer CF: A retrospective comparative analysis of Charcot ankle stabilization using an intramedullary rod with or without application of circular external fixator–utilization of the Retrograde Arthrodesis Intramedullary Nail database. J Foot Ankle Surg 2012;51:420–425.

61 Pinzur MS, Kelikian A: Charcot ankle fusion with a retrograde locked intramedullary nail. Foot Ankle Int 1997;18:699–704.

62 Bradley L, Lamm DP: Charcot neuroarthropathy of the foot and ankle in limb lengthening and reconstruction surgery; in Rozbruch SR, Ilizarov S (eds): Limb Length-Ening and Reconstruction Surgery. 1. London, Informa Healthcare, 2007, pp 221–232.

63 Wang JC: Use of external fixation in the reconstruction of the Charcot foot and ankle. Clin Podiatr Med Surg 2003;20:97–117.

64 Cooper PS: Application of external fixators for management of Charcot deformities of the foot and ankle. Foot Ankle Clin 2002;7:207–254.

65 Jolly GP, Zgonis T, Polyzois V: External fixation in the management of Charcot neuroarthropathy. Clin Podiatr Med Surg 2003;20:741–756.

66 Matsumoto T, Parekh SG: Midtarsal reconstructive arthrodesis using a multi-axial correction fixator in charcot midfoot arthropathy. Foot Ankle Spec 2015; 8:472–478.

67 Pinzur MS: Circular fixation for the nonplantigrade Charcot foot. Hosp Pract (1995) 2010;38:56–62.

68 Sayner LR, Rosenblum BI: External fixation for Charcot foot reconstruction. Curr Surg 2005;62: 618–623.

69 Hegewald KW, Wilder ML, Chappell TM, Hutchinson BL: Combined internal and external fixation for diabetic charcot reconstruction: a retrospective case series. J Foot Ankle Surg 2016;55:619–627.

70 Capobianco CM, Zgonis T: Soft tissue reconstruction pyramid for the diabetic charcot foot. Clin Podiatr Med Surg 2017;34:69–76.

71 Short DJ, Zgonis T: Circular external fixation as a primary or adjunctive therapy for the podoplastic approach of the diabetic charcot foot. Clin Podiatr Med Surg 2017;34:93–98.

72 Fitzgibbons TC, Hawks MA, McMullen ST, Inda DJ: Bone grafting in surgery about the foot and ankle: indications and techniques. J Am Acad Orthop Surg 2011;19:112–120.

73 McNally MA, Ferguson JY, Lau AC, Diefenbeck M, Scarborough M, Ramsden AJ, et al: Single-stage treatment of chronic osteomyelitis with a new absorbable, gentamicin-loaded, calcium sulphate/hydroxyapatite biocomposite: a prospective series of 100 cases. Bone Joint J 2016;98-B:1289–1296.

74 Wukich DK, Belczyk RJ, Burns PR, Frykberg RG: Complications encountered with circular ring fixation in persons with diabetes mellitus. Foot Ankle Int 2008;29:994–1000.

75 Lesens O, Desbiez F, Vidal M, Robin F, Descamps S, Beytout J, et al: Culture of per-wound bone specimens: a simplified approach for the medical management of diabetic foot osteomyelitis. Clin Microbiol Infect 2011;17:285–291.

76 Lavery LA, Sariaya M, Ashry H, Harkless LB: Microbiology of osteomyelitis in diabetic foot infections. J Foot Ankle Surg 1995;34:61–64.

77 Butalia S, Palda VA, Sargeant RJ, Detsky AS, Mourad O: Does this patient with diabetes have osteomyelitis of the lower extremity? JAMA 2008;299:806–813.

78 Crim BE, Wukich DK. Osteomyelitis of the foot and ankle in the diabetic population: diagnosis and treatment. J Diabetic Foot Complications 2010;1.

79 Ge Y, MacDonald D, Hait H, Lipsky B, Zasloff M, Holroyd K: Microbiological profile of infected diabetic foot ulcers. Diabet Med 2002;19:1032–1034.

80 Dinh MT, Abad CL, Safdar N: Diagnostic accuracy of the physical examination and imaging tests for osteomyelitis underlying diabetic foot ulcers: meta-analysis. Clin Infect Dis 2008;47:519–527.

81 Shank CF, Feibel JB: Osteomyelitis in the diabetic foot: diagnosis and management. Foot Ankle Clin 2006;11:775–789.

82 Kapoor A, Page S, Lavalley M, Gale DR, Felson DT: Magnetic resonance imaging for diagnosing foot osteomyelitis: a meta-analysis. Arch Intern Med 2007; 167:125–132.

83 Herbst SA, Jones KB, Saltzman CL: Pattern of diabetic neuropathic arthropathy associated with the peripheral bone mineral density. J Bone Joint Surg Br 2004;86:378–383.

84 Sinkin JC, Reilly M, Cralley A, Kim PJ, Steinberg JS, Cooper P, et al: Multidisciplinary approach to soft-tissue reconstruction of the diabetic Charcot foot. Plast Reconstr Surg 2015;135:611–616.

85 Hendricks KJ, Burd TA, Anglen JO, Simpson AW, Christensen GD, Gainor BJ: Synergy between Staphylococcus aureus and Pseudomonas aeruginosa in a rat model of complex orthopaedic wounds. J Bone Joint Surg Am 2001;83-A:855–861.

86 Armstrong DG, Lavery LA; Diabetic Foot Study Consortium: Negative pressure wound therapy after partial diabetic foot amputation: a multicentre, randomised controlled trial. Lancet 2005;366:1704–1710.

87 Armstrong DG, Lavery LA, Boulton AJ: Negative pressure wound therapy via vacuum-assisted closure following partial foot amputation: what is the role of wound chronicity? Int Wound J 2007;4:79–86.

88 Blume PA, Walters J, Payne W, Ayala J, Lantis J: Comparison of negative pressure wound therapy using vacuum-assisted closure with advanced moist wound therapy in the treatment of diabetic foot ulcers: a multicenter randomized controlled trial. Diabetes Care 2008;31:631–636.

89 Dalla Paola L: Diabetic foot wounds: the value of negative pressure wound therapy with instillation. Int Wound J 2013;10(suppl 1):25–31.

90 Kim PJ, Attinger CE, Oliver N, Garwood C, Evans KK, Steinberg JS, et al: Comparison of outcomes for normal saline and an antiseptic solution for negative-pressure wound therapy with instillation. Plast Reconstr Surg 2015;136:657e–664e.

91 Kim PJ, Attinger CE, Olawoye O, Crist BD, Gabriel A, Galiano RD, et al: Negative pressure wound therapy with instillation: review of evidence and recommendations. Wounds 2015;27:S2–S19.

92 Ha Van G, Siney H, Danan JP, Sachon C, Grimaldi A: Treatment of osteomyelitis in the diabetic foot. Contribution of conservative surgery. Diabetes Care 1996;19:1257–1260.

93 Aragon-Sanchez FJ, Cabrera-Galvan JJ, Quintana-Marrero Y, Hernandez-Herrero MJ, Lazaro-Martinez JL, Garcia-Morales E, et al: Outcomes of surgical treatment of diabetic foot osteomyelitis: a series of 185 patients with histopathological confirmation of bone involvement. Diabetologia 2008;51:1962–1970.

94 Aragon-Sanchez J: Treatment of diabetic foot osteomyelitis: a surgical critique. Int J Low Extrem Wounds 2010;9:37–59.

95 Griffiths GD, Wieman TJ: Metatarsal head resection for diabetic foot ulcers. Arch Surg 1990;125:832–835.

96 Patel VG, Wieman TJ: Effect of metatarsal head resection for diabetic foot ulcers on the dynamic plantar pressure distribution. Am J Surg 1994;167:297–301.

97 Armstrong DG, Fiorito JL, Leykum BJ, Mills JL: Clinical efficacy of the pan metatarsal head resection as a curative procedure in patients with diabetes mellitus and neuropathic forefoot wounds. Foot Ankle Spec 2012;5:235–240.

98 Dalla Paola L, Carone A, Morisi C, Cardillo S, Pattavina M: Conservative surgical treatment of infected ulceration of the first metatarsophalangeal joint with osteomyelitis in diabetic patients. J Foot Ankle Surg 2015;54:536–540.

99 Wukich DK: Pantalar arthrodesis for post-traumatic arthritis and diabetic neuroarthropathy of the ankle and hindfoot. Foot Ankle Int 2011;32:924.

100 Pinzur MS, Gil J, Belmares J: Treatment of osteo-myelitis in charcot foot with single-stage resection of infection, correction of deformity, and mainte-nance with ring fixation. Foot Ankle Int 2012;33: 1069–1074.
101 Ramanujam CL, Facaros Z, Zgonis T: External fixa-tion for surgical off-loading of diabetic soft tissue reconstruction. Clin Podiatr Med Surg 2011;28: 211–216.
102 Pinzur MS, Gurza E, Kristopaitis T, Monson R, Wall MJ, Porter A, et al: Hospitalist-orthopedic co-management of high-risk patients undergoing low-er extremity reconstruction surgery. Orthopedics 2009;32:495.
103 Schneekloth BJ, Lowery NJ, Wukich DK: Charcot neuroarthropathy in patients with diabetes: an up-dated systematic review of surgical management. J Foot Ankle Surg 2016;55:586–590.

Luca Dalla Paola, MD
Diabetic Foot Unit
Maria Cecilia Hospital
Via Corriera 1, IT–48010 Cotignola (Italy)
E-Mail ldallapaola@libero.it

Dalla Paola · Scavone · Carone · Vasilache · Boscarino

Piaggesi A, Apelqvist J (eds): The Diabetic Foot Syndrome.
Front Diabetes. Basel, Karger, 2018, vol 26, pp 131–146 (DOI: 10.1159/000480059)

Indications to Revascularization in the Ischaemic Diabetic Foot

Roberto Ferraresi[a] · Fabrizio Losurdo[b] · Roberto Lorenzoni[c] ·
Matteo Ferraris[d] · Maurizio Santi Caminiti[b] · Andrea Casini[b]

[a]Peripheral Interventional Unit, Humanitas Gavazzeni, Bergamo, [b]Diabetic Foot Care Center, Humanitas Gavazzeni, Bergamo, [c]Ospedale di Lucca, USL LU-2, Lucca, and [d]Vascular Surgery Unit, Ospedale di Legnano, Legnano, Italy

Abstract

Critical limb ischaemia is frequently associated to diabetic foot ulcers, and its recognition and timely treatment are crucial to achieve ulcer remission. Lower limb atherosclerosis in diabetic patients is characterized by having an earlier onset, a more aggressive pattern, a higher degree of arterial wall calcification and a multi-level lower limb arteries involvement, with frequent distal localizations. Foot ischaemia is usually diagnosed by integrating the clinical exam with non-invasive tests like ankle pressure measurement and Ankle Brachial Index, as well as, transcutaneous oximetry (TcPO2) or Colour-Doppler Ultrasound Scanning. Once the need for revascularization is established, the main artery to target is chosen in keeping with the foot angiosomal arrangement, so that a direct blood flow to the diseased area could be achieved. We usually favour an "angioplasty first" revascularization strategy, as this offers several advantages including better tolerability by the patient and repeatability in case of re-occlusion. We usually prefer surgical bypass as first choice in case of long femoropopliteal or infrapopliteal occlusions; however, this should be preceded by evaluating the patient's eligibility, considering his general status and expected procedure tolerability; foot conditions and planned foot surgery; presence of a suitable conduit and of an adequate distal vessel for anastomosis.
© 2018 S. Karger AG, Basel

Introduction

Peripheral artery disease (PAD) of the lower limb has been shown to be a contributing factor to foot tissue lesion in as much as 50% of diabetic foot ulcers [1].

Chronic hyperglycemia elicits endothelial cells damage yielding to atherosclerotic changes in several arterial districts, including the lower limb arteries [2]. This process results in narrowing and occlusions of the arterial lumen, leading eventually to reduced perfusion of distal territories. The progressive failure of the arterial system is clinically reflected by the development of symptoms and signs of impaired perfusion, ranging from claudication to critical limb ischaemia (CLI). Moreover, whenever a diabetic patient develops a skin ulcer, regardless of its primary cause, tissue healing may be severely delayed or actually hindered if the blood supply to the affected area is insufficient to provide an adequate amount of oxygen, nutrition molecules, leukocytes and antibiotics.

Therefore, recognizing and promptly addressing foot ischaemia is crucial to pursuing the healing of diabetic foot lesions. It is of utmost importance that the clinician involved in diabetic foot care is familiar with the most common patterns of PAD manifestations in diabetic patients as well as the available techniques for vascular assessment and the possible treatment strategies.

Patterns of PAD in Diabetic Patients

Although atherosclerotic arterial occlusive disease of the aortoiliac tract does not differ markedly between diabetic and non-diabetic individuals, PAD of the infra-inguinal vasculature has peculiar features in patients with long-standing diabetes.

While in non-diabetic patients PAD usually presents with single, unilateral and proximal arterial involvement, in diabetic subjects, obstructive lesions are often localized more distally and mostly in the below-the-knee (BTK) vessels, including foot vessels, with bilateral and multi-segmental involvement [3]. Moreover, diabetic patients have been reported to have an earlier disease clinical onset, higher average BMI and a high prevalence of peripheral neuropathy that could in turn result in paucity of subjective symptoms. In addition, PAD in diabetic patients is known to be more aggressive and rapid in its progression, and to have a quite silent onset in its earliest stages [4].

From the histopathological point of view, PAD in diabetic individuals typically manifests with a higher degree of arterial wall calcification leading to a higher incidence of mixed plaques mostly circumferential, in which the full lumen is involved [5].

Defining the type and extent of PAD is a crucial step when predicting the clinical prognosis of an ischaemic ulcerated foot, as infra-popliteal involvement is associated with a much higher risk of major amputation in diabetic subjects with ischaemic foot ulcers if not undergoing adequate revascularization.

As Faglia et al. [6] showed in 1998 that occlusion of BTK arteries can dramatically increase the risk of major amputation and therefore restoring a direct blood flow up to the foot is a fundamental condition to pursue limb salvage.

Our Experience in a Large Cohort of Diabetic Patients with CLI

Between 2009 and 2013, we performed more than 1400 baseline angiographic studies in diabetic patients with CLI and tissue lesion. Arterial segments were classified according to the DEFINE group [7]. The below-the-ankle (BTA) arteries were

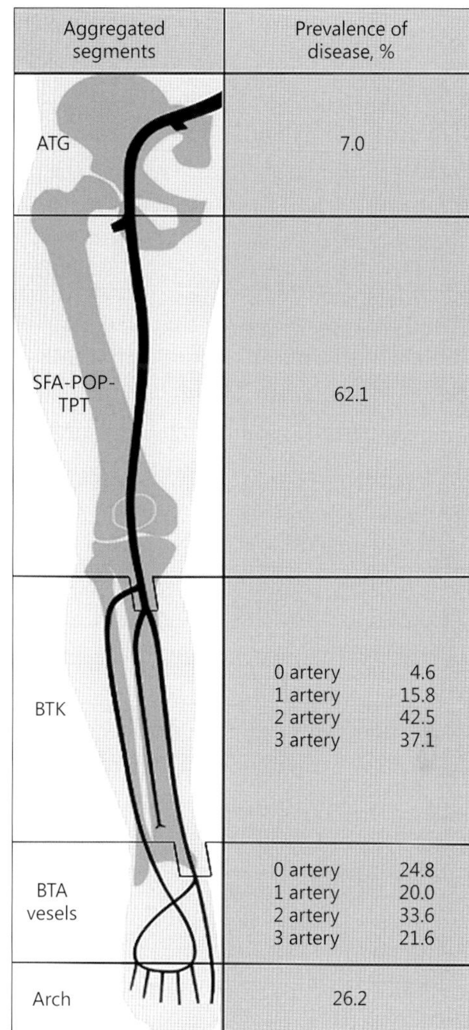

Fig. 1. Baseline angiographic studies (1,419 limbs – 1,212 patients) performed on diabetic patients with CLI and tissue lesions between 2009 and 2013.

considered dorsalis pedis artery (DPA); medial plantar artery; lateral plantar artery (LPA) and the plantar arch. The plantar arch was considered the distal arch originating from LPA, giving the metatarsal vessels and generally connecting to the DPA through the first perforating branch.

The distribution of PAD lesions in the lower limb among study subjects is reported in Figure 1. Most lesions occurred at distal sites (BTK and BTA arteries). Above-the-groin disease occurred in 7.0% of limbs; superficial femoral, popliteal and tibioperoneal artery disease occurred in 62.1%; BTK vessel disease was distributed as follows: no BTK vessels were involved in 4.6%, 1 BTK vessel in 15.8%, 2 BTK vessels in 42.5% and 3 BTK vessels in 37.1%. BTA vessels disease was distributed as follows: no BTA vessel in 24.8%, 1 BTA vessel disease in 20.0%, 2 BTA vessels in 33.6% and 3 BTA vessels in 21.6%. According to our data, the small vessel disease involving the arch was present in 26.2% of the patients.

Our data stresses the concept of a multilevel involvement of obstructive disease in diabetic patients with CLI. The obstructive disease was present in 62.1% of the superficial or popliteal arteries; 79.6% of the patients had 2 or 3 BTK vessels involved; 55,2% had 2 or 3 BTA vessels involved and 26.2% had an obstructive disease spreading to the small foot vessels.

Clinical Assessment of Foot Ischaemia

When a patient with a diabetic foot ulcer comes for treatment, a key step in patient evaluation is to assess whether the non-healing lesion has an ischaemic component or not.

The clinical assessment of foot ischaemia comprises several tools ranging from the basic clinical examination to more complex, invasive or expensive techniques, all of which could give the clinician different, and often complementary information, in diagnosing the presence and degree of foot ischaemia.

A point that should be emphasized is that the diagnosis of foot ischaemia is not an easy task, as it is not a YES or NO condition. Therefore, it is usually necessary to use more diagnostic tools together to answer the question "Is the blood supply to this lesion sufficient for healing or should it be improved?"

Clinical Examination
As with any medical condition, the evaluation of a patient with suspected foot ischaemia begins with history taking and a physical exam. A detailed lesion-related history should be taken to understand its location, when and how it developed and the presence of any associated symptoms like pain, tenderness or signs of co-existing infection. Moreover, the general patient history should elicit the presence or absence of CLI risk factors (e.g., smoking, renal failure, previous amputations, known coronary or carotid atherosclerosis, etc.) and patient co-morbidities, as reduced life expectancy due to reasons other than CLI could certainly influence therapeutic strategies.

Foot lesions with an ischaemic component are usually located very distally, mostly on toe tips or heel. Usually ischaemic lesions are painful (if nerve conduction is intact), with irregular margins and a necrotic or pale bed [8]; they can be spontaneous or triggered by a minor, often unnoticed, trauma, like improper nail trimming or use of an inadequate footwear. Moreover, a foot ulcer may develop because of reasons other than ischaemia (i.e. pressure, infection, trauma, burns, etc.) but persist and become non-healing due to poor perfusion. Therefore, ischaemia should be considered in any non-healing wound as a possible cause; however, history taking alone is not sufficiently accurate to rule it in or out.

		Ferraresi · Losurdo · Lorenzoni · Ferraris · Caminiti · Casini

Physical examination can be slightly more informative, particularly in excluding foot ischaemia. Khan et al. [9], found that the combination of normal posterior tibial artery (PTA) and DPA pulses in the absence of claudication was the most predictive feature in excluding PAD in diabetic patients. However, this study did not take into account the possibility of distal arterial disease, involving the plantar arch and the small forefoot vessels, which can easily lead to ischaemic lesions in diabetic patients despite normally palpable ankle pulses.

Moreover, absent pulses are not accurate enough to base therapeutic decision on, as DPA pulse may be absent in as much as 30% of PAD-free patients and may be poorly reproducible [10]; the PTA pulse seems to be more reliable; however, its detection may be difficult in case of ankle edema or large calf size. Furthermore, an absent pulse does not provide any information concerning how much the healing potential of the lesion itself is compromised by the impaired circulation and therefore cannot be used as a defining criterion for foot ischaemia.

Non-Invasive Diagnostic Tests

Several non-invasive tests are currently available to investigate blood supply to diabetic foot lesions. In a recent systematic review, Wang et al. [11] found that most of the available studies focused on Ankle Brachial Index (ABI) and Transcutaneous Oximetry (TcPO$_2$). However, several other tests like ankle blood pressure measurement, Toe-Brachial Index (TBI), toe Doppler arterial waveforms or duplex ultrasonography are currently available; more expensive techniques such as MR angiography or CT angiography (CTA) are also available.

Ankle Brachial Index

The ABI or Windsor Index is a simple and noninvasive test performed using a 10–12 cm sphygmomanometer cuff placed just above the ankle and a continuous wave 8 MHz Doppler instrument to measure systolic blood pressure at anterior and posterior tibial arteries of each foot [12]. The ABI of each leg is calculated by dividing the higher of the DPA pressure or PTA pressure by the higher of the right or left arm blood pressure; however, some studies have reported higher sensitivity to detect PAD if the ABI numerator is the lowest pressure in the arteries of both ankles [13, 14]. Most guidelines suggest using the ABI as a screening test for PAD in diabetic subjects or as the first step in evaluating patients with foot ulcers in suspected CLI [8, 10, 12]. The reference values proposed for ABI differ slightly among guidelines and are reported in Table 1. However, generally speaking, a very low ABI (<0.5) points towards CLI, while a higher-than-expected ABI suggests the presence of vascular calcifications that in turn make leg arteries poorly compressible by the sphygmomanometer cuff and thus falsely show a higher systolic pressure reading. The main pitfall with ABI use is, indeed, the risk of false negative results due to arterial calcifications, which is very common in diabetic and dialyzed patients, and that requires the necessity to generate with the

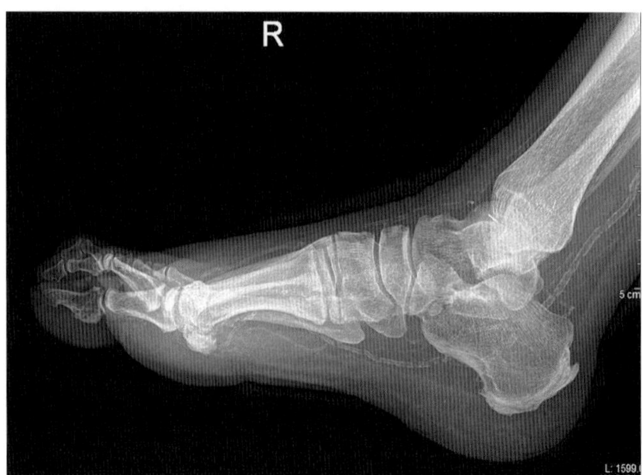

Fig. 2. Typical example of extensive leg calcifications. This condition makes tibial arteries uncompressible and, in turn, ABI measurement unreliable.

Table 1. ABI reference values according to different guidelines

Guideline	Normal ABI
ESC [12]	0.8–1.4
TASC [8]	0.9–1.4
AMD-SICVE [10]	0.7–1.3
IWGDF [31]	0.9–1.3
AHA [32]	0.9–1.4
ADA [33]	0.7–1.3

sphygmomanometer, a pressure much greater than the actual blood pressure to achieve complete compression and obliteration of the arterial lumen while measuring the ABI.

The picture in Figure 2 portrays a typical example of the kind of patient we often see in our practice, with extensive calcification of leg arteries.

In conclusion, the ABI is a good screening tool, particularly in the high-risk but asymptomatic patient with moderate to low pre-test probability of being affected by PAD, in whom a low ABI would suggest performing other tests to further investigate the patient's atherosclerotic load. Moreover, on the clinically symptomatic patient, with high pre-test probability of PAD, a very low ABI could confirm the diagnosis and prompt urgent vascular imaging or revascularization.

On the other hand, a non-suppressed ABI value cannot be enough to rule out PAD, particularly in the symptomatic patient in whom a high degree of arterial calcification is expected. Therefore, if the pre-test probability is high, a normal ABI should be followed by further tests like $TcPO_2$ and/or Duplex Ultrasound.

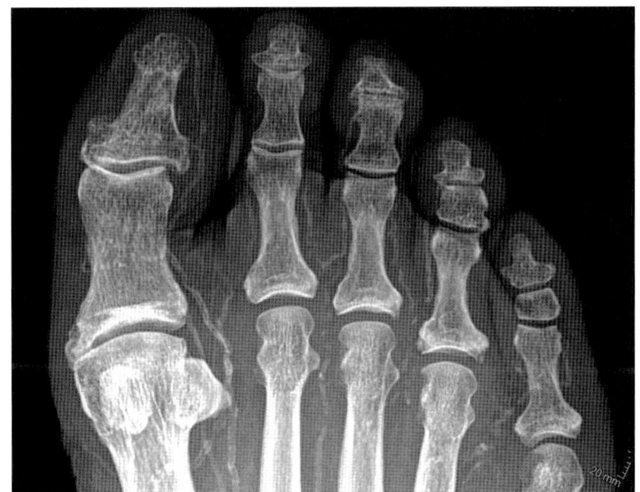

Fig. 3. Example of extensive digital arteries calcification causing unreliability in TBI measurement.

Ankle Pressure Measurement

Measurement of blood pressure at the ankle is part of the normal ABI testing and is performed as described above with a standard sphygmomanometer placed just above the malleoli and a handheld CW Doppler instrument. A value of ankle pressure below 50 mm Hg is usually considered diagnostic of CLI as ischaemic rest pain most commonly occurs below an ankle pressure of 50 mm Hg; however, values below 70 mm Hg in the presence of foot ulcers or gangrene are usually not enough to achieve healing of the lesion [8].

Toe Pressure Measurement and Toe Brachial Index

Measuring blood pressure at hallux digital artery level is possible using specific sphygmomanometers equipped with a toe-sized cuff and an 8 MHz handheld CW Doppler instrument. An absolute toe blood pressure below 50 mm Hg is usually considered to be insufficient to guarantee ulcer healing, and thus diagnostic of CLI.

Despite the presence of several guidelines reporting 0.7 as the cutoff value below which to consider TBI as pathologic, a recent systematic review by Høyer et al. [15] found that the evidence on which this choice has been based is quite poor and that the available literature at the time the review was conducted, was not sufficient to conclude a specific cutoff as diagnostic for PAD.

Moreover, toe digital arteries may, even though less frequently than leg arteries, develop arterial wall calcifications as well, therefore limiting the predictive role for a non-suppressed TBI reading for CLI (Fig. 3)

In conclusion, taking into account the costs for TBI testing equipment and the scant evidence available to support its results interpretation, TBI is not frequently used in most Diabetic Foot third-level centers; however, a pathologic TBI reading can certainly prompt urgent vascular imaging and possibly revascularization.

Transcutaneous Oximetry

$TcPO_2$, is a local, non-invasive technique measuring the amount of O_2 that has diffused from capillaries all the way through the epidermis. $TcPO_2$ provides information about the body's ability to deliver oxygen to the skin and therefore is dependent on oxygen uptake in the respiratory system, the oxygen transport/capacity of the blood and the general status of the circulatory system.

Technically, the test is performed applying an oxygen pressure sensor on the patient's skin that is heated by an electrode to create a local hyperemia that in turn maximizes local oxygen delivery. The electrode quantifies the local oxygen partial pressure in mm Hg and this value can provide information on the healing potential of a foot lesion.

The reference value is generally considered > 50 mm Hg, whereas values of below 30 mm Hg are associated with reduced healing potential and therefore are considered diagnostic for CLI. The test results should be interpreted cautiously in cases of marked edema or cellulitis as well as severe hyperkeratosis that can affect oxygen ability to travel to the external electrode.

A recent systematic review by Wang et al. [11] found 25 studies investigating the role of $TcPO_2$ in predicting ulcer healing. Even though based mostly on observational studies and therefore at high risk of bias, the results suggested a high diagnostic accuracy of the $TcPO_2$ test for predicting both ulcer healing and limb amputation [11].

In conclusion, $TcPO_2$ measurement provides an estimate of the amount of oxygen that is locally reaching the patient's skin, and this, in turn, may be very helpful in deciding whether or not limb revascularization is necessary. However, there are multiple interfering variables (i.e., severe anemia, respiratory disease, local edema or hyperkeratosis) that should be taken into account when interpreting $TcPO_2$ results.

Duplex Ultrasound

Duplex ultrasound scanning (DUS) and colour-Doppler ultrasound imaging combine classic B-mode ultrasound scanning with blood speed analysis using the pulsed wave Doppler mode and the colour-Doppler mapping, thus providing information on both arterial anatomy and blood flow.

A lower limb DUS investigates the arterial tree from the common iliac artery to the distal BTK and foot vessels, enabling detection and quantification of arterial stenosis or occlusions. Compared with angiography, several concordant meta-analyses estimated DUS sensitivity to detect >50% diameter angiographic stenosis at 85–90%, with a specificity of >95% [12]. However, performing a complete bilateral lower limb DUS mapping may be quite time consuming and requires a skilled and expert operator as well as a high-performance ultrasound system. Therefore, it is usually considered a second-line investigation to be used only in patients with positive results for quicker and less expensive screening tests, like the ABI, or in patients in which the clinical appearance is in contrast with the screening test results. A detailed description of how to perform and report lower limb arterial colour-Doppler ultrasound testing is beyond the scope of this chapter; however, it may be found elsewhere [16, 17].

Proposed Approach to Recognize Ischaemic Wounds Requiring Revascularization

In our practice, we usually base our choice whether to submit a patient to revascularization or not on a combination of the clinical and instrumental data.

The clinical gestalt, mostly based on wound location and presentation, as well as on the foot appearance as a whole, is usually the first step in suspecting foot ischaemia; however, it is not infrequent to have an ischaemic component in apparently purely neuropathic lesions.

Therefore, we perform an ABI as well as a $TcPO_2$ measurement on any diabetic patient with a foot ulcer, carefully positioning the electrode as close as possible to the ulcerated area. These tests provide information on two different arterial systems. The ABI is a proxy for the lower limb transmission system (i.e., from aorta to the ankle), while the $TcPO_2$ also takes into account the BTA vessel disease component, that we have found to be so important in our diabetic patients with CLI. If still in doubt regarding the need for revascularization, we complete the non-invasive evaluation with a DUS mapping in order to get more information regarding the localization and pattern of the disease. We do not perform TBI measurement, MR angiography or CTA on a regular basis, as we believe most of the information necessary to decide whether and how a patient needs to be revascularized can be obtained by a clinical exam integrated with ABI, $TcPO_2$ and DUS.

This approach is in keeping with most available guidelines that consider a $TcPO_2$ <30–40 mm Hg or an ABI <0.5 thresholds for undergoing revascularization in the presence of a foot lesion not responding to local therapy (i.e., infection control, proper dressing and offloading) [8, 10, 12]. Furthermore, we do not usually perform any prophylactic revascularization in clinically silent patients, as we believe that, in this case, the risk of revascularization procedure complications would greatly exceed the possible benefits of a successful procedure. This is in keeping with most guidelines that recommend against revascularization in asymptomatic patients, as the currently available evidence is insufficient to claim any benefit for such an approach [12, 34]. On the other hand, we favour a very close monitoring for patients with known limb arteries stenosis, based on a thorough vascular evaluation and a frequent clinical exam in order to pick up lesions, or clinically significant symptoms, as early as possible and to start timely and appropriate treatment. This is supported by a study by Faglia et al. [35] in which they found that about 50% of patients with a diagnosis of CLI in a single limb developed CLI in the contralateral limb over a 6-year period. However, the severity of foot lesions and the rate of amputations were both lower in contralateral limbs and this may be certainly explained by earlier diagnosis and treatment, both allowed by a close follow-up.

Targets of Revascularization

Once the need for revascularization of a patient's limb is established, it is necessary to decide which vessel should be targeted and subsequently which is the best strategy to achieve this task. In this section, we discuss our rationale in choosing the best revascularization targets.

Complete Revascularization or Wound-Related Artery Revascularization?
The possible goals of revascularization may be: "complete" revascularization or "wound-related artery" revascularization. Peregrin et al. [18] showed that "complete revascularization" with 3 revascularized leg arteries significantly reduces amputation risks. These data are in keeping with what Faglia et al. [19] found in a similar study in 2007. This is particularly true for patients with extensive ulcers or severe infections, where tissue damage extends over more angiosomes and where restoration of the best possible blood supply should always be pursued. Špillerová et al. [20] demonstrated that in CLI, the tissue lesion affects several angiosomes in the vast majority of the cases.

On the other hand, in patients with smaller and localized lesions, a wound-related strategy could be tried. This approach consists in revascularizing primarily the main feeding artery of the affected angiosome leading to direct blood flow to the wound and its neighbor tissues.

Four recent meta-analysis [21–24] showed that direct revascularization of the wound angiosome led to better wound healing and limb salvage rates compared to indirect revascularization. However, these data are based mostly on retrospective data and therefore subjected to a high risk of bias. Therefore, the main take-home message we could deduct from these studies is that during a revascularization procedure, it is preferable to try achieving complete revascularization, particularly in patients with extensive infection; however, if this turns out to be unrealistic, it is wiser not to waste time on unachievable tasks and to try to restore a direct blood flow to the affected area or, if this is still not possible, at least an indirect one. Moreover, neither of these tasks should be carried out uncritically; on the other hand, any revascularization procedure should always be tailored according to technical feasibility, patient's general conditions, planned foot surgery and possible further bypasses (i.e., respecting possible bypass graft landing zones).

Angiosomes of the Foot and Ankle
An angiosome is defined as a unit of skin and underlying tissues (fat, fascia, muscle, soft tissues and bones), supplied by a source artery through its distal arborizations, and drained by a venous plexus [25]. In treating patients with CLI, we must consider 5 major foot angiosomes:
- Dorsal: mostly supplied by the DPA
- Medial Plantar: supplied the medial plantar artery
- Lateral Plantar: supplied by the LPA

– Medial Calcaneal: supplied by the distal PTA
– Lateral Calcanear: supplied by the calcanear branch of the peroneal artery

It is important to keep in mind that contiguous angiosomes are usually linked to each other by "choke vessels," which are small distal tributaries of the main feeding artery. These vessels normally exist in a collapsed low flow state; however, when an adjacent angiosome becomes ischaemic, the pressure gradient generated activates them, thereby allowing blood to be diverted to the ischaemic tissue. Direct revascularization could have a different value depending on the presence or not of these vessels: Varela et al. [26] demonstrated that the restoration of blood flow to the ulcer through collateral vessels (pedal and distal peroneal branches) provided similar results to those obtained through its specific source artery in terms of healing and limb salvage.

Kawarada et al. [27] demonstrated that a single tibial artery revascularization, whether of the anterior or posterior tibial, yielded comparable improvements in microcirculation of the dorsal and plantar foot.

In diabetic and end-stage-renal-disease, patients' collateral vessels formation is reduced or absent and foot circulation becomes functionally terminal because of lack of collaterals [28, 29]. This is the reason why in feet with a poor distal vascular distribution system, the so called desert foot, we need to improve the most direct blood flow to the wounded area and the concept of angiosome gains importance: the value of an angiosome-oriented revascularization is inversely related to the function of collateral vessels. In conclusion, being familiar with foot and ankle angiosomes is very important in deciding which vessel to target in a revascularization procedure.

Revascularization Strategies

Treating CLI is a challenging task that should be pursued with a patient-centric approach trying to tailor the available strategies and techniques to the patient's clinical condition.

The evidence available on the effectiveness of each of the available techniques is quite heterogenous and frequently at high risk of bias [10]. Despite this, endovascular revascularization seems to offer some important advantages that led us to use, in our practice, an "Angioplasty first" strategy in most cases. A percutaneous approach offers favourable outcomes, in terms of feasibility, complications and limb salvage rates [30]. Moreover, angioplasty can be proposed for patients who cannot be good candidates for bypass surgery because of co-morbidities and high operative risk, as angioplasty does not require general anaesthesia and can usually be carried out quite straightforwardly even in patients with high surgical risk. Furthermore, complex procedures could be divided into different steps to decrease exposure to contrast media or could be performed with CO_2-based angiography.

Angioplasty also offers the important advantages of it being repeatable quite easily in case of early clinically significant restenosis or re-occlusion as well as not precluding possible further surgical treatments, as long as bypass "landing zones" are preserved during endovascular revascularization attempts.

Despite all this, surgery seems to achieve the best outcomes in some specific conditions, like in the presence of very long femoro-popliteal or infrapopliteal occlusions as well as in case of disease of the common femoral artery at its bifurcation, a location quite unusual for the typical diabetes-related PAD [10]. However, even before considering a surgical attempt, it is mandatory to carefully evaluate its feasibility considering the patient's general health and surgical risk, the state on inflow and outflow vascular tree and the availability of an adequate graft [10].

Once decided by clinical and instrumental investigations that an endovascular revascularization can be useful for wound healing and limb salvage for a specific patient, it is necessary to ascertain some key issues before and during the procedure.

As general targets, we must ascertain the condition of inflow vessels. In fact, significant lesions in the aorto-iliac or femoro-popliteal vessels must be corrected before approaching the BTK vasculature. The necessity of treating inflow vessels can also influence the access site. In fact, aorto-iliac lesions can be approached by an arm access (either radial or brachial) or by the transfemoral access (either retrograde or cross over). Conversely, proximal superficial femoral artery lesions are best treated by contralateral femoral access, while distal superficial femoral and popliteal artery lesions can be treated by antegrade femoral access. Therefore, the correct identification of the level of the lesions to be treated and the condition of the access site to be used are of paramount importance once the decision to proceed with an invasive treatment of ischaemic diabetic lesions is made.

However, the final decision on how to tackle BTK lesions is always made even during the revascularization procedure, with iodinated or CO_2 subtraction angiography. As a general rule, it is better to revascularize three vessels, instead of two and two vessels instead of one; similarly, it is better to revascularize a tibial artery, which reaches the foot directly, instead of the peroneal artery. Lastly, it is better to revascularize the angiosome-related artery instead of the non-wound-related artery.

Furthermore, the final strategy should be adapted based on information obtained from previous procedures that the patient has gone through. It is in fact increasingly common for our patients to undergo in their lifetime multiple revascularization procedures on the same leg, due to the chronic and progressive nature of the diabetes-related atherosclerotic disease. Therefore, knowing the results of previous angiographic studies is crucial to tailor the best revascularization strategy for the patient (i.e., best access site, amenable target vessels, type of balloon or stent needed).

In summary, our strategy in deciding if and how to revascularize a certain target territory can be summarized as follows:

1. Patients with a diagnosis of CLI, deemed to be in need of revascularization, undergo an imaging test that is capable of visualizing the whole arterial tree. This can be a complete colour-Doppler ultrasound mapping of lower limb's arteries (risk free but time consuming, technically difficult and not always definitive) or a diagnostic angi-

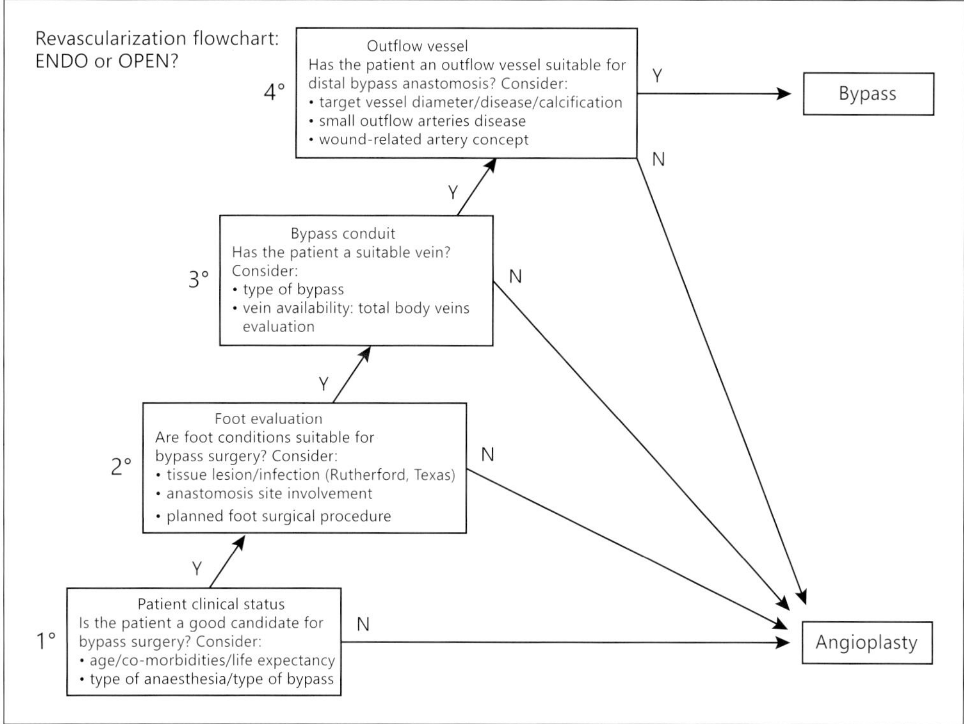

Fig. 4. Endovascular versus surgical revascularization decision strategy. If the answer to any of the 4 questions is a "Yes," then bypass should be considered first line; if any of the questions is answered by a "No," angioplasty could be chosen first.

ography (small risks, due mainly to the risk of arterial access haemorrhage, contrast-induced nephropathy and radiation burden, but definitive). In our CathLab, the angiography is made in a majority of the cases using a 4 French antegrade femoral approach and less than 20 mL of iodinated contrast dye.

2. Once the pattern of obstructive disease is completely defined, if we consider it better treatable by endovascular means, we proceed in the same session with a first endovascular attempt. However, if there are long vascular occlusions that could be possibly better treated with bypass surgery, we evaluate the patient's eligibility by answering 4 questions (Figure 4) [10]:

a. Is the patient's general status compatible with anaesthesia and a high surgical burden as expected for the planned bypass? Consider general surgical risk, ASA category and life expectancy.

b. Are foot conditions suitable for bypass surgery? Consider tissue infective burden, anastomosis site involvement and planned foot surgery.

c. Does the patient have a suitable vein for the bypass conduit?

d. Does the patient have a suitable distal target vessel for bypass anastomosis? Consider angiosome concept and small vessel outflow.

If the answer to all these 4 questions is a "Yes", we go ahead and consider surgery as a possible choice; otherwise, if any of these questions is answered by a "No," we prefer angioplasty as the revascularization procedure of choice.

3. If neither endovascular revascularization nor surgical bypass is possible, the patient is then considered "no-option patient" and candidate to either a trial of medical treatment with IV prostanoids or to major amputation (transtibial or transfemoral). However, this category of patients might still be offered unconventional or experimental treatment as an extreme trial of limb salvage, as long as this is safe and does not add any further risks. Examples of such treatments include foot vein arterialization, or in case of untreatable femoral occlusions with good collateral circuit to the popliteal, distal BTK endovascular revascularization only.

In conclusion, deciding if, when and how a diabetic foot patient needs to be revascularized is a task harder than it could apparently seem. The fundamental steps in this path include correct and precise diagnosis of CLI and thus of the need to be revascularized, by both clinical exam and non-invasive diagnostic tests. Once the need to revascularize has been established, the next step is to define the target arteries, keeping in mind the wound-related artery concept as well as its pitfalls. Eventually, the last step is to decide which approach to use in a tailored and patient-centered way.

It is still worthwhile to remind our readers that, unfortunately, saving a limb is often not possible despite putting into place the best available strategies, and therefore, it is important to always keep the patient informed of the constant high underlying risk of limb loss and to avoid being overoptimistic.

References

1 Prompers L, Schaper N, Apelqvist J, Edmonds M, Jude E, Mauricio D, Uccioli L, Urbancic V, Bakker K, Holstein P, Jirkovska A, Piaggesi A, Ragnarson-Tennvall G, Reike H, Spraul M, Van Acker K, Van Baal J, Van Merode F, Ferreira I, Huijberts M: Prediction of outcome in individuals with diabetic foot ulcers: focus on the differences between individuals with and without peripheral arterial disease. The EURODIALE Study. Diabetologia 2008;51;747–755.

2 Brownlee M: Biochemistry and molecular cell biology of diabetic complications. Nature 2001;414:813–820.

3 Jude EB, Oyibo SO, Chalmers N, Boulton AJ: Peripheral arterial disease in diabetic and nondiabetic patients: a comparison of severity and outcome. Diabetes Care 2001;24:1433–1437.

4 Graziani L, Silvestro A, Bertone V, Manara E, Andreini R, Sigala A, Mingardi R De Giglio R: Vascular involvement in diabetic subjects with ischemic foot ulcer: a new morphologic categorization of disease severity. Eur J Vasc Endovasc Surg 2007;33:453–460.

5 He C, Yang JG, Li YM, Rong J, Du FZ, Yang ZG, Gu M: Comparison of lower extremity atherosclerosis in diabetic and non-diabetic patients using multidetector computed tomography. BMC Cardiovasc Disord 2014;14:125.

6 Faglia E, Favales F, Quarantiello A, Calia P, Clelia P, Brambilla G, Rampoldi A, Morabito A: Angiographic evaluation of peripheral arterial occlusive disease and its role as a prognostic determinant for major amputation in diabetic subjects with foot ulcers. Diabetes Care 1998;21:625–630.

7 Diehm N, Pattynama PM, Jaff MR, Cremonesi A, Becker GJ, Hopkins LN, Mahler F, Talen A, Cardella JF, Ramee S, van Sambeek M, Vermassen F, Biamino G: Clinical endpoints in peripheral endovascular revascularization trials: a case for standardized definitions. Eur J Vasc Endovasc Surg 2008;36:409–419.

8 Norgren L, Hiatt WR, Dormandy JA, Nehler MR, Harris KA, Fowkes FG; TASC II Working Group: Inter-Society Consensus for the Management of Peripheral Arterial Disease (TASC II). J Vasc Surg 2007;45(suppl S):S5–S7.

   Ferraresi · Losurdo · Lorenzoni · Ferraris · Caminiti · Casini

9   Khan NA, Rahim SA, Anand SS, Simel DL, Panju A: Does the clinical examination predict lower extremity peripheral arterial disease? JAMA 2006;295:536–546.

10 Aiello A, Anichini R, Brocco E, Caravaggi C, Chiavetta A, Cioni R, Da Ros R, De Feo ME, Ferraresi R, Florio F, Gargiulo M, Galzerano G, Gandini R, Giurato L, Graziani L, Mancini L, Manzi M, Modugno P, Setacci C, Uccioli L: Treatment of peripheral arterial disease in diabetes: a consensus of the Italian Societies of Diabetes (SID, AMD), Radiology (SIRM) and Vascular Endovascular Surgery (SICVE). Nutr Metab Cardiovasc Dis 2014;24:355–369.

11 Wang Z, Hasan R, Firwana B, Elraiyah T, Tsapas A, Prokop L, Mills JL Sr, Murad MH: A systematic review and meta-analysis of tests to predict wound healing in diabetic foot. J Vasc Surg 2016;63(2 suppl):29S–36S.e1–e2.

12 European Stroke Organisation, Tendera M, Aboyans V, Bartelink L, Baumgartner I, Clement D, Collet JP, Cremonesi A, De Carlo M, Erbel R, Fowkes FG, Heras M, Kownator S, Minar E, Ostergren J, Poldermans D, Riambau V, Roffi M, Rother J, Sievert H, van Sambeek M, Zeller T: ESC Guidelines on the diagnosis and treatment of peripheral artery diseases: document covering atherosclerotic disease of extracranial carotid and vertebral, mesenteric, renal, upper and lower extremity arteries: the Task Force on the Diagnosis and Treatment of Peripheral Artery Diseases of the European Society of Cardiology (ESC). Eur Heart J 2011;32:2851–2906.

13 Schröder F, Diehm N, Kareem S, Ames M, Pira A, Zwettler U, Lawall H, Diehm C: A modified calculation of ankle-brachial pressure index is far more sensitive in the detection of peripheral arterial disease. J Vasc Surg 2006;44:531–536.

14 Tasci I: Best practice in ankle brachial index measurement. J Wound Ostomy Continence Nurs 2012;39:238.

15 Høyer C, Sandermann J, Petersen LJ: The toe-brachial index in the diagnosis of peripheral arterial disease. J Vasc Surg 2013;58:231–238.

16 Pellerito J, Pollak JF (ed 6): Introduction to Vascular Ultrasonography. Saunders, 2012.

17 Arger P, DeBari Iyoob S (ed 1). The Complete Guide to Vascular Ultrasound. Philadelphia, 2004.

18 Peregrin JH, Koznar B, Kovác J, Lastovicková J, Novotný J, Vedlich D, Skibová J: PTA of infrapopliteal arteries: long-term clinical follow-up and analysis of factors influencing clinical outcome. Cardiovasc Intervent Radiol 2010;33:720–725.

19 Faglia E, Clerici G, Clerissi J, Mantero M, Caminiti M, Quarantiello A, Curci V, Lupattelli T, Morabito A: When is a technically successful peripheral angioplasty effective in preventing above-the-ankle amputation in diabetic patients with critical limb ischaemia? Diabet Med 2007;24:823–829.

20 Špillerová K, Sörderström M, Albäck A, Venermo M: The feasibility of angiosome-targeted endovascular treatment in patients with critical limb ischemia and foot ulcer. Ann Vasc Surg 2016;30:270–276.

21 Huang TY, Huang TS, Wang YC, Huang PF, Yu HC, Yeh CH: Direct revascularization with the angiosome concept for lower limb ischemia: a systematic review and meta-analysis. Medicine (Baltimore) 2015;94:e1427.

22 Biancari F, Juvonen T: Angiosome-targeted lower limb revascularization for ischemic foot wounds: systematic review and meta-analysis. Eur J Vasc Endovasc Surg 2014;47:517–522.

23 Bosanquet DC, Glasbey JC, Williams IM, Twine CP: Systematic review and meta-analysis of direct versus indirect angiosomal revascularisation of infrapopliteal arteries. Eur J Vasc Endovasc Surg 2014;48:88–97.

24 Jongsma H, Bekken JA, Akkersdijk GP, Hoeks SE, Verhagen HJ, Fioole B: Angiosome-directed revascularization in patients with critical limb ischemia. J Vasc Surg 2017;65:1208–1219.

25 Agnew SP, Dumanian GA, Angiosomes of the calf, ankle and foot: anatomy, physiology and implications; in Sarrafian's Anatomy of the Foot and Ankle, 2011 Philadelphia, pp 668–677.

26 Varela C, Acín F, de Haro J, Bleda S, Esparza L, March JR: The role of foot collateral vessels on ulcer healing and limb salvage after successful endovascular and surgical distal procedures according to an angiosome model. Vasc Endovascular Surg 2010;44:654–660.

27 Kawarada O, Yasuda S, Nishimura K, Sakamoto S, Noguchi M, Takahi Y, Harada K, Ishihara M, Ogawa H: Effect of single tibial artery revascularization on microcirculation in the setting of critical limb ischemia. Circ Cardiovasc Interv 2014;7:684–691.

28 Weihrauch D, Lohr NL, Mraovic B, Ludwig LM, Chilian WM, Pagel PS, Warltier DC, Kersten JR: Chronic hyperglycemia attenuates coronary collateral development and impairs proliferative properties of myocardial interstitial fluid by production of angiostatin. Circulation 2004;109:2343–2348.

29 Azuma N, Uchida H, Kokubo T, Koya A, Akasaka N, Sasajima T: Factors influencing wound healing of critical ischaemic foot after bypass surgery: Is the angiosome important in selecting bypass target artery? Eur J Vasc Endovasc Surg 2012;43:322–328.

30 Alexandrescu V, Hubermont G, Philips Y, Guillaumie B, Ngongang C, Coessens V, Vandenbossche P, Coulon M, Ledent G, Donnay JC: Combined primary subintimal and endoluminal angioplasty for ischaemic inferior-limb ulcers in diabetic patients: 5-year practice in a multidisciplinary "diabetic-foot" service. Eur J Vasc Endovasc Surg 2009;37:448–456.

31 Hinchliffe RJ, Brownrigg JR, Apelqvist J, Boyko EJ, Fitridge R, Mills JL, Reekers J, Shearman CP, Zierler RE, Schaper NC: IWGDF guidance on the diagnosis, prognosis and management of peripheral artery disease in patients with foot ulcers in diabetes. Diabetes Metab Res Rev 2016;32(suppl 1):37–44.

32 Gerhard-Herman MD, Gornik HL, Barrett C, Barshes NR, Corriere MA, Drachman DE, Fleisher LA, Fowkes FG, Hamburg NM, Kinlay S, Lookstein R, Misra S, Mureebe L, Olin JW, Patel RA, Regensteiner JG, Schanzer A, Shishehbor MH, Stewart KJ, Treat-Jacobson D, Walsh ME: 2016 AHA/ACC guideline on the management of patients with lower extremity peripheral artery disease: executive summary. Circulation 2017;135:e686–e725.

33 Orchard TJ, Strandness DE Jr: Assessment of peripheral vascular disease in diabetes. Report and recommendations of an international workshop sponsored by the American Heart Association and the American Diabetes Association 18–20 September 1992, New Orleans, Louisiana. Diabetes Care 1993;16: 1199–1209.

34 Hingorani A, LaMuraglia GM, Henke P, Meissner MH, Loretz L, Zinszer KM, Driver VR, Frykberg R, Carman TL, Marston W, Mills JL Sr, Murad MH: The management of diabetic foot: a clinical practice guideline by the Society for Vascular Surgery in collaboration with the American Podiatric Medical Association and the Society for Vascular Medicine. J Vasc Surg 2016;63:3S–21S.

35 Faglia E, Clerici G, Mantero M, Caminiti M, Quarantiello A, Curci V, Morabito A: Incidence of critical limb ischemia and amputation outcome in contralateral limb in diabetic patients hospitalized for unilateral critical limb ischemia during 1999–2003 and followed-up until 2005. Diabetes Res Clin Pract 2007;77:445–450.

Roberto Ferraresi, MD
Peripheral Interventional Unit
Humanitas Gavazzeni Bergamo
Via Mauro Gavazzeni 21, IT–24125 Bergamo (Italy)
E-Mail roberto.ferraresi@gavazzeni.it

Ferraresi · Losurdo · Lorenzoni · Ferraris · Caminiti · Casini

Piaggesi A, Apelqvist J (eds): The Diabetic Foot Syndrome.
Front Diabetes. Basel, Karger, 2018, vol 26, pp 147–160 (DOI: 10.1159/000480060)

An Integrated Approach for the Effective Management of Limb-Threatening Ischaemia in the Diabetic Foot

Joseph L. Mills

Division of Vascular Surgery and Endovascular Therapy, Michael E. DeBakey Department of Surgery, Baylor College of Medicine, Houston, TX, USA

Abstract

Non-communicable diseases became the leading cause of global mortality almost a decade ago and the epidemic of diabetes is one of its major contributors. Diabetes affects more than 415 million people across the world and the diabetic foot ulcer (DFU) is one of its prime manifestations. The magnitude of this problem, which impacts 1 in 4 people with diabetes during his or her lifetime, necessitates an organized response to care delivery. It has been demonstrated repeatedly that amputation rates in people with diabetes can be dramatically reduced when patients with diabetes receive care from an integrated, coordinated team of dedicated clinicians from multiple disciplines, especially teams that include foot specialists and vascular specialists. This chapter begins with a brief outline of the history and evolution of the team approach. It then presents in detail an organized algorithm based on the underlying pathophysiology of the DFU and the skillsets needed to manage it to create a model for integrated diabetic foot care to prevent unnecessary amputations and improve quality of life for those affected.

Introduction

The 21st century is the era of non-communicable diseases (NCDs). In 2009, for the first time in the history of humankind, NCDs became the leading cause of mortality (60%) across the globe [1]. Diabetes has become a global epidemic, an unappreciated emergency. There is perhaps no better example than the diabetic foot to demonstrate the complexity involved when health care systems attempt to transition a structure that was designed to respond to trauma and acute problems to one that can manage chronic NCD. The diabetic foot is the canary in the mine, so to speak, and its emergence as a common, costly and morbid problem reflects the lack of coordinated political, socioeconomic and health care responses to the prevention and management of diabetes.

The prevalence of diabetes is increasing in almost every country from which reliable data have been reported [2–4]. More than 415 million people across the world have diabetes, which translates to a global prevalence of 1 in 11 adults [1, 5]. Diabetes afflicts the rich and poor alike, and is indifferent to race and gender. A diabetic foot ulcer (DFU) can be viewed as a manifestation of imperfections in our systems of NCD care. While often silent in onset because of underlying neuropathy and loss of protective sensation, DFUs constitute a major public health burden and are associated with startlingly high economic costs and significant reduction in quality and duration of life for those so afflicted [4]. It has been estimated that 20–25% of patients with diabetes will develop a DFU during their lifetime and that 25% of such DFUs will eventually result in major limb amputation. A recent report documented that at least in the United States, the annual direct costs of diabetic limb complications exceeded those of each of the 5 most common forms of cancer [3]. The primary risk factors for DFU and amputation risk include neuropathy, ischaemia (peripheral artery disease or PAD), tobacco use, nephropathy and poor glycaemic control.

The magnitude of this problem necessitates an organized response to care delivery. It has been demonstrated repeatedly that amputation rates in people with diabetes can be dramatically reduced when patients with diabetes receive care from an integrated, coordinated team of dedicated clinicians from multiple disciplines, especially teams that include foot specialists and vascular specialists. This chapter will begin by outlining briefly the history and evolution of the team approach, and present in detail an organized algorithm based on the underlying pathophysiology of the DFU and the skillsets needed to manage it to create a model for integrated diabetic foot care to prevent unnecessary amputations and improve quality of life for those affected.

Team Approach to Diabetic Foot Care

The evolution of the team approach to diabetic foot care includes a host of podiatrists, vascular surgeons, endocrinologists, internists and others, who from very early times recognized the risks for amputation associated with diabetic neuropathy and its frequent accompaniment, ischaemia. In the United States, Maurice Lewi, MD, founded the oldest school of podiatric medicine in New York City in the early 1900s. He recognized that "minor foot ills" were often neglected and felt to be pedestrian in nature. Importantly, he observed that neglected or poorly treated ulcers could eventually result in the formation of gangrene [6]. The discovery of insulin in 1922 by Frederick Banting and associates was both a blessing and a curse. The blessing was of course that children and young individuals affected by the diagnosis of diabetes were no longer condemned to death from diabetic coma. The curse was that as affected patients began living longer, complications that had not been seen previously began to develop.

Elliott Joslin, MD, a famous American diabetologist at the New England Deaconness Hospital in Boston noted that after the introduction of insulin, while mortality from coma had fallen in patients with diabetes from 60 to 5%, deaths from lower extremity gangrene had risen substantially. His astute clinical observations and fundamental understanding of the pathophysiology of DFU led him to establish what was most likely the first hospital diabetic foot clinic; it included chiropodists and a surgeon, Leland McKittrick, MD. It grew to include Frank Wheelock, Jr., MD, who was among the first American surgeons to perform a femoropopliteal bypass graft. These early beginnings grew under the subsequent leadership of Frank LoGerfo and Gary Gibbons, who pioneered distal revascularization, especially pedal bypass for patients with DFUs and severe limb ischaemia. They worked in close alignment with a dedicated group of podiatrists (the evolutionary descendants of chiropodists). Their work spawned the development of other multidisciplinary teams including ones led not only by vascular surgeons and podiatrists but also by orthopaedic surgeons. The interested reader is referred to a more complete history of diabetic foot team care, which is beyond the scope of the present chapter, but can be read in the recent, excellent monograph by Sanders et al. [6].

In Europe and the rest of the world, diabetic foot teams have most often been led by endocrinologists who were prescient to recognize the significance of DFUs for their patients, problems which were frequently neglected by other disciplines. Such programs include those established by Michael Edmonds at King's College Hospital in London; William Jeffcoate in Nottingham, UK; Andrew Boulton at the Manchester Royal Infirmary; Jan Apelqvist in Lund, Sweden; Max Spraul and Ernst Chanteleau at the University of Dussledorf in Germany; Kristien Van Acker at the University of Antwerp in Belgium; Ezio Faglia, Alberto Piaggesi, Luca Dalla Paola and Luigi Uccioli in Italy; and Per Hollstein in Copenhagen, Denmark. There are numerous reports of the excellent outcomes for DFU patients that can be obtained when teams are formed to work together [6–19].

Unfortunately, in the United States and many parts of Europe, such clinics are not the norm and the care received by a patient with a DFU in any given outpatient clinic or hospital is not routinely well organized and often quite haphazard. Many physicians and hospitals were ill prepared to deal with the epidemic of DFU that began in the 1990s and continues to explode into the 21st century. The problem was dramatically illustrated in 2 recent analyses of DFUs presenting for care either in the hospital emergency department of the hospital [4] or in the ambulatory setting [5]. A cross-sectional analysis of approximately 6.7 million patients with DFUs seen for ambulatory care visits from 2007 to 2013 across the United States reported the following striking findings: compared to ambulatory visits in patients without DFU, DFU visits were associated with a 3.4 times higher odds of direct emergency department or inpatient admission; double the number of previous visits during the past 12 months and double the odds of referral to another physician; and an outpatient visit length 1.4 times longer [5]. Among 1,019,861 cases of diabetic foot complications that presented to emergency departments in the United States from 2006 to 2010, 81.2% were admitted to the hospital. Among those admitted, estimated costs were USD 8.78 billion per annum; clinical outcomes included a sobering 2.0% mortality, 9.6% rate of sepsis and 10.5% minor or major amputation rate. Outcomes were significantly worse for patients residing in rural locations, Medicaid beneficiaries and for those residing in the lowest quartile of income regions [4].

Stratification of Amputation Risk: The Importance of Classification

From the perspective of a vascular surgeon, for nearly half a century, care for patients with threatened limbs due to chronic limb ischaemia from atherosclerosis was based upon the concept of "critical limb ischaemia" (CLI) [20] and either the Fontaine et al. [21] or Rutherford et al. [22] classification systems. But the concept of CLI was never intended to be applied to patients with diabetes [23, 24] and the Rutherford and Fontaine classifications do not adequately classify wound complexity and omit any mention of underlying infection. The rapid evolution of endovascular therapy expanded the number of patients and anatomic disease patterns that could be treated with an approach that was less invasive than open surgery. This technological revolution led to a lower extremity revascularization practice trend that focused extensively on angiographic findings and anatomic arterial disease extent, without adequate consideration of patient functional status, co-morbidities, and the physiologic state of the limb itself. The prevalence of PAD in patients with diabetes seems to have risen steadily since the 1990s, and PAD is now estimated to be present in as many as 50–60% of patients with DFUs [24, 25]. The estimated current prevalence rates of neuropathic, ischaemic and neuroischaemic ulcers in patients with diabetes are 35, 15 and 50% respectively [24, 25]. While one approach might be to aggressively perform angiography and endovascular therapy on all DFU patients thought to have a component of PAD, such an approach would likely generate enormous costs and perhaps unintended complications and morbidity. A more rational approach would stratify the risk of amputation for a given patient and predict the likelihood that revascularization would be helpful or needed to heal the DFU and prevent amputation. For these reasons, the Society for Vascular Surgery (SVS) developed and promulgated a new Threatened Limb Classification based simply upon grading each of the three major factors associated with limb threat status (Wound, Ischaemia and foot Infection or WIfI); these grades were then used to place a given limb into 4 stages of amputation risk ranging from very low (1) to high (4) [24]. This system evolved by merging and reorganizing key features of previous classification systems of PAD and ischaemia ("CLI", Fontaine and Rutherford) with foot ulcer classifications systems (Meggitt-Wagner [26, 27]; Texas [28] and PEDIS [29]) and using grades of each component to create stages of limb threat in a manner analogous to the Tumour, Nodes, Metastasis system for cancer. WIfI has been widely adopted and its applicability in clinical practice supported

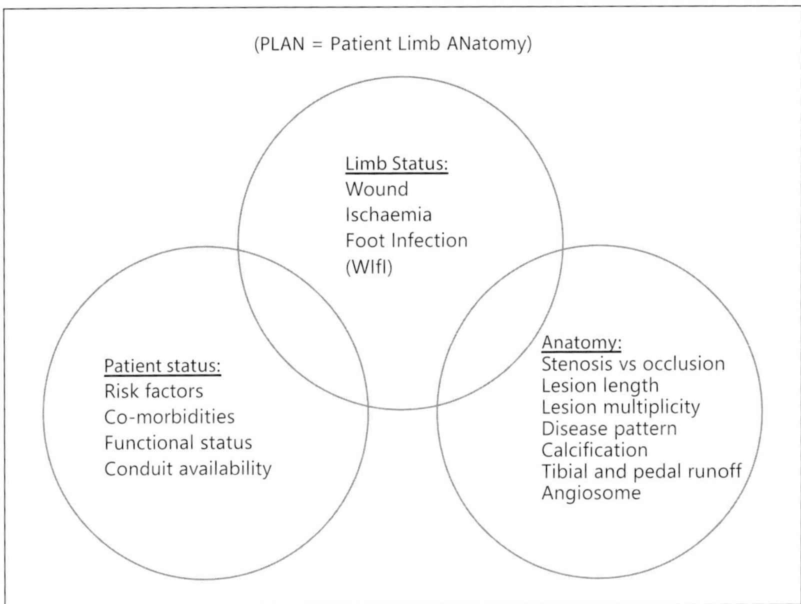

Fig. 1. Venn diagram on which to base individualized limb salvage care.

by least 8 published reports demonstrating that it predicts either amputation risk and/ or wound healing times [30–35]. The integrated team care model [7, 8], which we initially developed at the University of Arizona at SALSA (Southern Arizona Limb Salvage Alliance) employed this classification system to assess baseline risk and direct initial and subsequent care. Patient co-morbidities and arterial anatomic considerations must also be considered once limb risk is assessed and quantified (Fig. 1). We also base our foot and revascularization care at the Baylor College of Medicine (BCM) Save the Extremity Program (STEP) in Houston, for all patients with chronic limb threatening ischaemia, especially those with DFU, on the SVS WIfI classification.

One View of the Key Components of an Integrated Team

Providing outpatient and inpatient care for patients at risk of developing DFU or who have already developed DFU is a complex undertaking. As illustrated in Table 1, the provision of such care clearly lies beyond the confines of any one specialty. All patients with DFU or those at risk for developing DFU require the expertise and care of a foot specialist. In the United States, this role is most commonly filled by a podiatrist, while in Europe, it is often a diabetologist with a dedicated interest in problems of the diabetic foot who has received significant surgical training in the management of diabetic foot problems. This role could also be ably filled by an orthopaedic surgeon, general surgeon or plastic surgeon.

Table 1. Components of complete care for the diabetic foot

Metabolic know: general medical care; risk factor and diabetes management
Screening for DFU risk and preventive care
Gait analysis, biomechanics
Risk stratification (ADA foot risk class)
Pressure reduction and offloading
Vascular assessment and revascularization (SVS WIfI); long-term monitoring of the
    vascular intervention
Basic outpatient wound care
Surgical debridement, drainage complex infection
Postoperative monitoring of high risk foot
Amputation care, prostheses and rehabilitation for patients who require such

---

Regardless of specialty, such an individual must be dedicated to the training of assessing diabetic foot problems to become an expert and familiar with a wide array of non-surgical and surgical options for providing DFU care. Since ischaemia is increasingly a significant issue for people with DFUs and failure to diagnose and treat ischaemia a critical failure of care, it also seems mandatory to include a vascular surgeon or specialist in limb revascularization on the team. Studies by Goodney et al. [36] have strongly correlated the importance of vascular evaluation and revascularization with reduction in amputation rates in the United States. As part of national efforts in the United States to improve care for patients with DFUs, Dr. David Armstrong and I initiated efforts to build collaborations between the American Podiatric Medical Association and the SVS. This relationship has been sustained [37] and has remained productive [38] since its beginning in 2010 with the joint publication of a supplement dedicated to the diabetic foot entitled "Strategies to Prevent and Heal DFU: Building a Partnership for Amputation" (JVS 2010 52 supplement S). The introduction to that supplement noted that diabetic foot care was highly variable, often fragmented and lacked standardization. The supplement focused on the underlying pathophysiology and treatment of DFU and included several contributions on the importance of and means of creating an integrated limb salvage team [37]. In particular, the article by Rogers et al. [8] outlined the structure of a "toe and flow" team based on co-leadership by podiatrists and vascular surgeons (Fig. 2, 3). The remainder of this chapter will develop this theme and include lessons learnt, new components and suggestions for further improvement in structure.

Integrated Team Structure and Patient Management

Our version of an integrated DFU team is structured such that key members provide both inpatient and outpatient care. The core of the team consists of Podiatry and Vascular Surgery, but complex inpatients with multiple issues in addition to the foot re-

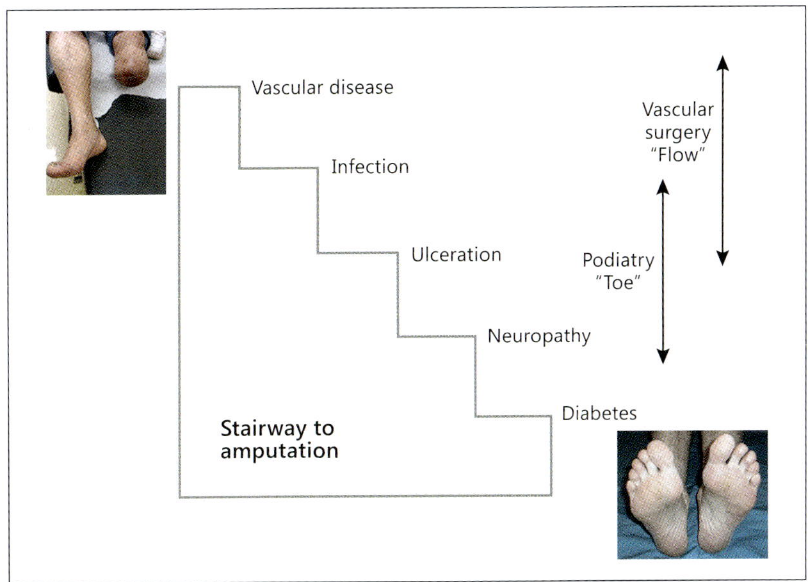

Fig. 2. The complementary care roles of podiatry and vascular surgery in preventing amputation; from Mills and Armstrong [37].

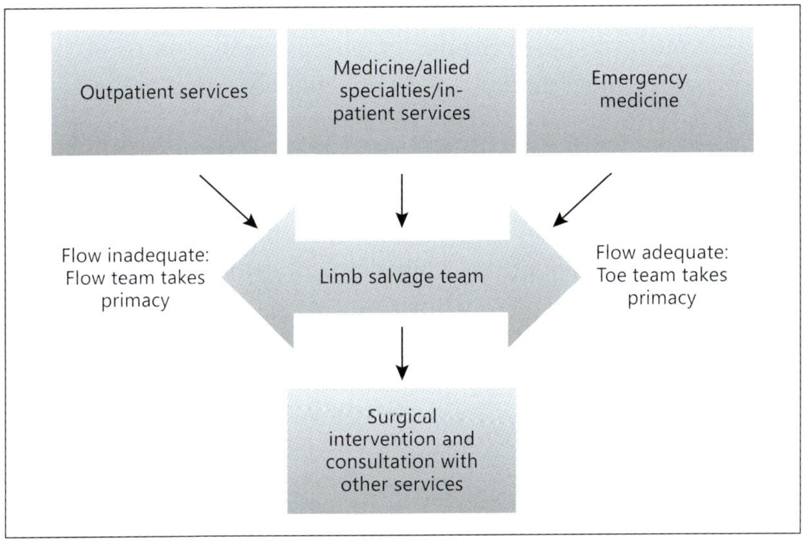

Fig. 3. Algorithm of toe and flow inpatient service; from Rogers et al. [8].

quire coordination of their care with Internal Medicine hospitalists, often with the active involvement of Nephrology and Cardiology. Infectious Disease is consulted for complex infections, resistant organisms, and recurrent infections. All inpatient DFU consults are seen initially by both Podiatry and Vascular Surgery. The initial care plan and its proper sequence are agreed upon after joint evaluation and open discussion.

In patients with DFU, infection has the highest priority among the three WIfI components. When present, it must be rapidly identified and controlled to salvage the limb. Prompt drainage of infection is essential. If moderate to severe infection is present and drainable, it should be drained first. Ischaemia is stratified by WIfI using ABI and TP, sometimes indocyanine green angiography. If there is no or minimal ischaemia, local care, debridement, offloading and digital amputations are performed aggressively, usually by podiatry. Either podiatry or vascular surgery performs "damage control" foot surgery depending on work load and availability. If there is failure to progress as expected, if wound healing stalls, or if the wound regresses, the team logically reviews the treatment sequence and questions the adequacy of offloading, re-evaluates for infection and reassesses vascular status with WIfI. Serial debridements in the presence of good vascularity are performed by podiatry specialists. Split thickness skin grafts when needed are performed by vascular surgeons with or without expertise in podiatry.

Once infection has been addressed, blood flow is the next factor that must be evaluated. A major tenet of vascular surgery is that perfusion deficits must be recognized and graded in an objective fashion based on haemodynamic data. The most reliable haemodynamic data in patients with DFUs are based on toe Doppler arterial waveforms and systolic pressures [39, 40], skin perfusion pressure [40, 41] and transcutaneous oxygen measurements [39, 40]. Newer techniques that measure perfusion rather than pressure such as indocyanine-green angiography also hold promise [42]. SVS WIfI stages 3 and 4 patients with grade 2 or 3 ischaemia undergo prompt revascularization as soon as evaluation and medical stabilization are complete.

The revascularization approach selected depends upon WIfI stage, particularly the degree of ischaemia and wound complexity. The precise level of perfusion needed to heal a foot ulcer is a complex issue that depends on a host of factors, including ulcer size location and depth, presence and extent of infection, nutritional status, oedema (whether a result of previous infection or CHF) as well as perfusion. The amount of blood flow improvement required to heal a small, shallow, non-infected ulcer in a compliant patient with well-controlled diabetes and a toe pressure of 35 mm Hg is likely to be less than that of a patient who requires open amputation of multiple toes for wet gangrene with poorly controlled diabetes and an identical toe pressure. Flow is undoubtedly important, but every patient and every ulcer do not require maximal reperfusion or angiosome driven complex endovascular therapy to heal the wound. Data suggests that wound healing times are shortened in anatomic scenarios in which it is possible to achieve angiosome targeted revascularization, particularly for endovascular therapy. However, a patient may have multiple wounds, the wound may border or include more than one angiosome, or angiosome-directed revascularization may not always be possible or practical. Thus, the experience and judgement of an experienced vascular specialist are crucial. While WIfI can be used to help predict a better approach, clinical judgement is still a key to estimate how far up the perfusion curve the wound must be pushed to achieve healing and whether long-term pa-

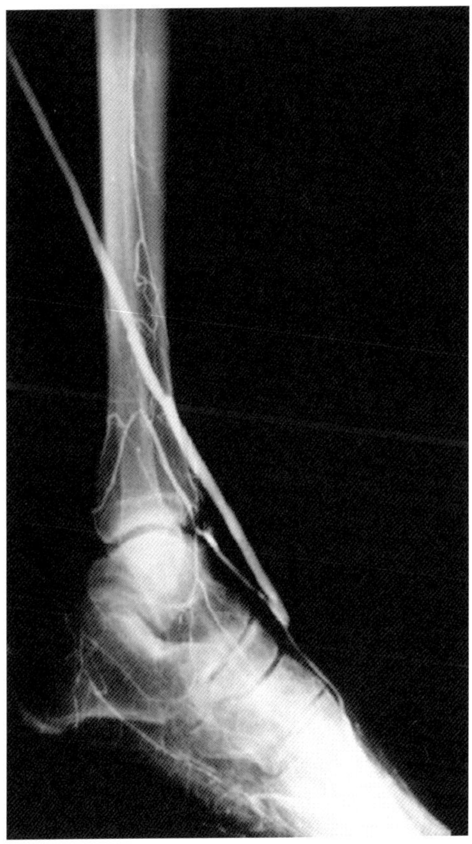

Fig. 4. Completion angiography of a reversed vein bypass to the dorsalis pedis artery. This is a very durable option for patients with DFU and severe ischaemia from long-segment tibial disease. The popliteal artery can frequently be used as the inflow source to shorten the bypass and reduce the length of high-quality autologous vein required.

tency of all components of the reconstruction (if multiple levels of disease are present, as is common) will be required to achieve durable healing and wound-free remission [43]. In low to moderate risk patients with good vein conduit, long-segment disease, and high WIfI wound and ischaemia grades, we still prefer vein bypass because of its reliability and durability (Fig. 4). If the autogenous vein is truly lacking, we generally prefer an aggressive endovascular approach including retrograde pedal access over prosthetic bypass [44]. In recent years, about 70% of our patients received endovascular therapy first, but endovascular therapy (Fig. 5) and open bypass should be viewed as complementary and not competitive approaches. The major current limitation to endovascular therapy for long-segment tibial disease is restenosis or reocclusion, occurring in 31–68% of patients within 3 months [45]. For patients with more complex, higher WIfI grade wounds, if an endovascular first approach is selected in such cases, meticulous surveillance and frequent clinical reassessment will be needed. Restenosis may require retreatment, sometimes more than once to achieve wound healing. Repetitive endovascular procedures have been shown to increase costs of care without reducing amputation risk [46]. Stratification of treatment based on WIfI classification by the San Francisco multidisciplinary group led by Michael

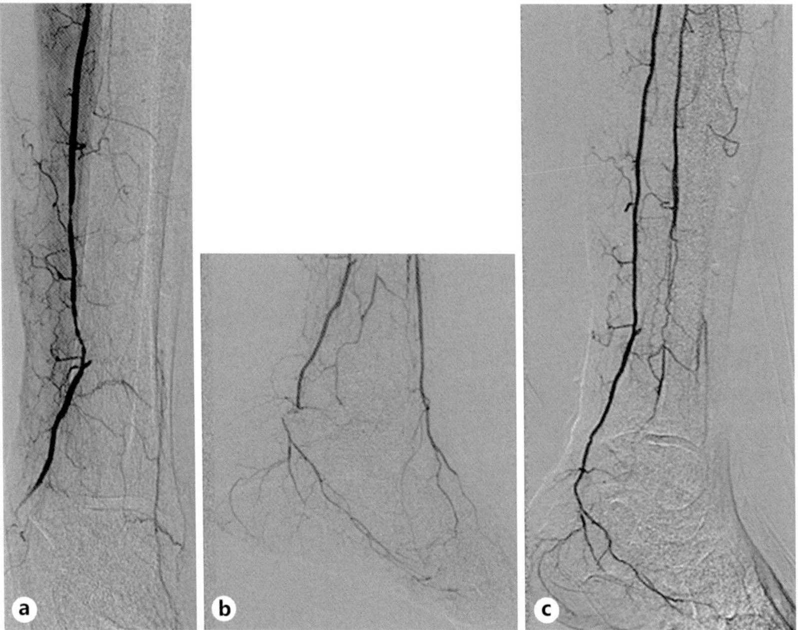

Fig. 5. Tibial angioplasty for multiple lesions and long-segment disease can be quite effective, particularly for lower grade WIfI wounds. Before (**a**, **b**) and after (**c**) posterior tibial artery angioplasty.

Conte [33] suggests improved limb salvage in WIfI stage 4 patients with a bypass as the first approach.

Wound care and eventual closure involve both podiatry and vascular surgery. The goal is to maintain a functional foot, preserve as much tissue as practical, expedite healing, and once healing is achieved, maintain remission. The latter requires good metabolic care of the patient, offloading, frequent foot checks, monitoring and surveillance of any vascular intervention that has been performed. Seeing patients repeatedly together with discussing and reviewing management options, and reassessing care when wound healing stalls or ulcers recur all require frequent, organized and face-to-face communication of the foot and flow specialists. Seeing inpatient consults together with joint visits for combined "toe and flow" patients in the outpatient clinic builds this teamwork over time and improves outcomes, as well as patient and physician/caregiver satisfaction.

Once an integrated team is built, there are always challenges and opportunities for improvement. The team leader should attempt to constantly drive efforts for improvement. Improvements being incorporated into our BCM STEP comprehensive, limb salvage program include the following: (1) all outpatient care will be under one roof at one site in one clinic and all specialists will see all wound and DFU patients at this site; (2) dedicated phone number with a dedicated receptionist and scheduler for all DFU patients; launching patient and physician friendly website; (3) dedicated and trained wound care nurses (RNs) help provide wound care following physician assessment and planning; (4) dedicated and certified wound-care specialists (includes internists, a geriatrician, an ID physician – non-surgeons); (5) improved collaboration with infectious disease by engaging one dedicated inpatient ID specialist and one primarily outpatient consultant with antibiotic algorithm and plans to perform weekly review (for inpatients) and monthly review (for outpatients) of antibiotic sensitivity patterns, review-specific patients with respect to organism, antibiotics and duration (quality review and catch potential errors in medication); (6) inclusion of orthopaedic expertise with 2 orthopaedist surgeons with substantial experience in Charcot and complex hind foot reconstruction; (7) incorporation of plastic surgery expertise with 2 plastic surgeons for complex wound management and flap coverage when needed. The BCM program is directed by a vascular surgeon with a clinical practice committee led by an internist and a Budget/Program Development Team co-led by a plastic surgeon, vascular surgeon and podiatrist with participation of other specialists including endocrinologists.

Challenges occur with respect to maintaining a cohesive team. The core group of podiatrists, vascular surgeons and nurse practitioners work together daily, but maintaining active participation by ad hoc members and those whose expertise is not required on a daily basis requires constant communication and frequent meetings to enforce the multidisciplinary scope of the effort. There are coverage and insurance issues after hospital discharge that will not permit or make it difficult to provide longitudinal patient care. We also work with many patients located at major distances from Houston and strive to coordinate some aspects of follow-up care with the patient's local wound care centre or primary care provider. Although our goal continues to be the provision of comprehensive care, we also continue to receive isolated referral for portions of a patient's care (e.g., a referring podiatrist who just desires vascular evaluation from vascular surgeon or a referring cardiologist/angiologist who only wants podiatric care). Our solution when such cases arise is to make every effort to work with patients and their referring physicians in any way we can, while striving to communicate the comprehensive nature of the STEP limb salvage programme. Over the past 2 years, we have increasingly been able to provide comprehensive care to a majority of patients referred to us since such an approach had been previously lacking in the region.

Conclusions

The latter years of the 20th century and the first 2 decades of the 21st century witnessed an alarming epidemic of NCDs of which diabetes mellitus has perhaps had the most profound impact. Physicians, in particular surgeons, as well as hospitals and health care systems, have evolved primarily over the ages to deal with trauma, disaster and acute emergencies. The door to catheterization laboratory time is a metric of provision of care for patients with an acute myocardial infarction. Level I trauma centres have evolved and must meet exacting standards of care for blunt and penetrating trauma victims to be so designated. Care at the best of these hospitals throughout the world for such emergencies is exemplary. However, physicians, hospitals and health care systems have been slow to adapt to the epidemic of NCD. Imperfect outpatient management of chronic conditions may convert them to emergencies and rather than comprehensive longitudinal care, patients often bounce from emergency to emergency for management of complications of their chronic disease.

The DFU provides an excellent window into the inadequacies of our current care systems. A patient who presents to the emergency room with sepsis [47], gas gangrene and a haemoglobin A1C of 14 with a history of a chronic neuropathic foot ulcer, which received poor outpatient management due to socioeconomic status [48, 49], insurance issues, and lack of standardized care represents our failure to manage and treat a chronic disease and serves as a poignant reminder of our need to improve care models. The care of the seemingly mundane foot ulcer offers the opportunity to develop integrated models of care for many NCDs. There are challenges to creating such adaptive and forward-thinking models, including lack of research funding [50]; lack of public education and awareness; lack of physician education; and reimbursement models that are procedure driven rather than disease management based. None of these challenges is insurmountable; team approaches that have been developed locally, regionally and nationally can be standardized, taught, learnt and implemented elsewhere. While they may require some regional variation [51], much like a good recipe, there is little doubt that integrated teams to treat DFU [52] are necessary to improve outcomes. Integrated teams have done much to improve care for patients with cancer and victims of trauma. Those afflicted by NCDs deserve as much.

References

1 Zarocostas J: Non-communicable diseases must have greater priority, says WHO. BMJ 2009; 339:b2857.
2 Boulton AJ, Vileikyte L, Ragnarson-Tennvall G, Apelqvist J: The global burden of diabetic foot disease. Lancet 2005;366:1719–1724.
3 Barshes NR, Sigireddi M, Wrobel JS, Mahankali A, Robbins JM, Kougias P, et al: The system of care for the diabetic foot: objectives, outcomes, and opportunities. Diabet Foot Ankle 2013;4.
4 Skrepnek GH, Mills JL Sr, Armstrong DG: A diabetic emergency one million feet long: disparities and burdens of illness among diabetic foot ulcer cases within emergency departments in the United States, 2006–2010. PLoS One 2015;10:e0134914.
5 Skrepnek GH, Mills JL Sr, Lavery LA, Armstrong DG: Health care service and outcomes among an estimated 6.7 million ambulatory care diabetic foot cases in the U.S. Diabetes Care 2017;40:1–7.
6 Sanders LJ, Robbins JM, Edmonds ME: History of the team approach to amputation prevention: pioneers and milestones. J Vasc Surg, 2010;52(3 suppl):3S–16S.
7 Armstrong DG, Bharara M, White M, Lepow B, Bhatnagar S, Fisher T, Kimbriel HR, Walters J, Goshima KR, Hughes J, Mills JL: The impact and outcomes of establishing an integrated interdisciplinary surgical team to care for the diabetic foot. Diabetes Metab Res Rev 2012;28:514–518.

8 Rogers LC, Andros G, Caporusso J, Harkless LB, Mills JL Sr, Armstrong DG: Toe and flow: essential components and structure of the amputation prevention team. J Vasc Surg, 2010;52(3 suppl):23S–27S.

9 Krishnan S, Nash F, Baker N, Fowler D, Rayman G: Reduction in diabetic amputations over 11 years in a defined U.K. population: benefits of multidisciplinary team work and continuous prospective audit. Diabetes Care 2008;31:99–101.

10 Edmonds ME, Blundell MP, Morris ME, Thomas EM, Cotton LT, Watkins PJ: Improved survival of the diabetic foot: the role of a specialized foot clinic. Q J Med 1986;60:763–771.

11 Fitzgerald RH, Mills JL, Joseph W, Armstrong DG: The diabetic rapid response acute foot team: 7 essential skills for targeted limb salvage. Eplasty 2009; 9:e15.

12 Van Houtum WH, Rauwerda JA, Ruwaard D, Schaper NC, Bakker K: Reduction in diabetes-related lower-extremity amputations in the Netherlands: 1991–2000. Diabetes Care 2004;27:1042–1046.

13 Eskelinen E, Eskelinen A, Albäck A, Lepäntalo M: Major amputation incidence decreases both in non-diabetic and in diabetic patients in Helsinki. Scand J Surg 2006;95:185–189.

14 Anichini R, Zecchini F, Cerretini I, et al: Improvement of diabetic foot care after the Implementation of the International Consensus on the Diabetic Foot (ICDF): results of a 5-year prospective study. Diabetes Res Clin Pract 2007;75:153–158.

15 Dargis V, Pantelejeva O, Jonushaite A, Vileikyte L, Boulton AJ: Benefits of a multidisciplinary approach in the management of recurrent diabetic foot ulceration in Lithuania: a prospective study. Diabetes Care 1999;22:1428–1431.

16 Aksoy DY, Gürlek A, Cetinkaya Y, et al: Change in the amputation profile in diabetic foot in a tertiary reference center: efficacy of team working. Exp Clin Endocrinol Diabetes 2004;112:526–530.

17 Rerkasem K, Kosachunhanun N, Tongprasert S, Khwanngern K, Matanasarawoot A, Thongchai C, et al: Reducing lower extremity amputations due to diabetes: the application of diabetic-foot protocol in Chiang Mai University Hospital. Int J Low Extrem Wounds 2008;7:88–92.

18 Viswanathan V, Madhavan S, Rajasekar S, Chamukuttan S, Ambady R: Amputation prevention initiative in South India: positive impact of foot care education. Diabetes Care 2005;28:1019–1021.

19 Campbell LV, Graham AR, Kidd RM, Molloy HF, O'Rourke SR, Colagiuri S: The lower limb in people with diabetes. Position statement of the Australian Diabetes Society. Med J Aust 2000;173:369–372.

20 Bell PRF, Charlesworth D, DePalma RG, Eastcott HHG, Eklöf B, Jamieson CW, et al: The definition of critical ischemia of a limb. Working party of the international vascular symposium. Br J Surg 1982; 69(suppl):S2.

21 Fontaine R, Kim M, Kieny R: [Surgical treatment of peripheral circulation disorders] Helv Chir Acta 1954;21:499–533.

22 Rutherford RB, Baker JD, Ernst C, Johnston KW, Porter JM, Ahn S, et al: Recommended standards for reports dealing with lower extremity ischemia: revised version. J Vasc Surg 1997;26:517–538.

23 Armstrong DG, Cohen K, Courric S, Bharara M, Marston W: Diabetic foot ulcers and vascular insufficiency: our population has changed, but our methods have not. J Diabetes Sci Technol 2011;52:1591–1595.

24 Mills JL, Conte MS, Armstrong DG, Pomposelli FB, Schanzer A, Sidawy AN, et al: The society for vascular surgery lower extremity threatened limb classification system: risk stratification based on Wound, Ischemia and foot Infection (WIfI). J Vasc Surg 2014; 59:220–234.

25 Ndip A, Jude EB: Emerging evidence for neuroischemic diabetic foot ulcers: model of care and how to adapt practice. Int J Low Extrem Wounds 2009;8: 82–94.

26 Meggitt B: Surgical management of the diabetic foot. Br J Hosp Med 1976;16:227–232.

27 Wagner FW Jr: The dysvascular foot: a system for diagnosis and treatment. Foot Ankle 1981;2:64–122.

28 Armstrong DG, Lavery LA, Harkless LB: Validation of a diabetic wound classification system. The contribution of depth, infection, and ischemia to risk of amputation. Diabetes Care 1998;21:855–859.

29 Schaper NC: Diabetic foot ulcer classification system for research purposes: a progress report on criteria for including patients in research studies. Diabetes Metab Res Rev 2004;20:S90–S95.

30 Mills JL Sr: The application of the Society for Vascular Surgery Wound, Ischemia, and foot Infection (WIfI) classification to stratify amputation risk. J Vasc Surg 2017;65:591–593.

31 Darling JD, McCallum JC, Soden PA, Guzman RJ, Wyers MC, Hamdan AD, et al: Predictive ability of the society for vascular surgery wound, ischemia, and foot infection (WIfI) classification system after first-time lower extremity revascularizations. J Vasc Surg 2017;65:695–704.

32 Zhan LX, Branco BC, Armstrong DG, Mills JL Sr: The society for vascular surgery lower extremity threatened limb classification system based on Wound, Ischemia, and foot Infection (WIfI) correlates with risk of major amputation and time to wound healing. J Vasc Surg 2015;61:939–944.

33 Causey MW, Ahmed A, Wu B, Gasper WJ, Reyzelman A, Vartanian SM, et al: Society for vascular surgery limb stage and patient risk correlate with outcomes in an amputation prevention program. J Vasc Surg 2016;63:1563–1573.

34 Ward R, Dunn J, Clavijo L, Shavelle D, Rowe V, Woo K: Outcomes of critical limb ischemia in an urban, safety net hospital population with high WIfI amputation scores. Ann Vasc Surg 2017;38:84–89.

35 Cull DL, Manos G, Hartley MC, Taylor SM, Langan EM, Eidt JF, et al: An early validation of the society for vascular surgery lower extremity threatened limb classification system. J Vasc Surg 2014;60:1535–1542.

36 Goodney PP, Holman K, Henke PK, Travis LL, Dimick JB, Stukel TA, Fisher ES, Birkmeyer JD: Regional Intensity of vascular care and lower extremity amputation rates. J Vasc Surg 2013;57:1471–1480.

37 Mills JL Sr, Armstrong DG (eds): Strategies to prevent and heal diabetic foot ulcers: building a partnership for amputation. JVS 2010;52(suppl S):1S–103S.

38 Hingorani A, LaMuraglia GM, Henke P, Meissner M, Loretz L, Zinszer KM, Driver VR, Frykberg R, Marston W, Mills JL Sr, Murad MH: The Management of diabetic foot: a clinical practice guideline by the society for vascular surgery in collaboration with the American podiatric medical association and the society of vascular medicine. J Vasc Surg 2016;63(2 suppl):3S–21S.

39 Wang Z, Hasan R, Firwana B, Elraiyah T, Tsapas A, Prokop L, Mills JL Sr, Murad MH: A systematic review and meta-analysis of tests to predict wound healing in diabetic foot. J Vasc Surg 2016;63(2 suppl):22S–28S.

40 Brownrigg JR, Hinchliffe RJ, Apelqvist J, Boyko EJ, Fitridge R, Mills JL, Reekers J, Shearman CP, Zierler RE, Schaper NC: Effectiveness of bedside investigations to diagnose peripheral artery disease among people with diabetes mellitus: a systematic review. Diabetes Metab Res Rev 2016;32(suppl 1):119–127.

41 Yamada T, Ohta T, Ishibashi H, et al: Clinical reliability and utility of skin perfusion pressure measurement in ischemic limbs – comparison with other noninvasive diagnostic methods. J Vasc Surg 2008; 47:318–323.

42 Braun JD, Trinidad-Hernandez M, Perry D, Armstrong DG, Mills JL Sr: Early quantitative evaluation of indocyanine green angiography in patients with critical limb ischemia. J Vasc Surg 2013;57:1213–1218.

43 Armstrong DG, Boulton AJM, Bus SA: Diabetic foot ulcers and their recurrence. N Engl J Med 2017;376: 2367–2375.

44 Bradbury AW, Adam DJ, Bell J, et al: Bypass versus Angioplasty in Severe Ischaemia of the Leg (BASIL) trial: an intention-to-treat analysis of amputation-free and overall survival in patients randomized to a bypass surgery-first or a balloon angioplasty-first revascularization strategy. J Vasc Surg 2010;51(5 suppl):5S–17S.

45 Schmidt A, Ulrich M, Winkler B, et al: Angiographic patency and clinical outcome after balloon-angioplasty for extensive infrapopliteal arterial disease. Catheter Cardiovasc Interv 2010;76:1047–1054.

46 Goodney PP, Travis LL, Brooke BS, et al: Relationship between regional spending on vascular care and amputation rate. JAMA Surg 2014;149:34–42.

47 Prompers L, Huijberts M, Apelqvist J, Jude E, Piaggesi A, Bakker K, et al: High prevalence of ischaemia, infection and serious comorbidity in patients with diabetic foot disease in Europe. Baseline results from the Eurodiale study. Diabetologia 2007;50:18–25.

48 Cavanagh P, Attinger C, Abbas Z, Bal A, Rojas N, Xu ZR: Cost of treating diabetic foot ulcers in five different countries. Diabetes Metab Res Rev 2012;28:107–111.

49 Gaskin DJ, Thorpe RJ Jr, McGinty EE, Bower K, Rohde C, Young JH, et al: Disparities in diabetes: the nexus of race, poverty, and place. Am J Public Health 2014;104:2147–2155.

50 Armstrong DG, Kanda VA, Lavery LA, Marston W, Mills JL Sr, Boulton AJ: Mind the gap: disparity between research funding and costs of care for diabetic foot ulcers. Diabetes Care 2013;36:1815–1817.

51 Mills JL: Lower limb ischemia in patients with diabetic foot ulcers and gangrene: recognition, anatomic patterns and revascularization strategies. Diabetes Metab Res Rev 2016;32(suppl 1):239–245.

52 Morbach S, Kersken J, Lobmann R, Nobels F, Doggen K, Van Acker K: The German and Belgian accreditation models for diabetic foot services. Diabetes Metab Res Rev 2016;32:(suppl 1):318–325.

Joseph L. Mills, Sr., MD
Division of Vascular Surgery and Endovascular Therapy
Michael E. DeBakey Department of Surgery, Baylor College of Medicine
One Baylor Plaza, MS BCM 390, Houston, TX 77030-2411 (USA)
E-Mail joseph.mills@bcm.edu

Piaggesi A, Apelqvist J (eds): The Diabetic Foot Syndrome.
Front Diabetes. Basel, Karger, 2018, vol 26, pp 161–166 (DOI: 10.1159/000480061)

Resistant Infections in the Diabetic Foot: A Frightening Scenario

Carlo Tascini

Department of Infectious Disease, Cotugno Hospital, Napoli, Italy

Abstract

In a world where both the prevalence of diabetes and resistance to antibacterial drugs are rapidly increasing, the emerging diabetic foot infection (DFI), which is caused by resistant and multi-resistant strains, is considered an emergency situation both from a clinical and from an organizative point of view. Both gram-positive and gram-negative strains show an increasing incidence of antibiotic resistance and both the morbidity and mortality of patients with DFI sustained by resistant strains are significantly higher than those of non-resistant DFIs. Besides well-known resistance to penicillin in gram-positive cocci, the new form of enzymatic resistance in gram-negative rods: extended-spectrum beta lactamases, ampicillinase-C and carbapenemase production, not to forget multi-drug resistance, are all creating a new and frightening scenario in DFI, to which only a paradigm shift in treatment strategies, like the atibacterial therapy stewardship programs, may give positive answers in the near future.

Introduction

Approximately one out of eight people with diabetes will develop an infected ulcer during their lifetime [1]. An adequate and timely treatment is important especially in infections caused by resistant bacteria and in infections that occur in frail individuals such as those with diabetic foot infection (DFI). *Staphylococcus aureus* is the most common infecting organism in DFI. Methicillin resistance confers resistance to all beta-lactams except ceftaroline and ceftobiprole. The rate of isolation of methicillin-resistant strains in DFI varies from 46% in Greece [2] to 22% at first visit in Tuscany, Italy [3]. We will try to analyze the complex relationship between the emerging resistant and multi-resistant strains and DFI in order to give an up-to-date and realistic picture of the changing DFI scenario, the problems that the DF specialists may encounter in addressing this issue and possible therapeutic solutions.

Methicillin-Resistant *Staphylococcus Aureus*

Methicillin-resistant *S. aureus* (MRSA) is more often isolated from patients who have been hospitalized in the previous 3 months, have received recently broad-spectrum antibiotic therapy, have had a recent amputation, whose nose is colonized by MRSA, who come from nursing home facility, although Lavery et al. [4] recently found that being a nursing home resident was not a risk factor for MRSA [5].

DFIs caused by MRSA have been thought to be associated with more severe infections, but not all authors agree to this; in fact, Richard et al. [6] did not find any association between MRSA and a longer hospitalization or more amputations, and a recent review found that patients with an isolation of MRSA had similar outcomes with respect to other pathogens [6, 7].

In many countries outside the United States, the distinction of community-acquired MRSA versus healthcare-associated MRSA strains has become less important because of the absence of an outbreak caused by community-acquired MRSA in these countries. The anxiety caused by MRSA forces doctors to prescribe more empiric therapy to treat DFI with coverage for MRSA, but if there is not a correct identification of patients at risk, unnecessary prescription of anti-MRSA therapy might be frequent. In fact, Reveles et al. [8] in a retrospective study, found that a total of 273 patients with DFI (86%) received MRSA antibiotic coverage, resulting in 71% unnecessary use. Therefore, physicians should recognize patients with risk factors for MRSA DFIs in a better manner; or the microbiological diagnosis should be more rapid and reliable using molecular and phenotypic tests to identify MRSA sooner and in an efficient way.

Extended-Spectrum Beta Lactamases, Ampicillinases C and KPC-Kp

In the past decade, other multidrug-resistant organisms have been increasing isolated from DFIs, especially gram-negatives with quinolones resistance, extended-spectrum beta-lactamases (ESBL) or ampicillinases C resistance [9, 10], and even carbapenamases [11].

Fluoroquinolones resistance in gram-negative strains is increasing worldwide: 10 years ago in the United States, Citron et al. [12] found that only 6% of gram-negative strains isolated from DFIs were resistant to levofloxacin, while recently we found that more than 50% of culture-positive samples obtained in DFI treated with levofloxacin were positive for gram-negative rods resistant to levofloxacin [3].

Therefore, in this study, fluoroquinolone monotherapy is seen as a much less effective therapy contrary to the findings of previous reports [13]. The reason for such a low eradication rate is probably due to the fact that many samples were found to be polymicrobial and many isolates showed a reduced susceptibility to this class of antibiotics compared to other classes, probably due to the wide use of these drugs in the general clinical practice. Fluoroquinolones are also likely to select resistant strains. Levofloxacin showed a higher capacity to select resistant strains, especially gram-negative. According to the "mutant selection window model," the window is a drug concentration range within which mutants are selectively enriched and the mutant prevention concentration is the upper boundary of the window for a single-step mutant. Levofloxacin might have a higher mutant prevention concentration than other fluoroquinolones; therefore, it is able to select more resistant isolates than other molecules of the same class active against gram-negative rods [14].

In developing countries, among diabetic patients, there is an increased rate of multi-drug resistant (MDR) gram-negative rods in the DFI. ESBL are enzymes capable of hydrolizing a third generation of cephalosporins and aztreonam; therefore, carbapenems are drugs utilized to treat these kinds of infections. Piperacillin/tazobactam or amoxicillin/clavulanate might be an alternative, although not all experts are confident with therapies different from carbapenem in curing ESBL infections [15–17].

In Africa, in diabetic patients with asymptomatic bacteruria, the rate of production of *Escherichia coli* ESBL is around 70% [18]. Rawat et al. [19], in India, found high rates of antibiotic resistance among all enterobacteria isolated in every kind of infection in diabetic patients: ESBL in 40% of cases and ampicillinases C β-lactamase (other class of enzyme capable to hydrolyze cephalosporins) in 32.5% of cases of Enterobacteria.

ESBL was found in 10% of DFI at first visit in Italy, where the rate of ESBL isolates is more than 25% in the hospitals and lower, but still high in the community [3]. ESBL strains diffusion has resulted in the overuse of carbapenem and selection of carbepenem-resistant *Klebsiella* spp and carbapenem-resistant non-fermenting gram-negative rods.

Carbapenemase-producing *Klebsiella pneumoniae* (KPC-Kp) is a strain resistant to all beta-lactams (except the new molecule ceftazidime avibactam, which is still not available in many European countries), quinolones and many other classes of antibiotics. The available antibiotic that is still active is colistin (but resistance is increasing), gentamicin and tigecycline. KPC might be advantaged by diabetes; in fact, in Israel, the risk of KPC-Kp infections in colonized patients is increased by 4.4-fold by the presence of diabetes [20].

We recently described an outbreak of colonization and infection of KPC-Kp in DFI patients in our Hospital Pisa, Italy. A subgroup of DFI patients with colonization and infection due to KPC-Kp had a particularly high risk for mortality. This risk was independent from the severity of the diabetic foot wound, determined on the basis of the University of Texas Score System and Charlson co-morbidity score [11]. More recently, an International multi-centric study confirmed that KPC-Kp colonization and DFI infection were independent risk factors for mortality (Fig. 1) [21].

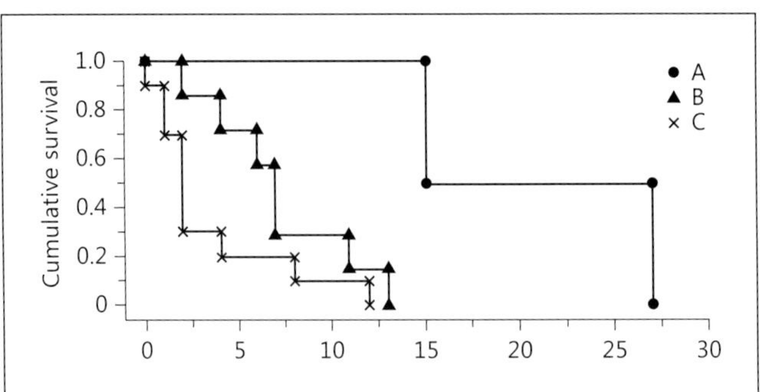

Fig. 1. Kaplan Meier curve of survival at 30 days of patients with DFI infections and gut colonization due to KPC-Kp, patients with DFI due to KPC-Kp but without gut colonization due to KPC-Kp and patients with DFI not due to KPC-Kp neither gut colonization due to KPC-Kp. Group A: patients with diabetic foot infection due to KPC-Kp; group B: patients with gut KPC-Kp colonization and DFI associated to micro-organisms different from KPC-Kp; group C: patients without KPC-Kp gut colonization and in which DFI is related to micro-organisms different from KPC-Kp.

MDR Strains

DFI caused by MDR *Pseudomonas aeruginosa* strains are difficult to treat because the available therapeutic options are limited and sometimes toxic. The therapeutic option is often represented by a single agent when the selection is guided by the susceptibility results. Therefore, monotherapy is often chosen. This may result in suboptimal treatment of the infections and sometimes failure [22]. Strains isolated from DFI in India are all MDR and showed resistance to all beta-lactam including cerbapenem in 20% of cases [23]. Another study from the same country demonstrated resistance to more than 8 antibiotics in 55% of cases [24].

We described the efficacy of a combination of colistin plus rifampin in DFI and osteomyelitis. Also, the addition of imipenem to the previous combination might be effective; colistin should always be used in combination, and adverse events (e.g., renal toxicity) were rare also in this setting of frail patients [25, 26].

The problem of increased antibiotic resistance in DFI is especially important in countries with low adherence to the national antibiotic policy and in hospitals without any antibiotic stewardship programs.

References

1   Lipsky BA, Berendt AR, Deery HG, Embil JM, Joseph WS, Karchmer AW, et al: Diagnosis and treatment of diabetic foot infections. Clin Infect Dis 2004; 39:885–910.

2   Tentolouris N, Petrikkos G, Vallianou N, Zachos C, Daikos GL, Tsapogas P, et al: Prevalence of methicillin-resistant *Staphylococcus aureus* in infected and uninfected diabetic foot ulcers. Clin Microbiol Infect 2006;12:186–189.

3   Tascini C, Piaggesi A, Tagliaferri E, Iacopi E, Fondelli S, Tedeschi A, Rizzo L, Leonildi A, Menichetti F: Microbiology at first visit of moderate-to-severe diabetic foot infection with antimicrobial activity and a survey of quinolone monotherapy. Diabetes Res Clin Pract 2011;94:133–139.

4   Lavery LA, Fontaine JL, Bhavan K, Kim PJ, Williams JR, Hunt NA: Risk factors for methicillin-resistant *Staphylococcus aureus* in diabetic foot infections. Diabet Foot Ankle 2014;5.

5   Ertugrul BM, Oncul O, Tulek N, et al: A prospective, multi-center study: factors related to the management of diabetic foot infections. Eur J Clin Microbiol Infect Dis 2012;31:2345–2352.

6   Richard JL, Sotto A, Jourdan N, Combescure C, Vannereau D, Rodier M: Risk factors and healing impact of multidrug-resistant bacteria in diabetic foot ulcers. Diabetes Metab 2008;34(4 pt 1):363–369.

7   Zenelaj B, Bouvet C, Lipsky BA, Uckay I: Do diabetic foot infections with methicillin-resistant *Staphylococcus aureus* differ from those with other pathogens?. Int J Low Extrem Wounds 2014;13:263–272.

8   Reveles KR, Duhon BM, Moore RJ, Hand EO, Howell CK: Epidemiology of methicillin-resistant *Staphylococcus aureus* diabetic foot infections in a large academic hospital: implications for antimicrobial stewardship. PLoS One 2016;11:e0161658.

9   Turhan V, Mutluoglu M, Acar A, et al: Increasing incidence of gram-negative organisms in bacterial agents isolated from diabetic foot ulcers. J Infect Dev Ctries 2013;7:707–712.

10   Islam S, Cawich SO, Budhooram S, et al: Microbial profile of diabetic foot infections in Trinidad and Tobago. Prim Care Diabetes 2013;7:303–308.

11   Tascini C, Lipsky B, Iacopi E, et al: KPC-producing *Klebsiella pneumoniae* rectal colonization is a risk factor for mortality in patients with diabetic foot infections. Clin Microbiol Inf 2015 21:790.e1–e3.

12   Citron DM, Goldstein EJ, Merriam CV, Lipsky BA, Abramson MA: Bacteriology of moderate-to-severe diabetic foot infections and in vitro activity of antimicrobial agents. J Clin Microbiol 2007;45:2819–2828.

13   Lipsky BA, Giordano P, Choudhri S, Song J: Treating diabetic foot infections with sequential intravenous to oral moxifloxacin compared with piperacillin – tazobactam/amoxicillin – clavulanate. J Antimicrob Chemother 2007;60:370–376.

14   Firsov AA, Vostrov SN, Lubenko IY, Drlica K, Portnoy YA, Zinner SH: In vitro pharmacodynamic evaluation of the mutant selection window hypothesis using four fluoroquinolones against *Staphylococcus aureus*. Antimicrob Agents Chemother 2003;47:1604–1613.

15   Retamar P, López-Cerero L, Muniain MA, Pascual Á, Rodríguez-Baño J; ESBL-REIPI/GEIH Group: Impact of the MIC of piperacillin-tazobactam on the outcome of patients with bacteremia due to extended-spectrum-b-lactamase-producing *Escherichia coli*. Antimicrob Agents Chemother 2013;57:3402–3404.

16   Ng TM, Khong WX, Harris PN, De PP, Chow A, Tambyah PA, Lye DC: Empiric piperacillin-tazobactam versus carbapenems in the treatment of bacteremia due to extended-spectrum-b-lactamase-producing Enterobacteriaceae. PLoS One 2016;11:e0153696.

17   Tamma PD, Han JH, Rock C, Harris AD, Lautenbach E, Hsu AJ, Avdic E, Cosgrove SE; Antibacterial Resistance Leadership Group: Carbapenem therapy is associated with improved survival compared with piperacillin-tazobactam for patients with extended-spectrum-β-lactamase-producing. Clin Infect Dis 2015;61:143.

18   Njunda AL, Assob NJC, Nsagha SD, et al: Uropathogen from diabetic patients with asymptomatic bacteriuria and urinary tract infections. Sci J Microbiol 2012;1:141–146.

19   Rawat V, Singhai M, Kumar A, Jha PK, Goyal R: Bacteriological and resistance profile in isolates from diabetic patients. N Am J Med Sci 2012;4:563–568.

20   Borer A, Saidel-Odes L, Eskira S, et al: Risk factors for developing clinical infections with carbapenem-resistant *Klebsiella pneumoniae* in hospital patients initially only colonized with carbapenem-resistant *Klebsiella pneumoniae*. Am J Infect Control 2012;40:421–425.

21   Iacopi E, Tascini C, Puerta Quintero J, Russo A, De Giglio R, Coppelli A, Bassetti M, Di Caprio G, Venditti M, Menichetti F, Piaggesi A: "Infection and gut colonization by KPC producing *Klebsiella Pneumoniae* as risk factors for mortality in patients with diabetic foot infections: a multicentre case-control study". Diabetes 2016:A167.

22   Paterson D, Cornaglia G, Mazzariol A, Lauretti L, Rossolini GM, Fontana R: Hospital outbreak of carbapenem-resistant *Pseudomonas aeruginosa* producing VIM-1, a novel transferable metallo-beta-lactamase. Clin Infect Dis 2000;31:1119–1125.

23   Vinodkumar CS, Hiresave S, Kandagal Giriyapal B, Bandekar N: Metallo beta lactamase producing *Pseudomonas aeruginosa* and its association with diabetic foot. Indian J Surg 2011;73:291–294.

24   Sivanmaliappan TS, Sevanan M: Antimicrobial susceptibility patterns of *Pseudomonas aeruginosa* from diabetic patients with foot ulcers. Int J Microbiol 2011;605–615.

25 Tascini C, Menichetti F, Gemignani G, Palumbo F, Leonildi A, Tedeschi A, Piaggesi A: Clinical and microbiological efficacy of colistin therapy in combination with rifampin and imipenem in multidrug-resistant *Pseudomonas aeruginosa* diabetic foot infection with osteomyelitis. Int J Lower Extremity Wounds 2006;5:213–216.

26 Tascini C, Gemignani G, Palumbo F, Leonildi A, Tedeschi A, Lambelet P, Lucarini A, Piaggesi A, Menichetti F: Clinical and microbiological efficacy of colistin therapy alone or in combination as treatment for multidrug resistant *Pseudomonas aeruginosa* diabetic foot infections with or without osteomyelitis. J Chemother 2006;18:648–651.

Carlo Tascini, MD
Department of Infectious Disease, Cotugno Hospital
Via Quagliariello 54
IT–80131 Napoli (Italy)
E-Mail carlo.tascini@libero.it

Piaggesi A, Apelqvist J (eds): The Diabetic Foot Syndrome.
Front Diabetes. Basel, Karger, 2018, vol 26, pp 167–183 (DOI: 10.1159/000480099)

Antibacterial Treatment in Diabetic Foot Infections

Eric Senneville[a, b]

[a] Department of Infectious Diseases, Gustave Dron Hospital, Tourcoing, and [b] French Reference Center for Osteo-Articular Infections (CRIOAC Lille-Tourcoing), Faculty of Medicine, Lille University 2, Lille, France

Abstract

Diabetic foot infections (DFIs) are very frequent conditions that lead to the prescription of antibiotics. Skin and soft tissue infections are distinct with regard to the management of osteomyelitis but are seen concomitantly in a high proportion of patients. The propensity of physicians to prescribe broad-spectrum intravenous antibiotics in a majority of patients presenting with an infection of the foot is responsible for an overuse of these agents in these settings and is likely to participate in the emergence of multiresistant bacterial strains. Current international guidelines insist on the necessity to first determine the existence of an infection by using validated diagnostic criteria and second distinguish some clinical entities in order to prescribe antibiotics in the most appropriate manner. The quality of the microbiological assessment is of major importance and avoiding swab sampling is now widely recommended. It is also important to keep in mind that antibiotics are used for the treatment of infection and therefore should not be continued until the wound is completely healed or more antibiotics should not be used in an attempt to help wound healing. A crucial contribution can be made by infectious disease specialists in the management of such complex and potentially severe infections.

Introduction

Antibiotics represent the vast majority of the anti-infectious agents prescribed for treating diabetic foot infections (DFIs). The difficulties in prescribing antibiotics to patients with DFIs reside in the necessity of respecting 2 objectives that are a priori incompatible: (I) reduce the risk of severe complications including limb loss and even death (i.e., the temptation to prescribe widely broad-spectrum antibiotics) and (ii) preserve the antibiotics activity (i.e., the obligation to prescribe narrow spectrum antibiotics and to avoid unjustified antibiotic prescriptions). The risk of the emergence of highly resistant strains represents indeed a global threat, which is discussed elsewhere in this book (see chapter 13). This threat has however promoted the development of antibacterial therapies not using systemic antibiotics, including topical treatment with antibiotics, antibacterial peptides and bacteriophages.

Different national and international guidelines currently available provide useful information on the indication, prescription and surveillance of antibiotic therapies (ATs) in patients with DFIs. This chapter aims to present the most recent recommendations in the field and to comment these recommendations in the light of the recent data published about the question of antibacterial therapies in patients with DFIs.

Soft Tissue Infections

Surgical management of DFIs is of paramount importance especially for the most severe of them. Surgery is indeed by far the most efficacious way to decrease the bacterial burden in the infected site to remove all the necrotic tissues and to obtain a decompression of the different infected compartments of the foot, which worsens the problems of blood supply of the infected foot. All these requirements justify the need for a multidisciplinary organization of medical and surgical complementary actions, which has proven efficacy for improving the outcome of such patients.

Indications for Antibiotic Therapy

The high frequency with which DFUs occur leads to a great number of potential opportunities to prescribe antibiotics in these patients. It is therefore essential to define an infected DFU, since this is the unique situation that requires antibiotics in these settings [1]. Since any chronic wound is colonized by bacteria from commensal flora and environmental origin, the development of a bacterial culture from superficial samples (e.g., swabs) cannot be used as an indication for prescribing antibiotics even in cases of virulent species like *Staphylococcus aureus* or *Escherichia coli*, for instance. This is also true for high bacteria load defined as $\geq 10^5$ colony forming units per gram of tissue in particular because this concept has not been verified in DFIs and quantitative microbiology is rarely available outside of research laboratories as well [2].

The diagnosis of DFI should therefore be based on clinical findings as proposed by both the Infectious Diseases Society of America (IDSA) and the International Working Group on the Diabetic Foot [1, 3]. The definition of DFI is based on the presence of a least 2 of the following classical signs of skin infection: redness, heat, pain (rare in infected DFUs), tenderness and pus discharge [1, 3]. The infection severity is classified into 3 grades (i.e., 2–4; 1 corresponding to a DFU without signs of infection) according to (i) the extension in surface (grade 2), (ii) to the extension in depth in particular with the extension to the underlying osteo-articular structures (grade 3), and (iii) to the existence of systemic signs of infection (grade 4). This classification is part of the global perfusion extension depth infection sensation classification that permits clinicians to categorize the patients with DFIs and is especially useful for conducting clinical research in this domain [1].

ATs for DFIs must obey the general rules of prescription of antibiotics, especially the following rules: (i) antibiotics should be limited to the patients with DFIs, (ii) the antibacterial spectrum of the antibiotics should be as narrow as possible, (iii) the duration should be as short as possible, including the intravenous part of the treatment, (iv) the choice of the antibiotic(s) should take into account its/their potential of selection of antibacterial resistance and, (v) the choice of the treatment should integrate the risk for potential severe antibiotic-related adverse effects due to the co-morbidities frequently encountered in these patients.

In this regard, to cure DFIs, the IDSA recommends the prescription of antibiotics with the following characteristics: (I) proven efficacy in treating DFI, (ii) must be able to act against the more common Gram-positive cocci encountered in DFIs and (iii) must have limited coverage of Gram-negative rods when these agents are unlikely. The IDSA also recommends that chronic DFIs, those previously treated with antibiotics and those with signs of infection severity should initially be treated with broad-spectrum antibiotics [1].

Once DFI is diagnosed, its outcome is usually difficult to predict and the potential consequences of delay in treating DFIs can be particularly severe including limb and even life loss. Taking these 2 elements into account, the current recommendations are to start the antibiotic treatment in these patients as early as possible after obtaining appropriate specimens for culture [1, 3], as molecular biological techniques to identify both the bacteria present in the samples and the presence of resistant strains are not yet available in the routine practice. Although these techniques exist at present, the AT is necessarily empirical in most patients presenting with DFIs. However, the empirical prescription of antibiotics for DFIs exposes the risk of overestimating the need for broad-spectrum antibiotics and therefore to overuse these agents. It is not yet clear in which situations physicians could wait for the results of samples culture before prescribing a targeted (as opposed to empirical) antibiotic treatment.

Microbiological Assessment

The aims of the microbiological assessment of DFIs are to identify the bacteria involved in the infectious process (i.e., the pathogens) and to determine their antibiotic susceptibility profile. Microbiological examination should be considered in a patient only with a DFI: DFUs should not be sampled, as these lesions are almost constantly colonized by bacteria and the microbiological results represent a clear incitation for prescribing ATs. Since no criteria can help in the routine practice to distinguish pathogens from contaminant agents cultured in a sample, the best way to identify the pathogen(s) is to obtain tissue material, provided the surface of the lesion has been cleansed before sampling. Bacteria cultured from a tissue sample are indeed very likely to have a pathogenic effect and not a contaminant that can only stay on the surface of the ulcer. The difficulty remains, however, to obtain these samples in the routine practice. It is indeed much easier to perform a swab than curettage or even a soft tissue biopsy (biopsy-punch) or a trans-cutaneous aspiration. The curettage of the ulcer surface after cleansing of the ulcer using sterile saline solution represents a satisfactory compromise [1, 3]. A recent cross-sectional multicentre large study compared the results of microbiology specimens for culture taken contemporaneously by swab and by tissue sampling from the same DFU; the 2 sampling techniques reported a difference in the identity and the number of pathogens for 58 and 50.4% of patients respectively [4]. It must be noted, however, that wound cultures may be difficult to obtain in the absence of an ulceration, which is however a rare situation in patients with DFIs and should rise the question of a non-infectious origin of the inflamed foot, especially an acute Charcot foot.

A Gram-stained smear of a wound specimen can help direct empiric AT, in particular, on the need of covering Gram-negative rods. New diagnostic molecular techniques, such as those using real-time polymerase chain reactions performed on tissue samples can also rapidly identify some multiresistant pathogens and potentially reduce empirical use of broad-spectrum antibiotics. These techniques, however, have not yet been proven to modify the outcome of those patients and are not yet implemented in the routine practice of most physicians [5]. Another question of importance is to define in which situations some patients with DFIs could be treated without any microbiological assessment of the ulcer. Patients with acute/superficial (A/S) DFIs, no previous antibiotic treatment within at least 6 months prior to the current episode of DFI and living in a region where the prevalence of resistant bacteria such as methicillin-resistant *S. aureus* (MRSA) or extended-spectrum beta-lactamase (ESBL) producing Enterobacteriaceae could probably be managed this way, but data on this point has never been reported so far.

Antibiotic Therapy

The multitude of parameters likely to influence the choice of the initial empirical antibiotic treatment makes this decision difficult to make. When the need for reducing the selection pressure on the microbiota is taken into account, this becomes particularly difficult. These aspects of the prescription of antibiotics in patients with DFIs justify the recommendations of both IDSA and International Working Group on the Diabetic Foot to seek advice from infectious diseases specialists in the settings of complex situations [1, 3].

Narrow versus Broad-Spectrum Antibiotic Therapy

It is generally believed that all DFIs are polymicrobial and therefore require broad-spectrum antibiotic regimens. This is a common false belief that is responsible for the over-prescription of unjustified broad-spectrum antibiotics in patients presenting with a DFI. It is indeed essential to distinguish (A/S) from chronic/deep (C/D) DFIs simply because the microbiome involved in these 2 entities are different and therefore should not always be treated with the same antibiotic regimens. Indeed, A/S DFIs are usually monomicrobial, caused by aerobic gram-positive cocci (i.e., *S. aureus* and beta-haemolytic streptococci [BHS]), whereas polymicrobial flora, including aerobic gram-negative (i.e., *E. coli*, *Klebsiella pneumoniae*, *Proteus* spp.,) and obligate anaerobic bacteria (i.e., *Finegoldia magna*,) are likely to be involved in C/D DFIs [1, 2]. The aspect of the ulcer including colour, odour and necrosis should be noted, as they can represent an orientation towards some particular microbiological aetiology. Overall, *S. aureus* is by far the most frequent pathogen isolated in patients with DFIs. This may not be true in warm climate countries especially in Africa and Asia where it is now well established that gram-negative organisms (especially *Pseudomonas aeruginosa*) are, for unclear reasons, the most frequent isolates in DFIs [1].

Of note, empirical antibiotic regimens that cover most, but not all, bacteria present on cultures, generally lead to clinical cure. For instance, although enterococci and *P. aeruginosa* are frequently identified from chronic wounds, especially if antibiotics such as cephalosporins with no activity against *P. aeruginosa* have been previously administered, it has been shown that the non-coverage of these bacteria is unlikely to decrease the chances for cure [6]. The severity of the infection including local and systemic signs is of great importance in the antibiotic choice, as the more severe situations should be managed with a minimum probability of inadequate initial treatment in order to limit the risk of deterioration of the infection, although this relation has not been clearly established in these settings. However, the decision to use broad-spectrum antibiotic regimens is not without consequences, as it exposes the patient to a high pressure of selection of resistant bacteria not only in his own microbiota but also in his environment due to the possible diffusion of the bacteria and/or the genetic material supporting the antibacterial resistance [7]. Other parameters such as the patient medical history relative to any previous hospitalization, systemic or local antibiotic administration and previous multiresistant infections or carriage are important to assess. Patient's characteristics regarding allergy or expected intolerance to antibiotics due to any co-morbid condition and/or possible drug-drug interaction are also likely to influence the choice of the antibiotic regimens.

Choice of Antibiotics

As discussed above, the antibiotic treatment for superficial and recent (i.e., less than 2 weeks) infected DFUs should target *S. aureus* and BHS. Beta-lactams are considered first-line antibiotics in these settings because of their favourable toxicity profile, their bactericidal activity and their good diffusion ability except in bone and joint structures. Of note, the need for bactericidal AT in skin and skin structure infections has been questioned in a recent meta-analysis conducted by Nemeth et al. [8]. Group A penicillin (e.g., ampicillin and amoxicillin) have no place as empirical treatment because of the secretion of a penicillinase by most staphylococci that inactivates these antibiotics. On the contrary, amoxicillin-clavulanic acid (co-amoxiclav) covers both MSSA and BHS. Two elements should, nevertheless, be taken into account: first, co-amoxiclav is inactive against MRSA and second this combination of antibiotics is likely to cause intestinal adverse effects especially *Clostridium difficile*-associated diarrhoea and to result in a high selection pressure on the gut microbiota probably because of its activity against the anaerobic bacterial flora.

Clindamycin may be indicated in case of allergy to beta-lactams; this antibiotic can cause *Clostridium difficile*-associated diarrhoea and dysgeusia. Clindamycin is usually active against community-acquired MRSA, but patients with MRSA-related DFIs are likely to be infected with hospital-acquired MRSA rather than community-acquired MRSA.

According to recent studies, the prevalence of MRSA in DFIs is estimated to range from 5 to 30% [9]. Risk factors for MRSA-related DFIs include prior long-term or inappropriate use of antibiotics, previous hospitalization, long duration of the foot wound, the presence of osteomyelitis and nasal carriage of MRSA. The most reliable predictor for MRSA as a cause of DFI is a previous history of MRSA infection [10]. The coverage of multiresistant MRSA is a matter of concern, as the number of antibiotic agents active against this bacteria are limited to a few classes such as glycopeptides (i.e., vancomycin and teicoplanin), and cyclic lipopeptides (i.e., daptomycin) and oxazolidinones (linezolid). The role of cephalosporins with anti-MRSA activity (i.e., ceftobiprole and ceftaroline) has only been evaluated in a few studies of patients with DFIs [11, 12]. The oxazolidinone agent linezolid has the advantage over the other cited drugs to be available as both oral and intravenous formulations, which helps decrease the duration of the hospital stay. The recommended duration of the antibiotic treatment for DFIs (i.e., less than 2 weeks) makes the risk of bone marrow toxicity, especially anaemia and thrombocytopenia unlikely to occur. However, the interaction with some drugs like mono-amine oxydative anti-depressors and some analgesics may limit the indication of this antibiotic. The new compound tedizolid is likely to have a better tolerance profile, but data in the treatment of DFIs is currently unavailable.

While the prevalence of MRSA is currently decreasing in the majority of western Europe countries and in the United States probably as a result of the improved hospital infection control measures, ESBL-producing Enterobacteriaceae, especially *E. coli* is out of control worldwide at least in part because of the incomplete efficacy of hygiene and infection control measures that are exactly opposite to the control measures observed with MRSA. The coverage of ESBL-producing Enterobacteriaceae poses many problems. The number of antibiotics active against these bacteria is indeed limited to some broad-spectrum beta-lactam agents, aminoglycosides, polypeptides, fosfomycine and phenicoles. Among BL agents, carbapenems display the best activity; however, the current spread of carbapenemases-producing Enterobacteriaceae calls for prudent decision making regarding the empirical use of these agents. The use of carbapenems should be considered only in the most severe patients (i.e., those presenting with septic shock) in combination with a complete coverage of Gram-positive cocci including MRSA (i.e., glyco/lipo-peptide agents) and amikacin in the absence of contraindications.

Polypeptide agents (colistine), fosfomycin and phenicoles have not proven their efficacy in treating the most severe DFIs and are limited by their potential toxicity in particular, on kidney (colistin), metabolic (fosfomycin) and bone marrow (phenicoles) regions. BL agents that can be used empirically in patients with DFIs suspected of being related to ESBL-producing organisms including carbapenems and cephalosporins of the 3rd and 4th generations, depending on the value of the MIC of the strains. Among the new cephalosporins-betalactamase inhibitor combinations, ceftolozane-tazobactam and ceftazidime-avibactam may also be active against these bacteria. These 2 antibiotics exhibit poor activity against gram-positive cocci including MRSA and against strict anaerobes and should therefore not be prescribed as empirical monotherapy in the setting of most severe DFIs.

The adjunction of aminoglycosides is likely to enhance the clearance of bacteria from blood and again may be beneficial for patients with the most severe DFIs. Aminoglycosides should be administered for short periods of time due to the potentially renal toxicity of these agents, especially in patients with chronic renal failure. The threat related to the spread of highly resistant bacteria in these settings, especially carbapenem resistant gram-negative rods and vancomycin-resistant enterococci, is discussed in Chapter 13.

Table 1 summarizes the empirical antibiotic regimens that can be proposed in patients presenting with DFIs based on the clinical situation and the risk of resistant bacteria.

Antibiotic Therapy and Microbiological Assessment

Whatever the AT used, it is recommended to assess the outcome of the patient, especially the local signs of infection within 2–3 days after the beginning of the AT in light of the culture results of the ulcer samples and to decide on the choice of treatment. It is recommended to narrow the spectrum of the AT as much as possible; in case of a satisfactory outcome, the treatment should not be modified even if the bacteria cultured from the samples are not covered by the empirical treatment. In cases where the initial empirical AT is too broad regarding the microbiological results and the patient condition is improving, it is recommended to de-escalate towards a narrower spectrum antibiotic. When the infection is worsening and the culture results indicate that the initial AT did not cover the pathogens, AT needs to be changed in order to cover

Table 1. Selecting an empiric antibiotic treatment for diabetic foot infections (modify from [3])

Infection Severity	Usual Pathogen(s)	Potential Empirical Regimens
Mild Acute infection (i.e., lasting ≤2 weeks)	*S. aureus* Beta-haemolytic streptococci	Group M penicillin (e.g., oxacillin, cloxacillin, …); 1st-generation cephalosporin (cephalexin)
Acute infection (i.e., lasting ≤2 weeks) and β-lactams known allergy and/or intolerance	*S. aureus* Beta-haemolytic streptococci	Clindamycin Trimethoprim-sulfametoxazole Doxycycline
Chronic infection (i.e., lasting >2 weeks) Recent antibiotic exposure	*S. aureus* Beta-haemolytic streptococci and Enterobacteriaceae (e.g. *E. coli*, *K. pneumoniae*, *P. mirabilis*, …)	Co-amoxiclav Trimethoprim-sulfametoxazole
High risk for MRSA	MRSA	Trimethoprim-Sulfametoxazole Add linezolid or lipo/glycopeptide if BL is considered
Moderate and Severe Acute infection (i.e., lasting ≤2 weeks)	*S. aureus* Beta-haemolytic streptococci	Co-amoxiclav 3rd-generation cephalosporin (cefotaxime, ceftriaxone)
Chronic infection (i.e., lasting >2 weeks) Recent antibiotic exposure	*S. aureus* Beta-haemolytic streptococci and Enterobacteriaceae (e.g., *E. coli*, *K. pneumoniae*, *P. mirabilis*, …) and Strict anaerobes (*Finegoldia magna.*, *Bacteroides* spp., *Clostridium* spp., etc.)	Broad spectrum B-IBL (piperacillin-tazobactam) or 3rd-generation cephalosporin (except ceftazidime) + metronidazole or carbapenem
Macerated ulcer, warm climate	GNB, including *Pseudomonas*	B-IBL (piperacillin-tazobactam) or Carbapenem (except ertapenem) +/− aminoglycoside (amikacin, tobramycin)
MRSA risk factors		Add linezolid or lipo/glycopeptide if BL is considered
Risk factors for resistant GNR	ESBL	Carbapenem (except ertapenem), aminoglycoside, colistin; in combination if feasible

B-IBL, beta-lactam plus betalactamase inhibitor; GNB, gram-negative bacilli.

Senneville

all isolated organisms. In case of worsening infection despite the initial AT covering all the identified pathogens, the cause of this discrepancy should be searched for and corrected. The causes could be any one of these factors: a collection that has to be drained, lack of blood supply to the limb, a problem in the compliance of the patient to the treatment especially in case of oral AT or a drug-drug interaction.

Route of Therapy

An important goal when prescribing antibiotics for DFIs is to achieve high blood concentrations, as there is no barrier between blood and infected foot tissues including bone. Intravenous administration is the most efficient way to rapidly obtain high blood concentrations. This mode of administration prevents under dosing due to problems in oral intake and/of oral bioavailability of the antibiotic. Intravenous administration, however, exposes patients to complications such as catheter-related infections including bacteraemia and thromboses and is likely to prolong the hospital stay and to augment the overall costs as well. This method of treatment should therefore be reserved to treat severe infectious cases where bacteraemia is likely and/or the prognosis of the foot/limb is being threatened, when there is no oral formulation of the molecule to administer or when the patient is unable to take it orally.

Oral antibiotic agents with complete bioavailability are limited to fluoroquinolones, especially levofloxacin and ofloxacin, oxazolidinones, clindamycin, trimethoprim-sulfametoxazole, metronidazole, rifampicin, doxycycline and fusidic acid [12]. These molecules also have the ability to achieve high tissue concentrations including bone with a bone/blood ratio exceeding 0.3 for all of them [13].

The use of systemic AT is responsible for the selection of resistant bacteria among the commensal flora especially in the gut and the skin. Topical AT has long been accused of promoting the selection of bacterial resistance at the site where the antibiotic is administered. However, due to insufficient diffusion into deep tissues, topical AT is indicated only in non-severe (i.e., low risk of systemic diffusion of the infection) and superficial infected wounds. Topical antibiotics such as gentamicin and neomycin can cause allergic contact dermatitis [14]. In order to alleviate the selection pressure of antibiotics on the bacterial flora present in the infected wound and at the periphery of the lesions, the use of non-antibiotic antibacterial agents is appealing. A topical antimicrobial peptide (Pexiganan) has been compared to an oral fluoroquinolone agent (ofloxacin) for the treatment of infected DFU in a randomized controlled study, which showed similar clinical improvement rates achieved in the 2 treatment group (85–90%) [15]. The in vitro activity of Pexiganan is not influenced by the resistance profile of the strains to antibiotics including those with a multiresistant profile [16]. Topical AT can also be used as an adjuvant to a systemic antibiotic treatment. One trial showed that daily application of a topical gentamicin-collagen sponge in addition to systemic levofloxacin was associated to a higher clinical cure rate at the test of cure visit (2 weeks after discontinuation of therapy) in patients with a moderate DFI [17]. Not only antibiotic-loaded sponges but also beads can be used in deep surgical wounds and they are particularly useful for filling dead spaces that may persist after surgical drainage of severe DFIs and/or (Diabetic Foot Osteomyelitis) DFOs [18, 19].

Bacteriophages represent an interesting research direction in the field of DFIs. These viruses can kill and lyse the infecting pathogenic bacteria, are self-replicating and have been proven to be safe in various animal models [20]. A cocktail of five lytic members of the family Myoviridae or Podoviridae showed antibacterial effects on both planktonic and biofilm cells including 3 bacteria frequently identified in DFIs (i.e., *S. aureus*, *P. aeruginosa* and *Acinetobacter baumannii*) [21]. In a recent report, a single administration of a lytic bacteriophage exhibited efficacy similar to that of linezolid in resolving the course of hind paw infection in diabetic animals and the combination of the 2 agents was more effective in arresting the entire infection process associated with a better tissue healing [22]. The current place of bacteriophages in the armamentarium for the treatment of DFIs is not yet clearly established in the absence of clinical human studies. Topical therapies could probably be considered in an attempt to reduce the consumption of antibiotics in patients with mild to moderate DFIs, whereas the use of bacteriophages should probably be restricted to infections due to difficult-to-treat infections related to highly resistant bacteria.

Duration of Therapy

The optimal durations of AT for DFIs is a subject of debate. Recent trends regarding the AT are to decrease as much as possible the length of exposition of the patient to antibiotics in an attempt to decrease the adverse effects among which the selection of resistance appears nowadays as one of the most important effects. The data from recent published studies suggests that 1 to 2 weeks seem sufficient in mild and moderate DFIs, whereas 2 to 3 weeks seem adequate for more severe infections [1, 3]. As antibiotics have not proven to promote wound healing, it is important to stop the antibiotic treatment once signs of infection have disappeared and not to wait for wound healing.

Diabetic Foot Osteomyelitis

DFO is a consequence of the spread of the skin tissue infection to the contiguous bone and joint structures underlying a DFU that may be present in up to 20% to more than 60% of DFIs according to the severity of the infection [1]. DFO augments the duration of AT, of hospital stay, of relapsing infection and the risk of amputation [23].

Microbiology

DFO is usually of polymicrobial origin and in almost all reported DFO series, *S. aureus* is the most common pathogen cultured from bone samples, followed by *S. epidermidis*, Enterobacteriaceae and *P. aeruginosa* [1]. The frequency of isolation of obligate anaerobes is generally low but depends on the method by which the bone fragments are sampled and transported to the laboratory. In a recent retrospective study, molecular techniques (16S rRNA sequencing) applied to the assessment of bone biopsies showed more anaerobes and more Gram-positive bacilli compared to conventional techniques (86.9 vs. 23.1%, $p = 0.001$ and 78.3 vs. 3.8%, $p < 0.001$ respectively) [24].

The concordance between superficial samples including swabs, needle aspiration and even tissue biopsies with bone cultures is low. It is therefore recommended that the choice of an antimicrobial agent for treating osteomyelitis should optimally be based on the results of a bone culture, especially because of the need for long-duration therapy [3]. Bone culture results allow to target the bone pathogens, especially in cases of uncertain diagnosis of osteomyelitis despite imaging evaluations, in cases where data from soft tissue cultures is non-informative, or when the infection has failed to respond to initial empiric antibiotic therapy [1, 3]. In addition, bone cultures permit to prescribe appropriate combinations of antibiotics with high potential for selecting resistant organisms such as rifampicin, fluoroquinolones, fusidic acid or clindamycin in decreasing the risk of selection of a resistant mutant that may occur if the pathogen(s) is(are) resistant to one component of the combination. As *S. aureus* is the most common pathogen responsible for DFI, it should be covered by any AT based on non-bone culture results.

Antibiotic Therapy

While DFO usually requires the resection of all or parts of the infected bone(s) (i.e., surgical approach), it is now well established that sustained remission can be obtained with antibiotic therapy only (i.e., medical approach). The clinical remission rates achieved with the medical approach are comparable to those reported in patients treated surgically (i.e., about two-thirds of cases) [25–29]. The majority of the patients reported in these series were treated with highly bioavailable oral agents like fluoroquinolones, clindamycin and rifampicin. These apparent satisfactory results are however limited by the retrospective design of the studies and doubt persists regarding the mode of selection of patients in whom the medical approach was applied.

The initial choice between medical and surgical management of DFO is of paramount importance, as failure of medical treatment of DFO could sometimes result in a more proximal level of amputation when compared to the initial surgical approach [30]. On the other hand, it is important to discuss the alternatives to surgery especially

Table 2. Medical (antibiotic treatment alone) versus surgical (resection of all or part of the infected bone) approaches for diabetic foot osteomyelitis (modified from [32])

Criteria in favour of the medical approach	Criteria in favour of the surgical approach
Patient too unstable for surgery	Substantial bone necrosis
Bad post-operative mechanics likely	Functionally non-salvageable foot
No other need for surgery	Patient is non-ambulatory
Small, forefoot lesion	Major risks of antibiotic problems
No skilled surgeon available	No available active antibiotic
Surgery costs prohibitive	Uncorrectable foot ischemia
Patient preference	Patient preference

when minor or major amputations are considered. In some selected patients with DFO (i.e., neuropathic forefoot ulcers complicated by osteomyelitis, but without ischaemia or necrotizing soft tissue infections which corresponded to only about a third of the patients they evaluated for the study), a prospective, randomized trial found that the outcomes of the treatment of DFO in patients who received exclusively antibiotic therapy (for up to 90 days) versus those who underwent limited resection of the osteomyelitic bone (accompanied by ~10 days of antibiotic therapy) were similar [31]. Some criteria that help choose between medical and surgical approaches are reported in Table 2 (modified from [32]).

Choice of Antibiotics

The currently available data is insufficient for supporting any recommendation on AT for DFO regarding the superiority of any specific antibiotic agent or treatment strategy, route, or duration of therapy [33]. Only one retrospective study of patients with DFO treated non-surgically suggests that AT chosen on the basis of bone culture is associated with a significantly better outcome when compared to empiric therapy [27].

AT chosen on the basis of non-bone tissues (swabs or deeper samples) and prescribed for longer durations than for soft-tissue infection has been classically used with apparently good results [34–36]. However, these studies were retrospective and did not include post-treatment follow-up (i.e., at least one year) enabling to detect late relapsing episodes of DFO.

A bone biopsy is generally obtained in patients with any sort of chronic osteomyelitis in order to best prescribe antibiotic regimens comprising agents with high bone/biofilm diffusion and sustained activity against bacteria in the stationary-growth phase as seen in these chronic infections. Antibiotics exhibiting such properties are limited to rifampicin, fluoroquinolones, clindamycin, linezolid and daptomycin, the latter being available only as intravenous formulation. The propensity of these antibiotics to select resistant mutants that are naturally present in the bacterial population justifies to prescribe these agents only in combination of active agents (i.e., both antibiotics of the combination are active against the pathogen[s]). This represents a strong argument for obtaining a reliable identification of the offending pathogens and their susceptibility profile to antibiotics when the prescription of such antibiotics is considered [1, 3]. The rules of AT for chronic osteomyelitis can be applied to patients with DFO, provided transcutaneous bone culture in patients who do not require surgery is routinely available [27].

It has long been stated that AT of chronic osteomyelitis should be administered parenterally and for prolonged periods of time [37]. These requirements are justified for beta-lactam AT but are questionable for those antibiotics that exhibit almost complete oral bioavailability and can achieve high bone concentrations such as fluoroquinolones, rifampicin (always combined with another agent), clindamycin, linezolid, fusidic acid and trimethoprim-sulfamethoxazole [13]. The switch to oral therapy can be done early with these antibiotics (after about a week of parenteral treatment to complete a course). Combinations of 2 agents with high oral availability and bone diffusion have been shown to arrest DFOs. Rifampicin-fluoroquinolone (oflo/cipro/levo or moxifloxacin) and BL-fluoroquinolones combinations seem appropriate for the treatment of, respectively, staphylococcal and gram-negative DFOs [27, 38]. The antibiotic combination should be continued until the completion of the treatment for staphylococcal DFOs because the risk of emergence of resistant mutants is particularly high with these bacteria [39].

Patients with DFO beyond any therapeutical solution to expect a sustained remission of the infection may receive either intermittent short courses of treatment in cases of recurrent signs of infection or even prolonged long-term suppressive AT. In case of intermittent AT, the changes in the microbiology and antibiotic susceptibility profile of the pathogen(s) should be assessed if the AT efficacy decreases over time. Antibiotics that can be used in these settings should be administrable by oral route, be well-tolerated even over prolonged treatment duration and should not exert a high selective pressure on bacterial resistance. In this regards, cycline agents, especially doxy or minocycline, appear to be suitable agents.

Routes of Administration

Parenteral administration of antibiotics should be considered only if the antibiotic has an incomplete oral bioavailability. This is the case for the glycopeptide agents, vancomycin and teicoplanin, the cyclic lipopeptide, daptomycin, colistin and the aminoglycosides. Oral administration of antibiotics in patients with DFO appears to be more convenient, better tolerated and less expensive than parenteral AT. Some studies have reported satisfactory outcome of patients treated orally for a DFO [27–29, 31]. Two recent reviews of the literature did not find any statistically significant difference

Table 3. Bone penetration of antibiotics that can be administered by both intravenous and oral routes (modified from [13])

Antibiotic, dose, route of administration	Cancellous/cortical concentrations, mg/g	Cancellous/cortical bone-serum ratios, %
Clindamycin 600 mg IV, SD	3.8/–	45/–
Levofloxacin 500 mg IV, SD	6/3	75/–
Ciprofloxacin 200 mg IV, SD	2/1.4	66/47
Ciprofloxacin 750 mg Oral, SD	2.9/1.4	48/–
Moxifloxacin 400 mg Oral, SD	1.9/1.3	39/27
Moxifloxacin 400 mg Oral, MD	2.9/2.5	48/40
Doxycycline 200 mg Oral, SD	2.6/–	86/–
Linezolid 600 600 mg, Oral MD	8.5/–	37/–
Metronidazole 500 mg, Oral, SD	14/–	100/–
Fusidic acid 500 mg, Oral, SD	12/–	44/–

Cancellous and cortical values are specified when known.
IV, intravenous; MD, multiple dose; SD, single dose; TMP-SMX, trimethoprim-sulfamethoxazole.

between oral versus parenteral antibiotics for the treatment of osteomyelitis if the bacteria are sensitive to the antibiotic used [13, 40].

Prolonged parenteral outpatient antibiotic treatment is usually difficult to administer, as some patients with DFO may receive anticoagulation following surgery and/or for any other reason. In this setting, antibiotics are generally administered through a central venous catheter or an implantable port that exposes the patient to catheter-related complications that may occur in up to 21% of patients [41]. Given their once-daily administration, antibiotic agents, such as ceftriaxone, ertapenem, teicoplanin and daptomycin, appear to be particularly suited for outpatient parenteral antibiotic therapy. Interestingly, the antibiotics that achieve highest bone to serum concentration ratios (i.e., fluoroquinolones, sulfamides, cyclines, macrolides, rifamycins, fusidic acid and oxazolidinones) are also those with the highest oral bioavailability making these agents good candidates for prolonged treatment of outpatients with osteomyelitis (Table 3). Antibiotics available as both parenteral and oral routes can be switched when the patient's condition has improved and this helps shorten the duration of the hospital stay.

Duration

Following surgical resection, the residual bone is likely to be vital (i.e., non necrotic) and therefore can be treated with shorter duration of AT than for necrotic infected bones. The IDSA recommends a short duration (2–5 days) when a radical resection leaves no remaining infected tissue, and a prolonged treatment (≥4 weeks) when there is persistent infected and/or necrotic bone [1]. Extending post-debridement antibiotic therapy beyond 6 weeks and giving IV treatment longer than 1 week do not appear to increase the remission rate. A recent randomized controlled trial that compared 6 vs. 12 weeks of antibiotic therapy for non-surgically treated DFO found no significant difference in the remission rate (60 vs. 70% respectively), but significantly fewer adverse effects with the shorter treatment option were observed [42].

Concomitant Skin and Soft Tissue Infection and Diabetic Foot Osteomyelitis of the Foot

While DFU skin and soft tissue infections (SSTI) need non-delayed AT because of the risk of worsening outcome that may lead to infectious gangrene, necrotizing cellulitis especially in case of streptococcal infections and sometimes bacteraemia, DFO as such is not an indication for urgent AT. This allows considering a sequential approach for patients presenting with a DFU SSTIS associated with a contemporary underlying DFO, which is the situation reported in 20 to up to 60% of DFIs [1, 3]. In brief, as bone biopsy cannot generally be performed at the time the diagnosis of DFI is made, it is possible to first treat the DFU SSTI for 7–14 days as recommended by using antibiotics unlikely to sterilize bone tissues and then to perform a transcutaneous bone biopsy after a 2-week antibiotic-free period in order to reduce the risk of false-negative results.

References

1 Lipsky BA, Berendt AR, Cornia PB, Pile JC, Peters EJ, Armstrong DG, Deery HG, Embil JM, Joseph WS, Karchmer AW, Pinzur MS, Senneville E: 2012 Infectious Diseases Society of America clinical practice guideline for the diagnosis and treatment of diabetic foot infections. Clin Infect Dis 2012;54:e132–e173.

2 Kallstrom G: Are quantitative bacterial wound cultures useful? J Clin Microbiol 2014;52:2753–2756.

3 Lipsky BA, Aragón-Sánchez J, Diggle M, Embil J, Kono S, Lavery L, Senneville É, Urbančič-Rovan V, Van Asten S; International Working Group on the Diabetic Foot, Peters EJ: IWGDF guidance on the diagnosis and management of foot infections in persons with diabetes. Diabetes Metab Res Rev 2016; 32(suppl 1):45–74.

4 Nelson EA, Wright-Hughes A, Brown S, Lipsky BA, Backhouse M, Bhogal M, Ndosi M, Reynolds C, Sykes G, Dowson C, Edmonds M, Vowden P, Jude EB, Dickie T, Nixon J: Concordance in diabetic foot ulceration: a cross-sectional study of agreement between wound swabbing and tissue sampling in infected ulcers. Health Technol Assess 2016;20:1–176.

5 Martin JM, Zenilman JM, Lazarus GS: Molecular microbiology: new dimensions for cutaneous biology and wound healing. J Invest Dermatol 2010;130:38–48.

6 Lipsky BA, Armstrong DG, Citron DM, Tice AD, Morgenstern DE, Abramson MA: Ertapenem versus piperacillin/tazobactam for diabetic foot infections (SIDESTEP): prospective, randomised, controlled, double-blinded, multicentre trial. Lancet 2005;366: 1695–1703.

7 National Institute for Health and Care Excellence: Evidence Summary: Medicines and Prescribing Briefing. Clostridium difficile Infection: Risk with Broad-Spectrum Antibiotics. 2015. https://www.nice.org.uk/advice/esmpb1/chapter/key-points-from-the-evidence.

8 Nemeth J, Oesch G, Kuster SP: Bacteriostatic versus bactericidal antibiotics for patients with serious bacterial infections: systematic review and meta-analysis. J Antimicrob Chemother 2015;70:382–395.

9 Eleftheriadou I, Tentolouris N, Argiana V, Jude E, Boulton AJ: Methicillin-resistant Staphylococcus aureus in diabetic foot infections. Drugs 2010;70:1785–1797.

10 Liu C, Bayer A, Cosgrove SE, Daum RS, Fridkin SK, Gorwitz RJ, Kaplan SL, Karchmer AW, Levine DP, Murray BE, J Rybak M, Talan DA, Chambers HF: Clinical practice guidelines by the infectious diseases society of america for the treatment of methicillin-resistant Staphylococcus aureus infections in adults and children. Clin Infect Dis 2011;52:e18–e55.

11 Lipsky BA, Cannon CM, Ramani A, Jandourek A, Calmaggi A, Friedland HD, Goldstein EJ: Ceftaroline fosamil for treatment of diabetic foot infections: the CAPTURE study experience. Diabetes Metab Res Rev 2015;31:395–401.

12 MacDonald A, Dow G: Ceftobiprole: first reported experience in osteomyelitis. Can J Infect Dis Med Microbiol 2010;21:138–140.

13 Spellberg B, Lipsky BA: Systemic antibiotic therapy for chronic osteomyelitis in adults. Clin Infect Dis 2012;54:393–407.

14 Powers JG, Higham C, Broussard K, Phillips TJ: Wound healing and treating wounds: chronic wound care and management. J Am Acad Dermatol 2016;74:607–625.

15 Lipsky BA, Holroyd KJ, Zasloff M: Topical versus systemic antimicrobial therapy for treating mildly infected diabetic foot ulcers: a randomized, controlled, double-blinded, multicenter trial of pexiganan cream. Clin Infect Dis 2008;47:1537–1545.

16 Flamm RK, Rhomberg PR, Simpson KM, Farrell DJ, Sader HS, Jones RN: In vitro spectrum of pexiganan activity when tested against pathogens from diabetic foot infections and with selected resistance mechanisms. Antimicrob Agents Chemother 2015;59:1751–1754.

17 Lipsky BA, Kuss M, Edmonds M, Reyzelman A, Sigal F: Topical application of a_gentamicin-collagen sponge combined with systemic antibiotic therapy for the treatment of diabetic foot infections of moderate severity: a randomized, controlled, multicenter clinical trial. J Am Podiatr Med Assoc 2012;102:223–232.

18 Roeder B, Van Gils CC, Maling S: Antibiotic beads in the treatment of diabetic pedal osteomyelitis. J Foot Ankle Surg 2000;39:124–130.

19 Barth RE, Vogely HC, Hoepelman AI, Peters EJ: 'To bead or not to bead?' Treatment of osteomyelitis and prosthetic joint-associated infections with gentamicin bead chains. Int J Antimicrob Agents 2011;38:371–375.

20 Kumari S, Harjai K, Chhibber S: Efficacy of bacteriophage treatment in murine burn wound infection induced by Klebsiella pneumoniae. J Microbiol Biotechnol 2009;19:622–628.

21 Mendes JJ, Leandro C, Mottola C, Barbosa R, Silva FA, Oliveira M, Vilela CL, Melo-Cristino J, Górski A, Pimentel M, São-José C, Cavaco-Silva P, Garcia M: In vitro design of a novel lytic bacteriophage cocktail with therapeutic potential against organisms causing diabetic foot infections. J Med Microbiol 2014;63:1055–1065.

22 Chhibber S, Kaur T, Sandeep Kaur: Co-therapy using lytic bacteriophage and linezolid: effective treatment in eliminating methicillin resistant Staphylococcus aureus (MRSA) from diabetic foot infections. PLoS One 2013;8:e56022.

23 Mutluoglu M, Sivrioglu AK, Eroglu M, Uzun G, Turhan V, Ay H, Lipsky BA: The implications of the presence of osteomyelitis on outcomes of infected diabetic foot wounds. Scand J Infect Dis 2013;45:497–503.

24 van Asten SA, La Fontaine J, Peters EJ, Bhavan K, Kim PJ, Lavery LA: The microbiome of diabetic foot osteomyelitis. Eur J Clin Microbiol Infect Dis 2016;35:293–298.

25 Game FL, Jeffcoate WJ: Primarily non-surgical management of osteomyelitis of the foot in diabetes. Diabetologia 2008;51:962–967.

26 Valabhji J, Oliver N, Samarasinghe D, Mali T, Gibbs RG, Gedroyc WM: Conservative management of diabetic forefoot ulceration complicated by underlying osteomyelitis: the benefits of magnetic resonance imaging. Diabet Med 2009;26:1127–1134.

27 Senneville E, Lombart A, Beltrand E, Valette M, Legout L, Cazaubiel M, Yazdanpanah Y, Fontaine P: Outcome of diabetic foot osteomyelitis treated non-surgically: a retrospective cohort study. Diabetes Care 2008;31:637–642.

28 Ulcay A, Karakas A, Mutluoglu M, Uzun G, Turhan V, Ay H: Antibiotherapy with and without bone debridement in diabetic foot osteomyelitis: a retrospective cohort study. Pak J Med Sci 2014;30:28–31.

29 Acharya S, Soliman M, Egun A, Rajbhandari SM: Conservative management of diabetic foot osteomyelitis. Diabetes Res Clin Pract 2013;101:e18–e20.

30 Aragón-Sánchez J: Treatment of diabetic foot osteomyelitis: a surgical critique. Int J Low Extrem Wounds 2010;9:37–59.

31 Lázaro-Martínez JL, Aragón-Sánchez J, García-Morales E: Antibiotics versus conservative surgery for treating diabetic foot osteomyelitis: a randomized comparative trial. Diabetes Care 2014;37:789–795.

32 Lipsky BA: Treating diabetic foot osteomyelitis primarily with surgery or antibiotics: have we answered the question? Diabetes Care 2014;37:593–595.

33 Peters EJ, Lipsky BA, Berendt AR, Embil JM, Lavery LA, Senneville E, Urbančič-Rovan V, Bakker K, Jeffcoate WJ: A systematic review of the effectiveness of interventions in the management of infection in the diabetic foot. Diabetes Metab Res Rev 2012;28(suppl 1):142–162.

Senneville

34 Venkatesan P, Lawn S, Macfarlane RM, Fletcher EM, Finch RG, Jeffcoate WJ: Conservative management of osteomyelitis in the feet of diabetic patients. Diabet Med 1997;14:487–490.

35 Game FL, Jeffcoate WJ: Primarily non-surgical management of osteomyelitis of the foot in diabetes. Diabetologia 2008;51:962–967.

36 Embil JM, Rose G, Trepman E, Math MC, Duerksen F, Simonsen JN, Nicolle LE: Oral antimicrobial therapy for diabetic foot osteomyelitis. Foot Ankle Int 2006;27:771–779.

37 Waldvogel FA, Medoff G, Swartz MN: Osteomyelitis: a review of clinical features, therapeutic considerations and unusual aspects. 3. Osteomyelitis associated with vascular insufficiency. N Engl J Med 1970;282:316–322.

38 Senneville E, Yazdanpanah Y, Cazaubiel M, Cordonnier M, Valette M, Beltrand E, Khazarjian A, Maulin L, Alfandari S, Caillaux M, Dubreuil L, Mouton Y: Rifampicin-ofloxacin oral regimen for the treatment of mild to moderate diabetic foot osteomyelitis. J Antimicrob Chemother 2001;48:927–930.

39 Kaye KS, Engemann JJ, Fraimow HS, Abrutyn E: Pathogens resistant to antimicrobial agents: epidemiology, molecular mechanisms, and clinical management. Infect Dis Clin North Am 2004;18:467–511.

40 Conterno LO, da Silva Filho CR: Antibiotics for treating chronic osteomyelitis in adults. Cochrane Database Syst Rev 2009;8:CD004439.

41 Pulcini C, Couadau T, Bernard E, Lorthat-Jacob A, Bauer T, Cua E, Mondain V, Chichmanian RM, Dellamonica P, Roger PM: Adverse effects of parenteral antimicrobial therapy for chronic bone infections. Eur J Clin Microbiol Infect Dis 2008;27:1227–1232.

42 Tone A, Nguyen S, Devemy F, Topolinski H, Valette M, Cazaubiel M, Fayard A, Beltrand É, Lemaire C, Senneville É: Six-week versus twelve-week antibiotic therapy for nonsurgically treated diabetic foot osteomyelitis: a multicenter open-label controlled randomized study. Diabetes Care 2015;38:302–307.

Eric Senneville, MD, PhD
Department of Infectious Diseases, Gustave Dron Hospital
135 rue du Président Coty
FR–59200 Tourcoing (France)
E-Mail esenneville@ch-tourcoing.fr

Piaggesi A, Apelqvist J (eds): The Diabetic Foot Syndrome.
Front Diabetes. Basel, Karger, 2018, vol 26, pp 184–199 (DOI: 10.1159/000480101)

The Role of Surgery in the Management of the Infected Diabetic Foot

Javier Aragón-Sánchez

Department of Surgery and Diabetic Foot Unit, La Paloma Hospital, Las Palmas de Gran Canaria, Spain

Abstract

Surgery is frequently required to treat diabetic foot infections (DFIs) as part of the comprehensive approach of providing treatment to the patient. The goal is to evacuate pus, remove necrotic tissue and minimize the risk for further spread, thereby creating a good wound bed to achieve total healing. Surgical interventions will range from minor debridement to major resection, amputation or revascularization when necessary. Delay in the implementation of appropriate surgery may be responsible for the high percentage of amputations because it allows the infection to proliferate and destroy tissue. This is especially true in cases of infections in ischaemic feet. The level of experience of the surgeon also conditions the outcomes after surgical treatment due to DFIs. Surgeons must have a thorough knowledge of the compartmental anatomy of the foot and the basis of surgical debridement in these cases. Optimal treatment of the patient with diabetic foot osteomyelitis (DFO) is still controversial. Even though recent evidences support the treatment of DFO exclusively with antibiotics, surgery still has an important role in treating such patients. The combination of antibiotics with surgical removal of the infected bone, sometimes without amputation, may cure most cases of DFO.   © 2018 S. Karger AG, Basel

Surgery is frequently required to treat diabetic foot infections (DFIs) as part of the comprehensive approach in providing treatment to the patient. The goal of surgical treatment is to evacuate pus, remove necrotic tissue and minimize the risk for further spread [1]. Surgical interventions will range from minor debridement to major resection including amputation. It is very important for clinicians and surgeons dealing with these complicated patients to have a comprehensive knowledge of the compartmental anatomy of the foot and the basis of surgical debridement in these cases.

Clinical Presentation of DFIs

DFIs can be classified into 2 main groups: soft tissue and bone infections. Soft tissue infections are then classified as cellulitis, abscesses, tenosynovitis and necrotizing soft tissue infections (NSTIs) [2]. Cellulitis is a diffuse inflammation of the skin and subcutaneous tissue. Abscesses are purulent collections in soft tissues, beneath the epidermis, in subcutaneous tissue or beneath the fascia. Subepidermal abscesses and paronichia should be considered mild infection. Abscesses can be confined to subcutaneous tissue. In such cases, the infection is not deep, but if it is not adequately treated, the infection may lead to severe complications. A deep abscess is located below the fascia. NSTIs are associated with extensive tissue destruction. Necrotizing cellulitis is diagnosed when the necrotizing changes only involve the skin and subcutaneous tissue. Necrotizing fasciitis is diagnosed when there is involvement of the fascia, necrotizing tensynovitis is diagnosed when there is involvement of the tendons and their sheaths and myonecrosis is diagnosed when the necrotizing process involves the muscle. The typical signs of NSTIs are foul smell, extensive cellulitis, skin necrosis, bluish patches and haemorrhagic bullae. In one series involving 223 patients with diabetes foot infections, necrotising tendovaginitis/fasciitis affected 20% of the patients [3].

Diabetic foot osteomyelitis (DFO) is always associated with ulceration due to polyneuropathy, peripheral arterial disease, or both, and/or penetrating injury inoculating bacteria from the skin into the bone. This means that soft tissues, periostium, cortical bone and bone marrow are sequentially affected by the infection before reaching the bone. The clinical presentation of osteomyelitis may vary considerably when associating with soft tissue infection and ischaemia [4]. An attempt to characterize the grading of the severity of osteomyelitis was made recently. Osteomyelitis was classified as follows: osteomyelitis without ischaemia and without soft tissue involvement (class 1), osteomyelitis with ischaemia without soft tissue involvement (class 2), osteomyelitis with soft tissue involvement (class 3), and osteomyelitis with ischaemia and soft tissue involvement (class 4). The characterization of osteomyelitis into four classes showed a statistically significant trend towards increased severity and increased amputation rate and mortality [4]. No amputation was required in a subgroup of 25 out of 81 patients without ischaemia and soft tissue infections (class 1). Although such classification could be useful in order to determine the type of patients to be included in clinical studies, it does not assist the clinicians to determine the need for surgery.

Evaluation of a Patient with Diabetes and Foot Infection

Non-infectious causes of inflammation, such as acute Charcot joint changes, superimposed gouty arthritis, inappropriate footwear, and excessive weight bearing on an area, can cause localized changes mimicking infection [5]. Suppuration and local signs of inflammation are necessary in order to make a diagnosis of infection.

General symptoms, such as fevers and chills, general malaise, nausea and vomiting, may suggest a more serious infection, but ≥50% of patients with a limb-threatening infection do not manifest systemic signs or symptoms [6]. DFIs are classified according to their severity as mild, moderate and severe [6]. The International Working Group on Diabetic Foot has proposed the PEDIS scheme (Perfusion, Extent, Depth, Infection and Sensation) for classifying foot ulcers. Infection is divided into 4 types. Classification of the severity of the infections according to IDSA and the International Consensus are similar and are very useful for the clinicians in order to decide the need for hospitalization and the route of administration of antibiotics but do not indicate clearly the need for surgical treatment. International Working Group on Diabetic Foot recommends hospitalization in cases of severe infection, metabolic or hemodynamic instability, in cases in which intravenous therapy is needed (and not available/appropriate as outpatient), when diagnostic tests are needed and not available as outpatient, when critical ischaemia is present and when surgical procedures (more than minor) are required. Admission is also necessary in cases of failure of outpatient management; when the patient is unable or unwilling to comply with outpatient-based treatment, there is a need for more complex dressing changes than patient/caregivers can provide or when a careful, continuous observation is needed [7].

The point of entry of the infection is frequently an ulcer but may be another type of lesion, for example a nail puncture. The location of the ulcer, whether it is plantar, dorsal, medial, lateral or interdigital, must be defined. The evaluation of the depth of the infection is important because this has been a significant factor in the outcome of the treatment of foot ulcers. Ulcers with callus and necrosis should be debrided as soon as possible to facilitate determination of the depth. The Halsted-mosquito is very useful for detecting fistulous tracks, cavities and paths of spreading of the infection through the foot. Ideally, clinicians would like to determine if a soft tissue infection also involves bone at the time the patient presents with a foot wound. Osteomyelitis should be suspected when a foot ulcer does not heal after 6 weeks of appropriate treatment, when the ulcer is deep or has an area >2 cm (especially if overlying a bony prominence) and when there is a visibly exposed bone. The probe-to-bone (PTB) test [8, 9] is a potentially useful tool for diagnosing osteomyelitis underlying a foot ulcer. This test was originally described using a sterile, blunt, 14.0-cm, 5F, stainless steel eye probe [8]. A metal forceps (Halsted-mosquito) has also been used by other authors [9]. The surgical instrument is gently introduced through the wound and the PTB is considered "positive" if bone (a hard or gritty surface) is touched. When first described 15 years ago, this test showed a positive predictive value of 0.89 in detecting bone involvement in patients with limb-threatening infections [8]. However, subsequent studies dealing with this manoeuvre showed a considerably lower predictive value. The usefulness of the PTB test is highly affected by the prevalence of osteomyelitis in the population studied, as well as by the criterion standard used for diagnosis.

The basic imaging study required for evaluating diabetic patients with foot infections is the simple X-ray in 2 standard views. This should be part of the initial consultation whenever foot infection is suspected in a diabetic patient. Three important signs should be looked for in the simple X-ray: a foreign body, free gas in the soft tissues and bone destruction. The presence of gas in an X-ray alerts the clinician to the presence of a severe, limb-threatening infection, which should be treated immediately with surgical intervention. In cases of osteomyelitis, X-rays show cortical disruption, periosteal elevation, a sequestrum or involucrum or gross destruction of bone. However, these radiological changes do not appear until 10–14 days after the onset of the bone infection [10]. For this reason, the reported sensitivity of plain radiography in the diagnosis of osteomyelitis is usually low, especially in the early stages of infection. Furthermore, the radiological diagnosis of bone infection in diabetic patients is difficult because of complications due to neuroarthropathy, previous bone and/or soft tissue infections, previous bone trauma and bone deformities. In cases where no positive findings are found, follow-up radiography is usually done 2–6 weeks later, although there is no agreed upon best interval. MRI has been suggested as the most useful imaging study to evaluate both soft tissue and bone-related infections, especially in the early stages [10]. Abscesses associated with osteomyelitis, necrosis and tendon involvement are also identified effectively using MRI. Despite the generalized opinion that MRI may help surgeons to plan the surgical procedure, the exact role of advanced imaging studies in order to determine the level of resection minimizing the recurrence of the infection has still not been clarified. Few studies have been carried out on this topic. One study reported that 13 out of 21 diabetic feet were operated upon and that the level of amputation/resection was limited to the specific region of infection demonstrated at MRI [11]. There were no recurrences at the surgical margins during 9 months of follow-up. However, no information about the type of resection, that is, whether the wound was closed or open in order to heal by secondary intention, was provided [11]. Furthermore, the author recognized that the extent of infection could have been overestimated at MRI and the authors did not find any histologic correlation with regard to the extent of involvement. Furthermore, preoperative MRI in cases of DFO with ischaemia may be less effective for distinguishing osteomyelitis from bone marrow oedema than in cases of neuropathic ulcers [12]. Recently, a group of authors suggested a surgical strategy based on MRI. They recommended that the appropriate surgical margin performing amputations should be set in the area of bone marrow oedema based on MRI examination after revascularization if needed [13]. However, it is very difficult to extract definitive conclusion in a very short retrospective study.

Newer hybrid imaging techniques (SPECT/CT, positron emission tomography [PET]/CT, and PET/MRI) look to be useful but more research is needed. When MRI is not available or contraindicated, white blood cell-labelled radionuclides scan, or possibly SPECT/CT or 18 F-FDG PET scans should be considered [7].

Who Is the Appropriate Surgeon?

Diabetic foot surgery must not be considered a "minor procedure" that can be performed by anyone. It has been reported that the level of experience of the surgeon influences the outcomes after amputations due to DFIs [14]. The outcome of surgery largely depends on the skill and experience of the surgeon and the degree of care taken. The consequences of performing diabetic foot surgery without experience and appropriate training may be disastrous for the patient. Taylor et al. [15] were aware of this issue and they stated in their report that senior surgeons carried out the procedures and the operations were not delegated to unsupervised junior house officers. Surgeons who have to treat patients with diabetic foot problems must be aware that debridement should not be done before knowing the etiology of the ulcer. Debridement in a foot with critical ischaemia should be done only in cases of severe infections and when revascularization has been scheduled. Because inadequate debridement rarely achieves the resolution of the problem, the patient should quickly be referred to a specialized multidisciplinary team. Referring the patient to a centre specialized in treating diabetic foot problems may be the best way to achieve limb salvage. Specialized teams handling acute diabetic foot problems may result in a reduction of lower limb amputations [16, 17]. Previous procedures may condition the proper surgery that the patient should undergo [2].

Timing for Performing Surgery

Non-vascular surgical interventions due to acutely infected diabetic foot are classified as class III or curative (procedures performed to assist in healing open wound) or class IV or emergency (procedures performed to limit progression of acute infection) [18]. They include drainage, debridement, bone resections and minor or major amputations. However, no classification exists in order to determine either the point at which surgery becomes absolutely necessary or when surgery is likely to produce a better outcome than further prolonged treatment with antibiotics. There is agreement that when the infection is potentially life threatening (severe or PEDIS 4), immediate surgery should be indicated [19]. Delay in the implementation of appropriate surgery may be responsible for the high percentage of amputations. Early surgical treatment including extensive use of revascularization may reduce the need for above-ankle amputations [15, 20]. Delay in referral is considered a risk factor for amputation and this is especially true in cases of ischaemic foot in which "time is tissue."

Guidelines for treating DFO suggest urgent surgery for necrotising fasciitis, deep soft-tissue abscesses, or gangrene accompanying osteomyelitis. Non-urgent surgery may be necessary if there is a significant compromise of the soft-tissue envelope [21]. Based on the clinical presentation of osteomyelitis, surgery is required when the bone is protruding through the ulcer, when there is extensive bone destruction seen on

X-ray or progressive bone damage on sequential X-ray while undergoing antibiotic treatment, when the soft tissue envelope is destroyed and when there is gangrene or spreading soft tissue infection [22].

The optimum timing for vascular surgery in diabetic patients with ischaemia and foot infection has not yet been identified. In cases of severe infections, it is important to proceed with surgical debridement as soon as possible with the intention of performing revascularization after debridement. For a patient with a severely infected dysvascular foot, it is preferable to perform revascularization within 1–2 days of the initial surgical debridement [23]. When the patient is metabolically stable and osteomyelitis is not accompanied by necrotising changes, deep abscesses or systemic response to infection, it is preferable to start antibiotic treatment and perform revascularization as soon as possible. Thus, increased distal flow can be attained to promote wound healing after a surgical procedure on the infected bone. A team in Rome monitoring transcutaneous oxygen tension (TcPO2) after percutaneous transluminal angioplasty in diabetic patients concluded that when it is possible to delay surgery, the best time to perform a more aggressive debridement or minor amputations is 3–4 weeks after successful revascularization [24].

Soft Tissue Debridement

The surgeon who treats patients with diabetes and foot infections should have a thorough knowledge of the anatomy of the foot and should be able to identify the ways in which infections spread through the foot [2]. Acute DFI will follow the path of least resistance, which in the foot is comprised of the tendons [25]. Many patients must undergo more than one surgical procedure in order to save the infected foot and re-operations should be based on the same anatomical principles.

The foot is anatomically divided into rigid compartments. When an infection penetrates into a compartment, oedema appears then increasing the compartmental pressure. Oedema can also be caused by the sorbitol pathway and disturbances in the capillary permeability. When compartmental pressure exceeds the capillary pressure, necrosis occurs. Bacterial growth, toxins and leucocyte response may also produce necrosis. The aim of the surgical treatment is to decompress the compartments and remove all the devitalized and infected tissue in order to create a healthy wound bed. Surgical procedures to achieve this aim include surgical debridement, minor and major amputations.

In Figure 1, we can see a cross-section of the compartments of the foot. The floor of the compartments is the plantar fascia, which is attached to the calcaneus and spreads distally to the toes. The plantar aponeurosis is the outermost fascia and it is the anatomical layer located beneath the subcutaneous tissue. The medial and central compartments are separated by the medial intermuscular septum, which extends from the medial calcaneal tuberosity to the first metatarsal head. The central and

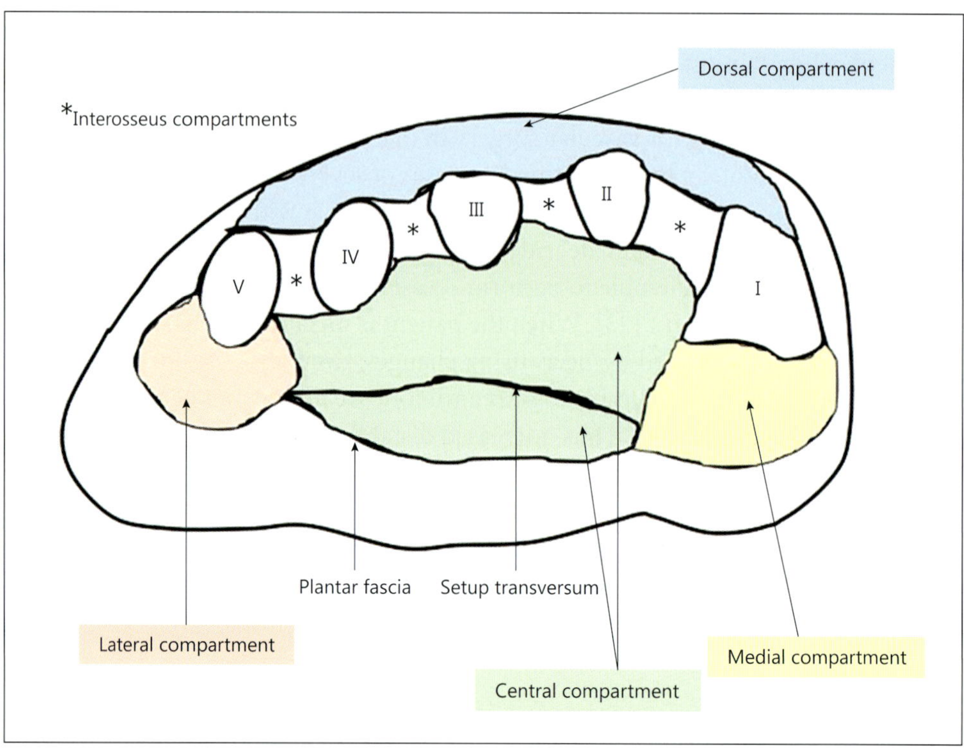

Fig. 1. Cross-section of the compartments of the foot.

lateral compartments are separated by the lateral intermuscular septum, which extends from the calcaneus to the fifth metatarsal head. The interosseus compartment is located between the metatarsal bones and contains the interossei muscles. The dorsal compartment has a thin layer of subcutaneous tissue, and the tendons contained in this space can be easily exposed in the presence of a lesion. Most commonly than not, the incisional approach will follow the extensor or flexor tendon of the foot, since infections may spread proximately through the tendons located in the compartments. There is a relationship between the point of entry to the infection and the compartment in which the infection spreads. Infections arising from the big toe and first metatarsal head spreads through the medial compartment, those arising in the second, third and fourth toes and metatarsal heads spread through the central compartment and those arising from the fifth toe and fifth metatarsal head spread through the lateral compartment. Mixed infections involving soft tissues and bone are very common. In such cases, the bone infection should be treated during the procedure according to the experience of the surgeon. We show in Figure 2a, a patient with infected neuropathic plantar ulcer below second metatarsal head spreading distally to the toe and proximately along flexor tendons. Second toe amputation and opening of the central compartment was carried out (Fig. 2b).

Aragón-Sánchez

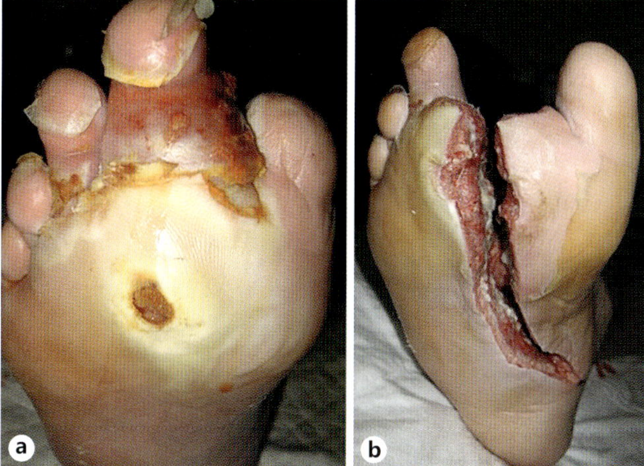

Fig. 2. a Foot ulcer complicated by osteomyelitis and severe soft tissue infection. **b** Extensive debridement of the central compartment of the foot.

Removing Bone Infection without Amputation

Surgical treatment of DFO without amputation is an attractive option to remove infected bone while conserving the soft tissue envelope and maintaining the external appearance of the foot. This option is named as "conservative surgery," which was defined as any procedure in which only the infected bone and non-viable soft tissue are removed, but no amputation of any part of the foot is undertaken [26]. Surgery without amputation may be more acceptable than amputation for a patient with diabetes, although the impact of this type of surgery on the quality of life has not been addressed. In theory, a conservative surgical approach removing bone fragments also changes the foot biomechanics. Osteomyelitis of the distal phalanx can be easily removed, thereby eliminating the high-pressure point. Percutaneous tenotomy can be performed in an outpatient clinic in cases of claw toe deformities with distal phalanx osteomyelitis [27]. In cases of involvement of the interphalangeal joint, a resection arthroplasty can be carried out [22, 26, 28]. Other authors have reported using modified arthroplasty to treat osteomyelitis. The bone was removed through a dorsal wound, the wound was irrigated and a Kirschner wire 1.2 mm in diameter was placed [28]. Healing was achieved in 25.6 ± 6.2 days. Metatarsal head resection is a very useful procedure employed in cases with or without osteomyelitis.

Osteomyelitis involving hallux is a serious problem because it has an important role in the biomechanics of the foot. One-stage resection and pin stabilization were reported in a retrospective series consisting of 15 patients (18 feet) with an average follow-up of 48.8 months [29]. Another option is to use external fixation after removing the infected bone [30]. The authors used staged surgical procedures consisting of ulcer excision, removal of all necrotic soft tissue and bone, followed by pulse lavage irrigation, culturing and polymethylmethacrylate antibiotic cement administration. After that, a mini-external fixator was placed in 4 out of 6 cases. When the infection was cleared, they subsequently used allogenic bone graft, iliac crest bone graft or arthroplasty without bone grafting with the external fixator. None of the surviving subjects developed recurrent ulceration or required amputation after 14 months of follow-up [30]. Another group reported a cohort including 28 patients with osteomyelitis of the first ray treated by a technique requiring a one-stage surgical approach [31]. After surgical debridement with removal of the infected bone, the authors placed antibiotic-loaded bone cement and stabilized the treated area with an external fixator. Four patients developed a relapse of the ulceration after the procedure. During the follow-up period, no ulceration recurrences, transfer ulcerations, shoe fit problems, or gait abnormalities were detected in the other 24 patients [31].

Minor Amputation

Several types of amputation have been classically used to remove infected bone in patients with diabetes and forefoot infections. Toe and ray resections allow the patient to use fairly normal shoes. However, these amputations may produce biomechanical disturbances resulting in new high-pressure points and predisposing patients to subsequent re-ulceration. In a retrospective study of 90 patients undergoing amputation of the big toe, 60% underwent a second amputation and 17% of these had a below-the-knee amputation [32]. However, the number of re-ulcerations and re-amputations could probably be reduced with a specialized multidisciplinary postoperative treatment based on custom-made shoes and foot care [33].

Mid and Rearfoot Osteomyelitis

Cases involving midfoot osteomyelitis are frequently associated with underlying Charcot deformity. It has been suggested that repeat bone resection is followed by using antibiotic cement spacer or beads in such cases [34]. As a consequence of bone resection, the foot becomes destabilized and immobilization has to be enforced. Several ways of immobilizing an unstable foot have been reported, including internal fixation, external fixation or both. Internal fixation is contraindicated in an area of previous osteomyelitis. Circular fixation based on Ilizarov principles provides stabilization following correction of deformities [35].

Saving the foot in cases of heel ulcers and calcaneus osteomyelitis is a challenge because failure frequently leads to a major amputation. A systematic review of partial or total calcanectomy as an alternative to below-the-knee amputation was recently reported [36]. The combined data represented 100 patients who had undergone 76 partial and 28 total calcanectomy, giving a total of 104 calcanectomies. Forty-nine out of 76 partial calcanectomies (64.4%) did not have complications. Total calcanectomy was carried out without complications in 14 out of 28 cases (50%). Seven cases of partial calcanectomy (9.2%) and four cases of total calcanectomy (14.3%) subsequently required a major amputation (14.3%). Patients with diabetes had a fivefold greater risk of undergoing a major amputation [36].

A group of authors reported a series that was not included in the aforementioned review, which consisted of 24 patients who had undergone a partial calcanectomy [37]. Using a midline incision, they removed the necrotic soft tissue and bone. Resection of the insertion of the Achilles tendon was sometimes required when it was involved in the infection. If primary closure was possible, they closed in a single layer with 2/0 nylon. If not possible, the wound was left open and repeat debridement with secondary closure was planned. Only one patient out of 24 underwent a below-the-knee amputation. Only in 1 out of the 8 patients with diabetes, the infection was not controlled and required further resection. Mean hospital stay in patients with diabetes was 56.7 days and healing was achieved in 118 days. There was no major difference in the failure rate between patients with and without diabetes. All patients were able to walk with our without external support [37]. When the wound healed, the patient needed regular podiatric care, customized insoles and adequate footwear to minimize the risk of re-ulceration. Orthotic devices, custom shoes, ankle-foot orthosis and Charcot-restraint orthotic walker were used to assist the patients to maintain their ambulatory status after total or partial calcanectomy [36].

Outcomes of Surgical Treatment of DFIs

A group of authors included in their series 114 diabetic patients who underwent emergency surgery for indications of infection, gangrene or infected neurotrophic ulcers [15]. Surgery was always performed within 48 h of admission in the operating room under regional (never local) anaesthesia. Forty-seven percent of those patients underwent 2 or more surgical procedures. They stated that early aggressive drainage, debridement, and local foot amputations combined with liberal use of revascularization resulted in cumulative limb salvage of 74% at 5 years [15]. Eneroth et al. [3] published a series involving 223 patients treated for foot infections. They reported that 43% of their patients healed after an amputation (major or minor). The total rate of major amputations was 10.7% [3]. Another group reported the outcomes of patients with presumed adequate circulatory status undergoing digit amputations. Complete healing was achieved only in 34%, and infection persisted in 36% of the operated limbs. Twenty-four percent of the patients underwent a major amputation [38]. An Italian group reported that when aggressive revascularization was carried out, deep foot infections in ischaemic patients had the same prognosis as in non-ischaemic patients [39]. Early surgical debridement of deep foot abscesses and revascularization were the keys to achieving good results. Only 4.7% in a group of 106 patients with deep foot infections underwent major amputation. Revascularization was performed in 60.3% of the patients [39]. Other authors have also reported high short-term limb salvage with aggressive treatment of invasive foot infection during a period of less than 48 h from admission followed by autogenous bypass [40]. These reports remark the fact that careful vascular status determination must be made before performing amputation. The possibility of the presence of ischaemia should always be completely ruled out in diabetic patients with infected foot ulcers. In cases where pedal pulses are absent, a vascular surgeon should always be consulted. Minor amputation in a foot without adequate foot perfusion may be complicated by non-healing wounds, the spread of infection and necrosis, with major amputation subsequently being required. Failure of treatment was linked to values of ankle systolic blood pressure <50 mm Hg, toe systolic blood pressure <30 mm Hg, ankle/brachial index <0.5 and transcutaneous oxygen pressure <20 mm Hg in a prospective series of DFIs, including 58% of osteomyelitis [41]. Other authors also reported peripheral vascular disease as a risk factor for failure of conservative surgery and amputation [4, 26, 42]. Henke et al. [43] demonstrated that peripheral arterial disease was associated with a lower rate of wound healing and limb salvage. In their sample, bypass surgery was linked to wound healing and limb salvage.

In an analysis of randomized controlled trials of antibiotic treatment, methicillin-resistant *Staphylococcus aureus* (MRSA) isolation was described as a significant factor associated with the failure of treatment in patients with DFIs [44]. In one study dealing with surgery of DFO, MRSA was isolated in 35 cases (36.8% of *S. aureus* isolated and 18% of the total bacteria isolated) and was the only pathogen on 22 occasions. Here, MRSA osteomyelitis was associated with a higher temperature, raised white blood cell counts, fetid odours and cutaneous necrosis than the methicillin-sensitive *S. aureus*. Moreover, MRSA osteomyelitis was not associated with a worse prognosis in this study [45]. Another group of authors found that MRSA osteomyelitis was associated with poor prognosis [46].

The location of osteomyelitis is related to the outcome of treatment. Karchmer and Gibbons [47] reported the outcomes of the surgical treatment of DFO in 110 patients, with diagnosis proven by biopsy in 96% of the cases. In this group, 88% of minor and 12% of major amputations were performed in 86 cases of forefoot osteomyelitis. Another study reported that 48.5% of 167 patients with forefoot osteomyelitis underwent conservative surgery without amputation, 45.5% with minor amputations and 6% with major amputations [26]. Faglia et al. [48] stated that toe or ray amputation was performed in 198 out of 234 patients with forefoot osteomyelitis (84.6%), while the rest underwent 25 transmetatarsal and one Lisfranc amputations. Mid- and hindfoot osteomyelitis were associated with worse prognosis than forefoot osteomyelitis [22, 26, 47]. The outcome of conservative surgery treating DFO is not well defined. One report investigated a group of 185 patients, including those with severe soft-tissue infections accompanying osteomyelitis. After excluding the patients for whom conservative surgery was found to be impossible on admission, 111 patients underwent conservative surgery as the first choice. Of those, only 20 (18%) required subsequent amputations: 13 minor (11.7%) and 7 major amputations (6.3%). Conservative surgery was successful in 82% of the cases [26]. The same working group reported a new cohort of 81 patients with the same characteristics. Forty-eight patients (59.3%) had conservative surgery, 32 (39.5%) minor amputations and 1 underwent a (1.2%) major amputation [49]. The presence of limb ischaemia and soft tissue infections associated to osteomyelitis is associated with a worse prognosis and amputation in cases of DFO [4, 26]. Patients with osteomyelitis and deep tissue infections have worse prognosis than those with isolated bone infections [3].

When ischaemia is not present, the outcomes reported in the literature are optimal. A group of authors [50] retrospectively compared the results of the treatment of osteomyelitis without ischaemia over 2 different periods. Thirty-two patients belonged to a historical group (1986–1993) of patients treated with antibiotic therapy, offloading and local wound care. The second group consisted of 32 patients who underwent conservative surgery followed by the same regime of care (September 1993 to March 1995). Healing rates were 57% for the former group and 78% for the latter ($p < 0.008$); there was also a significant difference in healing time: 462 +/– 98 days and 181 +/– 30 days ($p < 0.008$) for the first and second groups respectively. In the group that underwent conservative surgery, only 2 patients (6.25%) required a minor amputation. In the antibiotic group, failure of the medical management resulted in 40% of patients undergoing amputations: 9 toe, 3 transmetatarsal and 2 below-the-knee. These authors concluded that in the case of osteomyelitis of the foot in diabetic patients, conservative surgery reduced healing time, the duration of antibiotic therapy and the number of secondary surgical procedures. Healing was achieved in 181 +/– 30 days [50]. Other authors reported that open wounds healed by secondary intention over a median period of 90 days. The median wound-healing times in patients with successful conservative surgery was 80 days (12–365) compared to 120 days (21–365) for those who had minor amputations ($p = 0.003$). Median wound-healing times were longer in cases where there was associated soft-tissue infection ($p = 0.0005$) and limb ischaemia ($p = 0.001$) [26]. Another investigation assessed 157 patients with complicated foot ulcers and 51 patients had osteomyelitis. Forty-five patients had osteomyelitis without foot ischaemia and 41 of these (91%) underwent surgical treatment: 28 conservative surgery (68%) and 13 minor amputations (32%) [17].

Little information is currently available on osteomyelitis remission in the feet of diabetic patients, although its potential to recur is widely accepted [51]. One study dealt specifically with the issue of DFO recurrence after surgery. Recurrence of osteomyelitis was defined as the appearance of bone infections at the same or adjacent site after healing of both the ulcer and the surgical wound. In cases of recurrence, the ray, bone and/or joint affected was the same as that operated on in the first attempt. Reulceration was defined as any ulcer, whatever depth, appearing during follow-up at the same or other sites including the contra-lateral foot. A new episode of osteomyelitis was defined in cases where the new ulcer was complicated by bone infection, but this was not considered a recurrence [49]. Osteomyelitis was located on the forefoot in 74 patients (91.3%), midfoot in 4 patients (4.9%) and hindfoot in 3 patients (3.7%).

Forty-eight patients (59.3%) underwent conservative surgery, 32 (39.5%) had minor amputations including 9 open transmetatarsal amputations and there was 1 (1.2%) major amputation. Recurrence was diagnosed in 3 out of 65 patients (4.6%) 75, 51 and 105 days after healing. No recurrences were observed after this period. Twenty-four out of 65 patients developed re-ulceration (36.9%) at a new site after a median period of 46.5 weeks. Re-ulceration was associated with plantar location of the ulcer during the first episode ($p = 0.02$, HR 2.4, 95% CI 1.1–5.1) and Charcot deformity ($p = 0.002$, HR 4.3, 95% CI 1.6–10.9). A new episode of osteomyelitis was diagnosed in 11 patients (17%). There was no doubt about the new site of infection in all the cases and limb salvage was achieved in each case [49]. Recent works have highlighted the fact that patients with bone margins affected by infection after undergoing amputation for osteomyelitis have poor prognosis. Wide excision of necrotic and infected bone with 5 mm or greater of clearance has been shown to reduce the risk for recurrence in cases of chronic osteomyelitis [52] but in this study only 7 out of 50 patients (14%) had chronic osteomyelitis, which had spread from an overlying ulcer. It is difficult to extract any conclusion from this study for the treatment of bone infection in the feet of patients with diabetes. A group of researchers reported a retrospective series of 111 patients, evaluating the impact of residual osteomyelitis on surgical margins after surgical resection of the infected bone [53]. Forty-seven patients underwent digital amputation, 21 partial ray (metatarsal) resections, 38 ray resections and 5 other procedures. Of the 111 patients included in the study, 39 (35.14%) had pathologically confirmed margins positive for residual osteomyelitis. Patients with positive margins presented significantly higher rates of proximal amputations, as well as skin and soft tissue infections. The authors concluded that residual osteomyelitis at the pathologic margin was associated with a higher rate of treatment failure, despite the longer duration of antibiotic therapy [53]. Another retrospective observational study involving 27 patients with diabetes showed that the overall rate of residual osteomyelitis was 40.7% (11/27). Nine out of eleven patients (81.8%) with positive margins had poor outcomes, including 3 re-amputations, 3 wound dehiscences, 1 re-ulceration, 1 death and 1 chronic wound that required skin grafting [54].

Conclusions

Surgery is necessary for treating DFIs in many occasions especially in cases of severe infections. Despite the fact that many patients may require amputations to control the infection, several groups have demonstrated that a more conservative surgical approach is possible. Achieving successful outcomes of the surgery require specialized surgeons and prompt surgery after a quick stabilization of the patient. New surgical techniques and materials may help the surgeons to achieve limb salvage.

References

1 Fisher TK, Scimeca CL, Bharara M, Mills JL Sr, Armstrong DG: A step-wise approach for surgical management of diabetic foot infections. J Vasc Surg 2010; 52(3 suppl):72S–75S.

2 Aragon-Sanchez J: Seminar review: a review of the basis of surgical treatment of diabetic foot infections. Int J Low Extrem Wounds 2011;10:33–65.

3 Eneroth M, Larsson J, Apelqvist J: Deep foot infections in patients with diabetes and foot ulcer: an entity with different characteristics, treatments, and prognosis. J Diabetes Complications 1999;13:254–263.

4 Aragon-Sanchez J: Clinical-pathological characterization of diabetic foot infections: grading the severity of osteomyelitis. Int J Low Extrem Wounds 2012; 11;107.

5 Joseph WS, Tan JS: Infections in diabetic foot ulcerations. Curr Infect Dis Rep 2003;5:391–397.

6 Lipsky BA, Berendt AR, Deery HG, Embil JM, Joseph WS, Karchmer AW, LeFrock JL, Lew DP, Mader JT, Norden C, Tan JS: Diagnosis and treatment of diabetic foot infections. Clin Infect Dis 2004;39:885–910.

7 Lipsky BA, Aragon-Sanchez J, Diggle M, Embil J, Kono S, Lavery L, Senneville E, Urbancic-Rovan V, Van Asten S, Peters EJ; International Working Group on the Diabetic Foot: IWGDF guidance on the diagnosis and management of foot infections in persons with diabetes. Diabetes Metab Res Rev 2016; 32(suppl 1):45–74.

8 Grayson ML, Gibbons GW, Balogh K, Levin E, Karchmer AW: Probing to bone in infected pedal ulcers. A clinical sign of underlying osteomyelitis in diabetic patients. JAMA 1995;273:721–723.

9 Aragon-Sanchez J, Lipsky BA, Lazaro-Martinez JL: Diagnosing diabetic foot osteomyelitis: is the combination of probe-to-bone test and plain radiography sufficient for high-risk inpatients? Diabet Med 2011; 28:191–194.

10 Dinh T, Snyder G, Veves A: Current techniques to detect foot infection in the diabetic patient. Int J Low Extrem Wounds 2010;9:24–30.

11 Morrison WB, Schweitzer ME, Wapner KL, Hecht PJ, Gannon FH, Behm WR: Osteomyelitis in feet of diabetics: clinical accuracy, surgical utility, and cost-effectiveness of MR imaging. Radiology 1995;196: 557–564.

12 Fujii M, Armsrong DG, Terashi H: Efficacy of magnetic resonance imaging in diagnosing diabetic foot osteomyelitis in the presence of ischemia. J Foot Ankle Surg 2013;52:717–723.

13 Fujii M, Terashi H, Yokono K: Surgical treatment strategy for diabetic forefoot osteomyelitis. Wound Repair Regen 2016;24:447–453.

14 Wong YS, Lee JC, Yu CS, Low BY: Results of minor foot amputations in diabetic mellitus. Singapore Med J 1996;37:604–606.

15 Taylor LM Jr, Porter JM: The clinical course of diabetics who require emergent foot surgery because of infection or ischemia. J Vasc Surg 1987;6:454–459.

16 Faglia E, Favales F, Aldeghi A, Calia P, Quarantiello A, Barbano P, Puttini M, Palmieri B, Brambilla G, Rampoldi A, Mazzola E, Valenti L, Fattori G, Rega V, Cristalli A, Oriani G, Michael M, Morabito A: Change in major amputation rate in a center dedicated to diabetic foot care during the 1980s: prognostic determinants for major amputation. J Diabetes Complications 1998;12:96–102.

17 Hartemann-Heurtier A, Ha Van G, Danan JP, Koskas F, Jacqueminet S, Golmard JL, Grimaldi A: Outcome of severe diabetic foot ulcers after standardised management in a specialised unit. Diabetes Metab 2002;28(6 pt 1):477–484.

18 Armstrong DG, Frykberg RG: Classifying diabetic foot surgery: toward a rational definition. Diabet Med 2003;20:329–331.

19 Frykberg RG, Wittmayer B, Zgonis T: Surgical management of diabetic foot infections and osteomyelitis. Clin Podiatr Med Surg 2007;24:469–482, viii–ix.

20 Tan JS, Friedman NM, Hazelton-Miller C, Flanagan JP, File TM Jr: Can aggressive treatment of diabetic foot infections reduce the need for above-ankle amputation? Clin Infect Dis 1996;23:286–291.

21 Berendt AR, Peters EJ, Bakker K, Embil JM, Eneroth M, Hinchliffe RJ, Jeffcoate WJ, Lipsky BA, Senneville E, Teh J, Valk GD: Specific guidelines for treatment of diabetic foot osteomyelitis. Diabetes Metab Res Rev 2008;24(suppl 1):S190–S191.

22 Aragon-Sanchez J: Treatment of diabetic foot osteomyelitis: a surgical critique. Int J Low Extrem Wounds 2010;9:37–59.

23 Zgonis T, Stapleton JJ, Rodriguez RH, Girard-Powell VA, Cromack DT: Plastic surgery reconstruction of the diabetic foot. AORN J 2008;87:951–966; quiz 967–970.

24 Caselli A, Latini V, Lapenna A, Di Carlo S, Pirozzi F, Benvenuto A, Uccioli L: Transcutaneous oxygen tension monitoring after successful revascularization in diabetic patients with ischaemic foot ulcers. Diabet Med 2005;22:460–465.

25 La Fontaine J, Bhavan K, Talal TK, Lavery LA: Current concepts in the surgical management of acute diabetic foot infections. Foot (Edinb) 2014;24:123–127.

26 Aragon-Sanchez FJ, Cabrera-Galvan JJ, Quintana-Marrero Y, Hernandez-Herrero MJ, Lazaro-Martinez JL, Garcia-Morales E, Beneit-Montesinos JV, Armstrong DG: Outcomes of surgical treatment of diabetic foot osteomyelitis: a series of 185 patients with histopathological confirmation of bone involvement. Diabetologia 2008;51:1962–1970.

27 Tamir E, McLaren AM, Gadgil A, Daniels TR: Outpatient percutaneous flexor tenotomies for management of diabetic claw toe deformities with ulcers: a preliminary report. Can J Surg 2008;51:41–44.

28 Kim JY, Kim TW, Park YE, Lee YJ: Modified resection arthroplasty for infected non-healing ulcers with toe deformity in diabetic patients. Foot Ankle Int 2008;29:493–497.

29 Johnson JE, Anderson SA: One stage resection and pin stabilization of first metatarsophalangeal joint for chronic plantar ulcer with osteomyelitis. Foot Ankle Int 2010;31:973–979.

30 Schweinberger MH, Roukis TS: Salvage of the first ray with external fixation in the high-risk patient. Foot Ankle Spec 2008;1:210–213.

31 Dalla Paola L, Carone A, Morisi C, Cardillo S, Pattavina M: Conservative surgical treatment of infected ulceration of the first metatarsophalangeal joint with osteomyelitis in diabetic patients. J Foot Ankle Surg 2015;54:536–540.

32 Murdoch DP, Armstrong DG, Dacus JB, Laughlin TJ, Morgan CB, Lavery LA: The natural history of great toe amputations. J Foot Ankle Surg 1997;36:204–208; discussion 256.

33 Dalla Paola L, Faglia E, Caminiti M, Clerici G, Ninkovic S, Deanesi V: Ulcer recurrence following first ray amputation in diabetic patients: a cohort prospective study. Diabetes Care 2003;26:1874–1878.

34 Capobianco CM, Stapleton JJ, Zgonis T: Surgical management of diabetic foot and ankle infections. Foot Ankle Spec 2010;3:223–230.

35 Pinzur MS: Circular fixation for the nonplantigrade Charcot foot. Hosp Pract (Minneap) 2010;38:56–62.

36 Schade VL: Partial or total calcanectomy as an alternative to below-the-knee amputation for limb salvage: a systematic review. J Am Podiatr Med Assoc 2012;102:396–405.

37 Van Riet A, Harake R, Stuyck J: Partial calcanectomy: a procedure to cherish or to reject? Foot Ankle Surg 2012;18:25–29.

38 Nehler MR, Whitehill TA, Bowers SP, Jones DN, Hiatt WR, Rutherford RB, Krupski WC: Intermediate-term outcome of primary digit amputations in patients with diabetes mellitus who have forefoot sepsis requiring hospitalization and presumed adequate circulatory status. J Vasc Surg 1999;30:509–517.

39 Faglia E, Clerici G, Caminiti M, Quarantiello A, Gino M, Morabito A: The role of early surgical debridement and revascularization in patients with diabetes and deep foot space abscess: retrospective review of 106 patients with diabetes. J Foot Ankle Surg 2006;45:220–226.

40 Chang BB, Darling RC 3rd, Paty PS, Lloyd WE, Shah DM, Leather RP: Expeditious management of ischemic invasive foot infections. Cardiovasc Surg 1996; 4:792–795.

41 Diamantopoulos EJ, Haritos D, Yfandi G, Grigoriadou M, Margariti G, Paniara O, Raptis SA: Management and outcome of severe diabetic foot infections. Exp Clin Endocrinol Diabetes 1998;106:346–352.

42 Aragon-Sanchez J, Lazaro-Martinez JL: Impact of perioperative glycaemia and glycated haemoglobin on the outcomes of the surgical treatment of diabetic foot osteomyelitis. Diabetes Res Clin Pract 2011; 94:e83–e85.

43 Henke PK, Blackburn SA, Wainess RW, Cowan J, Terando A, Proctor M, Wakefield TW, Upchurch GR Jr, Stanley JC, Greenfield LJ: Osteomyelitis of the foot and toe in adults is a surgical disease: conservative management worsens lower extremity salvage. Ann Surg 2005;241:885–892.

44 Vardakas KZ, Horianopoulou M, Falagas ME: Factors associated with treatment failure in patients with diabetic foot infections: an analysis of data from randomized controlled trials. Diabetes Res Clin Pract 2008;80:344–351.

45 Aragon-Sanchez J, Lazaro-Martinez JL, Quintana-Marrero Y, Hernandez-Herrero MJ, Garcia-Morales E, Cabrera-Galvan JJ, Beneit-Montesinos JV: Are diabetic foot ulcers complicated by MRSA osteomyelitis associated with worse prognosis? Outcomes of a surgical series. Diabetic Medicine 2009;26:552–555.

46 Couret G, Desbiez F, Thieblot P, Tauveron I, Bonnet R, Beytout J, Laurichesse H, Lesens O: [Emergence of monomicrobial methicillin-resistant Staphylococcus aureus infections in diabetic foot osteomyelitis (retrospective study of 48 cases)]. Presse Med 2007; 36(6 pt 1):851–858.

47 Karchmer AW, Gibbons GW: Foot infections in diabetes: evaluation and management. Curr Clin Top Infect Dis 1994;14:1–22.

48 Faglia E, Clerici G, Caminiti M, Curci V, Somalvico F: Prognostic difference between soft tissue abscess and osteomyelitis of the foot in patients with diabetes: data from a consecutive series of 452 hospitalized patients. J Foot Ankle Surg 2012;51:34–38.

49 Aragon-Sanchez J, Lazaro-Martinez JL, Hernandez-Herrero C, Campillo-Vilorio N, Quintana-Marrero Y, Garcia-Morales E, Hernandez-Herrero MJ: Does osteomyelitis in the feet of patients with diabetes really recur after surgical treatment? Natural history of a surgical series. Diabet Med 2012;29:813–818.

50 Ha Van G, Siney H, Danan JP, Sachon C, Grimaldi A: Treatment of osteomyelitis in the diabetic foot. Contribution of conservative surgery. Diabetes Care 1996;19:1257–1260.
51 Berendt AR, Peters EJ, Bakker K, Embil JM, Eneroth M, Hinchliffe RJ, Jeffcoate WJ, Lipsky BA, Senneville E, Teh J, Valk GD: Diabetic foot osteomyelitis: a progress report on diagnosis and a systematic review of treatment. Diabetes Metab Res Rev 2008;24(suppl 1):S145–S161.
52 Simpson AH, Deakin M, Latham JM: Chronic osteomyelitis. The effect of the extent of surgical resection on infection-free survival. J Bone Joint Surg Br 2001; 83:403–407.
53 Kowalski TJ, Matsuda M, Sorenson MD, Gundrum JD, Agger WA: The effect of residual osteomyelitis at the resection margin in patients with surgically treated diabetic foot infection. J Foot Ankle Surg 2011;50: 171–175.
54 Atway S, Nerone VS, Springer KD, Woodruff DM: Rate of residual osteomyelitis after partial foot amputation in diabetic patients: a standardized method for evaluating bone margins with intraoperative culture. J Foot Ankle Surg 2012;51:749–752.

Javier Aragón-Sánchez, MD, PhD
Department of Surgery and Diabetic Foot Unit
La Paloma Hospital, C/Maestro Valle, 20
ES–35005 Las Palmas de Gran Canaria (Spain)
E-Mail drjaviaragon@gmail.com, javiaragon@telefonica.net

Piaggesi A, Apelqvist J (eds): The Diabetic Foot Syndrome.
Front Diabetes. Basel, Karger, 2018, vol 26, pp 200–209 (DOI: 10.1159/000480102)

Local Management of Diabetic Foot Ulcers, Dressings and Other Local Treatments

Frances L. Game

Department of Diabetes and Endocrinology, Derby Teaching Hospitals NHS Foundation Trust, Derby, UK

Abstract

The outcome of ulcers of the foot in diabetes is generally poor with prolonged healing times and a marked increase in the risk of amputation compared with patients without diabetes. There is therefore an urgent need for the development of interventions to improve outcomes. The evidence base to support many of the interventions in common use, including wound dressings and applications is poor, and these are described here. The available data suggests that while some therapies show promise, more work is needed to substantiate their role in day-to-day clinical practice and their cost effectiveness. It should not be forgotten, however, that there is effective evidence for a number of simple interventions with proven efficacy including frequent wound inspection, sharp debridement of the ulcer with a scalpel to remove necrotic tissue and callous, and offloading of plantar neuropathic ulcers.
© 2018 S. Karger AG, Basel

Background

Foot problems complicating diabetes are a source of major suffering and costs, costing approximately GB 1 billion in England between 2014 and 2015 [1] and is estimated to add between. US USD 9 billion to USD 13 billion to the annual costs associated directly with diabetes [2].

Diabetic foot ulcers (DFUs) are often slow to heal, with observational studies from a number of specialist centres suggesting that only 50% heal without surgery in 6 months, and only two-thirds ever heal at all. Unfortunately, approximately 1 in 10 of all ulcers results in a major (above ankle) amputation.

It is clear therefore that any intervention that improves the speed or probability of ulcer healing would be of major benefit both socially and financially.

Factors that May Delay Healing of Ulcers of the Foot in Diabetes
Delayed healing of foot ulcers in patients with diabetes results from a number of different pathologies, usually acting in combination, but occasionally alone.

Tissue ischaemia is caused by macrovascular or microvascular disease or the functional hypoxia resulting from the autonomic dysregulation of capillary perfusion. Distal neuropathy causes loss of neural regulation of tissue regeneration as well as continued trauma secondary to loss of protective sensation, and increased tissue glucose may lead to abnormal leucocyte function with defective phagocytosis, and infection of the wound. However, the way in which these factors lead to disordered regulation of the healing cascade is not completely understood.

Research into the causes and treatment of ulcers of the foot in diabetes has increased considerably over the last few decades. Types of studies vary from in vitro work looking at the details of pathological processes affecting wound healing, right through to full clinical studies focussing on wound healing or amputation prevention. Unfortunately, many compounds that show promise in basic in vitro work fail to translate into positive outcomes in the clinical studies either because the studies are too poorly performed to be certain that they are of clinical as well as economic benefit, or because a single biochemical or molecular defect is unlikely to be the sole cause of impaired healing in such a complex system. This review therefore concentrates on clinical studies.

Evaluation of Studies into Wound Healing in Patients with Diabetes and Ulcers of the Feet
Repeated systematic reviews of evidence in this area have unfortunately drawn attention to the lack of good quality evidence of this type [3–5], despite the escalating size of the clinical problem as described above. In terms of the quality of evidence for any intervention into wound healing, those shown to be of benefit in a well-conducted randomised controlled trial (RCT) with appropriate and well-described outcome measures may be considered of most relevance [6].

Clinical trials should ideally, therefore, be randomized and the results compared with a control group that is not exposed to the treatment being assessed, although all other aspects of care should be according to best practice and identical. The outcome measures should be of direct clinical relevance (e.g., healing, survival, limb salvage) or surrogate measures must be consistent with clinical improvement (e.g., change in wound area, improvement in the appearance of the wound or a person-related outcome such as pain, well-being or function).

Non-randomized studies may be essential in some circumstances and involve comparing similar groups that either have or have not been exposed to the treatment being assessed. It is essential however that the populations are described and matched as far as possible. Studies that do not include a control population are of little value but may be used for hypothesis generation for future controlled trials.

Evidence of the Value of Local Treatments of Ulcers of the Feet in Diabetes

Debridement
The term debridement refers to the removal of surface debris, slough and infected matter with the aim of leaving a clean, viable tissue that may then heal by secondary intention. Debridement may be undertaken surgically (sharp debridement), biologically (larvae), biochemically (enzymes) or chemically.

Expert opinion is that debridement is an essential first step prior to the application of any type of dressing to the wound; however, the data to support this is surprisingly sparse.

Sharp Debridement
In one systematic review, only 2 studies of sharp debridement were identified [3]; one that was a subgroup analysis of cases from an RCT of another intervention. This reported that healing at 12 weeks was more likely following a more vigorous debridement assessed retrospectively from images of the wounds. The other was too difficult to assess due to lack of published detail.

Larval Therapy
Despite widespread use, evidence to support the use of larval therapy in improving the outcome of DFUs is poor. Only 4 controlled studies were identified in a series of systematic reviews [3–5]. None of the studies were randomized, however. Only one, a case-control study in elderly, non-ambulant people with peripheral arterial disease, reported an apparent significant decreased time to healing and amputation rates in those patients for whom 6-month follow-up data was available; however, the design of the study meant there was a high risk of bias. None offered any analysis on the possible cost effectiveness of the therapy above best practice standard care, which was poorly described in all the studies.

Hydrotherapy
Only one small controlled study reported on this therapy in this patient group [7] and reported no benefit of healing at 12 weeks.

Clostridial Collagenase
The use of Clostridial collagenase ointment used daily as a debriding agent has been examined in one small study [8]. This un-blinded study of non-ischaemic wounds showed an apparent improvement in area reduction from baseline in the treated group after 4 weeks, whereas there was no improvement seen in the control group. There were no between-group comparisons made, however, and usual care was not described for the control arm, whose wounds actually deteriorated.

In general, it is accepted that sharp debridement is an essential part of routine care but that without more evidence there is no justification for using other approaches.

Game

Local Treatment of Infection/Bacterial Colonization

It is clear that clinical infection such as described by the Infectious Diseases of Society of America classification [9] should be treated with systemic antibiotics. However, topical antiseptics/antimicrobial dressings are also widely used with a view to promoting healing or preventing clinical infection.

The Effect Dressing Products with an Apparent Antimicrobial/Antiseptic Action
The commonest marketed products with antiseptic properties contain iodine, silver or honey. None of the 3 reviews undertaken by the International Working Group of the Diabetic Foot (IWGDF) [3–5], a recent review on dressings (10), or a Cochrane review [11] found any evidence that these dressing products had an impact on wound healing. The only large RCT undertaken of a silver-containing dressing in DFUs was an un-blinded RCT and hence subject to bias. Even so, there was no difference in healing between the 2 study groups, and no improvement in the incidence of secondary infection although this was not a primary outcome. The only study of any methodological quality of iodine containing dressings, which compared an iodine containing dressing with a simple non-adherent gauze dressing and a modern hydrofibre in an observer blinded RCT, found no difference in healing between the 3 groups at 24 weeks, and similarly no reduction in secondary infections.

Surprisingly, given the widespread use of honey containing dressings, only 3 controlled studies of this intervention have been published. None are of good methodological quality, all non-blinded and only 2 of the 3 were randomized [3–5]. A recent Cochrane review suggested that the use of honey dressings should not be encouraged for economic reasons [11].

Wound Applications That May Encourage Healing by the Use of Collagen or Collagen Containing Preparations
Collagen containing wound dressings are an appealing therapeutic target for improving outcomes of DFUs especially if combined with the normal cellular components of skin development such as fibroblasts or keratinocytes. Collagen can be obtained from a variety of sources including living and non-living bovine, porcine and equine skin, following which a bioscaffold matrix can be created, which potentially acts as a framework for the growth of new blood vessels and extravascular tissue into a wound.

Collagen containing dressings exist in several forms; as bioengineered skin/skin substitutes or in a more standard dressing or application.

Bioengineered Skin/Skin Substitutes
Several reviews have described the details of the studies evaluating the possible benefit of bioengineered skin comprising cultured fibroblasts (Dermagraft®) and bilayered bioengineered skin (fibroblasts and keratinocytes: Graftskin®, Apligraf®).

The first RCT of Dermagraft® [12] demonstrated a significant improvement in healing of the intervention group compared with controls, but it is relevant that the rate of healing in the control group was very poor (8% at 12 weeks), despite the fact that the study group comprised a cohort of none-infected, non-ischaemic, neuropathic DFUs. It should also be noted that the rate of healing of the control group in the first RCT of Apligraf® was similar to that of the intervention group of the Dermagraft® study [13] – even though the 2 studies were conducted in equivalent populations.

The decision to study these dressings in this population group is understandable in as much as there are fewer pathological confounders. These healing results need to be set in the context of studies of offloading in a similar patient group however, where there have been reports of a much greater rate of healing [14] than those achieved, and yet off-loading was not standardized in these trials. A later publication of a non-completed study using Apligraf in a UK population [15] suggested benefit of only borderline significance. Thus, the data to justify the use of bioengineered skin products for the ulcer types for which they are currently recommended – those with ulcers that have persisted despite management according to the best standards of routine practice – is not convincing.

More recently, studies involving the use of amniotic membrane have been described. One was included in the IWGDF reviews [5], but a large RCT has been published more recently [16]. The first trial reported was a small, non-blinded trial and was once again marred by the observation of a very low healing rate in the control arm despite those consisting non-infected, non-ischaemic neuropathic ulcers. The most recent study was, however, a well-conducted single blind randomized multicentre trial and showed a significant improvement in patients allocated to the intervention group. Although the rate of healing in the control group was not as high as expected, the difference between groups was so marked that recruitment was halted on the advice of a blinded review committee who undertook a pre-planned interim analysis. Although very encouraging, it would be advisable for studies to be repeated in other populations to confirm these findings with a full health economic analysis, before widespread adoption.

Other Collagen Products
Various attempts have been made to modulate the activity of matrix metalloproteinases with dressings. These are enzymes that if over-expressed, may result in excessive breakdown of tissue proteins, but attempts to do so with dressing products or applications have been disappointing. Combining collagen with oxidized regenerated cellulose has been shown to reduce the presence of matrix metalloproteinases in the wound tissue [17]; however, their use has been studied in only a few small poorly performed trials, either through the lack of blinding of outcome, per protocol analysis or by the lack of clear definition of outcome measures [3–5], leading to no clear evidence of any advantage of their use.

Growth Factors

(a) Platelet-Derived Growth Factor-BB

Two initial studies led to the regulatory approval of platelet-derived growth factor-BB (Becaplermin) in the United States. The first, a small RCT in non-infected neuropathic ulcers followed by a later definitive phase III study [18], has not been confirmed in later studies [3–5]. An equally large European study has never been published, the reasons for which are unclear.

The product is expensive, and in 2008, the FDA issued a safety warning alerting prescribers to an increased risk of death from cancer in those who had who used three or more tubes of platelet-derived growth factor-BB compared with patients who had had no exposure. The incidence of new cancer could not be established however and they concluded that the product should be used only when the benefits are expected to outweigh the risks.

(b) Basic Fibroblast Growth Factor-β

A good-quality RCT has demonstrated that basic fibroblast growth factor [19] has no obvious clinical benefit in this field, although the per protocol analysis of a later trial suggested promise. Preliminary results of another trial published in the clinical trial registry suggest there is no difference between intervention and control arms of the study in terms of healing after 12 weeks.

(c) Epidermal Growth Factor

An early dose-ranging study of topical epidermal growth factor (EGF) cream suggested benefit at the highest dose used which may imply that there is a role for recombinant EGF in terms of healing at 12 weeks, but the numbers in this study were very small [3]. Other studies have failed to confirm this finding [3], although an RCT of intra-lesional injection of EGF reported a highly significant difference between groups in the prevalence of granulation tissue after just 2 weeks [20]. Unfortunately, this latter study was marred by switching those in the control group to an intervention arm after the first 2 weeks and no conclusion about healing can be made.

(d) Vascular Endothelial Growth Factor

A number of studies on the intramuscular administration of vascular endothelial growth factor have suggested a significant benefit in terms of peripheral arterial blood supply, and in one RCT [21], there was a significant improvement in healing in the intervention group of the subset with DFUs. This interesting result needs repeating however.

(e) Platelets and Platelet Supernatant

There have been a number of studies published over the last 10 years to suggest that the administration of either platelets (blood bank, ABO matched or autologous) or the supernatant derived from platelet suspension may enhance wound healing [3–5]. Platelet products have not yet, however, been widely adopted because of the difficulty experienced in handling the product and the associated costs.

(f) Stem Cells

Although the administration of bone marrow-deprived stem cells may improve distal circulation in people with diabetes complicated by peripheral arterial disease, good placebo-controlled data indicating an effect on healing is awaited.

Compression or Negative Pressure Wound Therapy

Compression

A small number of controlled studies have been published on the use of compression of DFUs (3 RCTs and a cohort study). All had methodological problems, with one allowing patients to choose therapy, or outcomes being non-blinded. Thus, the evidence to support this therapy even in the postoperative wound is poor [3–5].

Topical Negative Pressure Wound Therapy

Negative pressure wound therapy (NPWT) may assist in wound management by collecting high volumes of wound exudate, thus enabling a reduction in the frequency of dressing, and reducing odour. There have also been suggestions, however, that the application of mechanical force to the wound provides biologically plausible processes by which wound healing is promoted, for example, the physical approximation of wound edges, increased perfusion, and the removal of infectious material and exudate. NPWT might also have a beneficial effect by encouraging offloading, as devices, even when apparently portable will limit ambulation.

Once again, despite the very widespread use of NPWT, the evidence to support effectiveness and cost effectiveness are poor. The repeated systematic reviews of the IWGDF [3–5] found only 9 studies, a majority of which were small, un-blinded, non-randomized or of otherwise poor methodological quality.

In 2005, however, a relatively large study reported a significant benefit of NPWT in both time to, and proportion of persons, healing in those who had recently undergone foot surgery [22] even though the definition of "healing" used included those who were healed after repeat surgeries were performed, and this weakens the conclusions to be drawn from the results. A second RCT (342 patients) also showed a reduced time to wound closure, an increased incidence of healing by 16 weeks, a greater reduction in cross-sectional area by 8 weeks and reduced incidence of minor amputation. It is not clear from this study, however, how many of the wounds were postoperative; the mean baseline area of the ulcers being 11 and 13.5 cm^2 in the control and intervention groups respectively [23].

A cohort study published in 2007 attempted to confirm the effectiveness of NPWT through the analysis of reimbursement claims, but the results could potentially be explained by confounding factors.

An interesting recent small, non-blinded RCT compared the use of NPWT after split skin graft with a non-adherent dressing over the graft, which suggested that the proportion of the split skin grafts that developed successfully was significantly higher in those who had the NPWT. Lack of blinding and information on baseline wound characteristics makes this result difficult to interpret [5]. This novel use of NPWT is, however of interest, even though the study needs confirmation.

Despite the above information, the risk of bias in the published studies (and known publication bias), a recent Cochrane review [24] concluded that further robust evidence is required.

RCT research is needed to help to reduce the uncertainty regarding the effectiveness of this therapy and in which clinical situation it may be most effective and cost-effective.

Conclusions

Speeding up healing of ulcers on the foot of patients with diabetes and reducing amputations remains difficult. It is, however, important that the effectiveness and cost effectiveness of new treatments are rigorously assessed, and that treatments should not be used without strong evidence of both effectiveness and cost-effectiveness. The conclusion of almost all systematic reviews [3–5, 25] of the subject is similar that the evidence to support many of the therapies that are in routine use is poor. While some new therapies are showing promise in clinical trials, their place in the wound-healing process remains to be confirmed.

By contrast, it is important that clinicians bear in mind that there is good evidence to support the use of interventions other than advanced wound care products. The IWGDF has developed a set of simple guidelines [26] for local management of ulcers and these include:

- Frequent inspection of the ulcer
- Debridement of the ulcer with a scalpel to remove necrotic tissue and callous
- The selection of dressings to control excess exudation and maintain a moist wound-healing environment

The National Institute of Health and Clinical Care Excellence in the UK (NICE) guideline [25] also suggests that dressings should be of the lowest acquisition cost to perform these tasks in order to ensure that, in a cash-limited health care system, every patient has access to the above-mentioned tasks in an expert multi-professional setting.

Disclosure Statement

The author has no conflicts of interest to declare.

References

1 Diabetes UK: Improving Footcare for People with Diabetes and Saving Money: An Economic Study in England. https://www.diabetes.org.uk/Upload/Shared%20practice/Improving%20footcare%20economic%20study%20(January%202017).pdf (accessed April 2, 2017).

2 Rice JB, Desai U, Cummings AK, Birnbaum HG, Skornicki M, Parsons NB: Burden of diabetic foot ulcers for medicare and private insurers. Diabetes Care 2014;37:651–658.

3 Hinchliffe RJ, Valk GD, Apelqvist J, Armstrong DG, Bakker K, Game FL, Hartemann-Heurtier A, Löndahl M, Price PE, van Houtum WH, Jeffcoate WJ: A systematic review of the effectiveness of interventions to enhance the healing of chronic ulcers of the foot in diabetes. Diabetes Metab Res Rev 2008;24(suppl 1):S188–S189.

4 Game FL, Hinchliffe RJ, Apelqvsit J, Armstrong DG, Bakker K, Hartemann A, Löndahl M, Price PE, Jeffcoate WJ: A systematic review of interventions to enhance the healing of chronic ulcers of the foot in diabetes. Diabet Metab Res Rev 2012;28(suppl 1):119–141.

5 Game FL, Apelqvist J, Attinger C, Hartemann A, Hinchliffe RJ, Löndahl M, Price PE, Jeffcoate WJ: Effectiveness of interventions to enhance healing of chronic ulcers of the foot in diabetes: a systematic review. Diabetes Metab Res Rev 2016;32(suppl 1):154–168.

6 Jeffcoate WJ, Bus SA, Game FL, Hinchliffe RJ, Price PE, Schaper NC; International Working Group on the Diabetic Foot and the European Wound Management Association: Reporting standards of studies and papers on the prevention and management of foot ulcers in diabetes: required details and markers of good quality. Lancet Diabetes Endocrinol 2016;4:781–788.

7 Caputo WJ, Beggs DJ, DeFede JL, Simm L, Dharma H: A prospective randomized controlled trial comparing hydrosurgery debridement with conventional surgical debridement in lower extremity ulcers. Int Wound J 2008;5:288–294.

8 Tallis A, Motley TA, Wunderlich RP, Dickerson JE Jr, Waycaster C, Slade HB; Collagenase Diabetic Foot Ulcer Study Group: Clinical and economic assessment of diabetic foot ulcer debridement with collagenase: results of a randomized controlled study. Clin Ther 2013;35:1805–1820.

9 Lipsky BA, Berendt AR, Deery HG, Embil JM, Joseph WS, Karchmer AW, LeFrock JL, Lew DP, Mader JT, Norden C, Tan JS: Diagnosis and treatment of diabetic foot infections. Clin Infect Dis 2004;39:885–910.

10 Dumville JC, Soares MO, O'Meara S, Cullum N: Systematic review and mixed treatment comparison: dressings to heal diabetic foot ulcers. Diabetologia 2012;55:1902–1910.

11 Jull AB, Cullum N, Dumville JC, Westby MJ, Deshpande S, Walker N: Honey as a topical treatment for wounds. Cochrane Database Syst Rev 2015;3:CD005083.

12 Gentzkow GD, Iwasaki SD, Hershon KS, et al: Use of Dermagraft, a cultured human dermis, to treat diabetic foot ulcers. Diabetes Care 1996;19:350–354.

13 Veves A, Falanga V, Armstrong DG, Sabolinski ML: Graftskin, a human skin equivalent, is effective in the management of noninfected neuropathic diabetic foot ulcers: a prospective randomized multicenter clinical trial. Diabetes Care 2001;24:290–295.

14 Armstrong DG, Lavery LA, Wu S, Boulton AJ: Evaluation of removable and irremovable cast walkers in the healing of diabetic foot wounds: a randomized controlled trial. Diabetes Care 2005;28:551–554.

15 Edmonds M: Apligraf in the treatment of neuropathic diabetic foot ulcers. Int J Low Extrem Wounds 2009;8:11–18.

16 Lavery LA, Fulmer J, Shebetka KA Regulski M, Vayser D, Fried D, Kashefsky H, Owings TM, Nadarajah J; Grafix Diabetic Foot Ulcer Study Group: The efficacy and safety of Grafix(®) for the treatment of chronic diabetic foot ulcers: results of a multi-centre, controlled, randomised, blinded, clinical trial. Int Wound J 2014;11:554–560.

17 Motzkau M, Tautenhahn J, Lehnert H, Lobmann R: Expression of matrix-metalloproteases in the fluid of chronic diabetic foot wounds treated with a protease absorbent dressing. Exp Clin Endocrinol Diabetes 2011;119:286–290.

18 Wieman TJ, Smiell JM, Su Y: Efficacy and safety of a topical gel formulation of recombinant human platelet-derived growth factor-BB (becaplermin) in patients with chronic neuropathic diabetic ulcers. A phase III randomized placebo-controlled double-blind study. Diabetes Care 1998;21:822–827.

19 Richard JL, Parer-Richard C, Daures JP, Clouet S, Vannereau D, Bringer J, Rodier M, Jacob C, Comte-Bardonnet M: Effect of topical basic fibroblast growth factor on the healing of chronic diabetic neuropathic ulcer of the foot. A pilot, randomized, double-blind, placebo-controlled study. Diabetes Care 1995;18:64–69.

20 Fernandez-Montequin JI, Valenzuela- Silva CM, Diaz OG, Savigne W, Sancho-Soutelo N, Rivero-Fernández F, Sánchez-Penton P, Morejón-Vega L, Artaza-Sanz H, García-Herrera A, González-Benavides C, Hernández-Cañete CM, Vázquez-Proenza A, Berlanga-Acosta J, López-Saura PA: Intra-lesional injections of recombinant human epidermal growth factor promote granulation and healing in advanced diabetic foot ulcers: multicentre, randomised, placebo controlled, double-blind study. Int Wound J 2009;6:432–443.

21 Kusumanto YH, Van Weel V, Mulder NH, Smit AJ, van den Dungen JJ, Hooymans JM, Sluiter WJ, Tio RA, Quax PH, Gans RO, Dullaart RP, Hospers GA: Treatment with intramuscular vascular endothelial growth factor gene compared with placebo for patients with diabetes mellitus and critical limb ischemia: a double-blind randomized trial. Human Gene Ther 2006;17:683–691.

22 Armstrong DG, Lavery LA; Diabetic Foot Study Consortium: Negative pressure wound therapy after partial diabetic foot amputation: a multicentre, randomised controlled trial. Lancet 2005;366:1704–1710.

23 Blume PA, Walters J, Payne W, Ayala J, Lantis J: Comparison of negative pressure wound therapy using vacuum assisted closure with advanced moist wound therapy in the treatment of diabetic foot ulcers. Diabetes Care 2008;31:631–636.

24 Dumville JC, Hinchliffe RJ, Cullum N, Game F, Stubbs N, Sweeting M, Peinemann F: Negative pressure wound therapy for treating foot wounds in people with diabetes mellitus. Cochrane Database Syst Rev 2013;10:CD010318.

25 NICE Guideline (NG19): Diabetic Foot Problems: Prevention and Management. https://www.nice.org.uk/guidance/ng19 (accessed April 6, 2017).

26 Schaper NC, Van Netten JJ, Apelqvist J, Lipsky BA, Bakker K; International Working Group on the Diabetic Foot: Prevention and management of foot problems in diabetes: a summary guidance for daily practice 2015, based on the IWGDF guidance documents. Diabetes Metab Res Rev 2016;32(suppl 1):7–15.

Prof. Frances L. Game, FRCP
Department of Diabetes and Endocrinology
Derby Teaching Hospitals NHS Foundation Trust
Uttoxeter Road, Derby DE22 3NE (UK)
E-Mail frances.game@nhs.net

Piaggesi A, Apelqvist J (eds): The Diabetic Foot Syndrome.
Front Diabetes. Basel, Karger, 2018, vol 26, pp 210–218 (DOI: 10.1159/000480104)

Towards Extending Ulcer-Free Days in Remission in the Diabetic Foot Syndrome

Jano A. Boghossian[a] · John D. Miller[b] · David G. Armstrong[a]

[a]Southwestern Academic Limb Salvage Alliance (SALSA), Department of Surgery, Keck School of Medicine, University of Southern California, Los Angeles, CA, and [b]DVA Maryland Healthcare System, Baltimore, MD, USA

Abstract

Management of the diabetic foot is multifaceted and requires constant monitoring from patients and health care providers. The alarmingly high rates of diabetic foot ulcer recurrence are an indication for a change that we need to bring about in our approach to care and to the use of vernacular in the medical literature. With its high rates of morbidity and recidivism, care of the complex diabetic foot may be aptly comparable to many forms of cancer. Therefore, our efforts should be not only to achieve rapid healing of open wounds but also to maximize the number of ulcer-free days for the patient in diabetic foot remission. Novel approaches in surgical techniques and advances in wearable technology appear to show promise in measuring inflammation and modulating dangerous pressures to extend remission and improve quality of life for these most complex patients.

Diabetes and other non-communicable diseases of decay are now the leading cause of global mortality both in the developed and developing world [1]. As the continuously growing epidemic of diabetes further expands, it inflicts affected patients with a myriad of subsequent diabetic complications and co-morbidities that necessitate further financial investments in managing these patients in a multidisciplinary setting to save limbs from amputation. There are several well-known guidelines for prolonging remission from ulceration in the diabetic foot with the mindset of "active prevention," including having a heightened awareness of these risk factors associated with ulceration, patient education, staying active, frequent inspection of the feet, reducing friction by wearing diabetic socks and proper footwear, avoiding self-injurious behavior such as walking barefoot and long-term management of the various co-morbid systemic diseases associated with diabetes [2, 3].

Due to the economic, physical and psychological cost of diabetic foot ulcers (DFUs), efforts to delay or prevent their development are a prudent use of medical resources. Remarkably, people with DFUs have a risk of hospitalization that is comparable to or exceeding the risk of having heart failure, pulmonary disease, renal disease and most cancers [4]. Patients with diabetes mellitus undergoing treatment of DFUs often present with confounding factors and subsequently experience high rates of recurrence. Of the individuals who successfully heal a DFU, the risk of ulcer recurrence within the first year of healing a prior ulceration is likely 40% [5, 6]. Naturally, these devastating rates of recurrence lend themselves to comparison with rates of the deadliest of cancers and warrant a change in terminology and format of communicating and counseling this patient population [7]. We believe a change in the syntax of resolved DFUs from the past tense of "healed" to the active "in remission" best represents the threat to the patient and the need for ongoing preventative care. This has the added benefit of preventing patients from being lost to follow-up or prudent at-home care, as patients are now given the task of increasing their own "ulcer-free days" and reducing the severity of recurrences rather than simply "remaining healed" [6–8].

Reducing Peak Plantar Pressures

The Use of Custom Footwear for Extending Ulcer-Free Days
In treating DFU, alleviating pressure at areas of high vertical and shear stress can be achieved by offloading the foot with various techniques, starting with total contact casts or irremovable offloading devices (Fig. 1, 2) for those with active wounds to custom therapeutic footwear for people with post-ulcerative lesions in remission. Patients with diabetes have an association with elevated peak plantar pressures [9] (Fig. 3). Coupled with repetitive pedal stress caused by osseous and structural abnormalities of the foot in the presence of neuropathy and peripheral arterial disease, these risk factors are some of the strongest predictors of ulcer development [9]. As a result, redistribution of constant plantar pressure is of utmost importance in managing a diabetic in remission [10]. In quantifying an in-shoe peak plantar pressure threshold, 200 kPa has been suggested as a meaningful value below which ulceration may be prevented, as seen from patients whose previous ulceration sites have remained in remission. This number, of course, is a compromise, as other ingredients (shear stress, duration of standing, cycles of repetitive stress) may also increase risk for those with lower peak plantar stress numbers [11, 12].

Surgical Methods to Extend Ulcer-Free Days

While wound care and ulcer management are crucial in this patient population, it is akin to treating neither the symptom not its underlying cause-pressure [13]. Surgical methods for maintaining the DFU in remission is of paramount

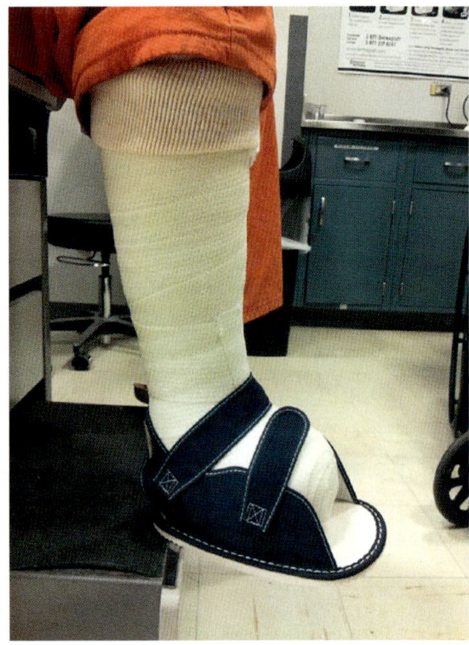

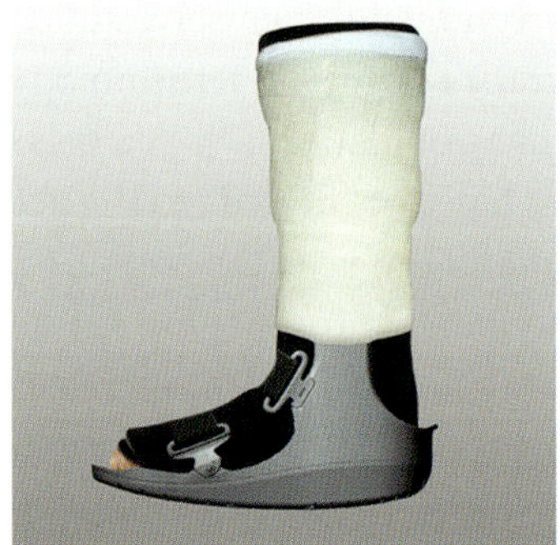

Fig. 1. Total contact casts are the gold standard for offloading diabetic neuropathic wounds, yet are quite cumbersome for patients and take significant time and expertise to apply properly in the clinical setting.

Fig. 2. The instant total contact cast. A removable cast walker rendered irremovable due to wrapping the upper portion with a layer of fibre glass.

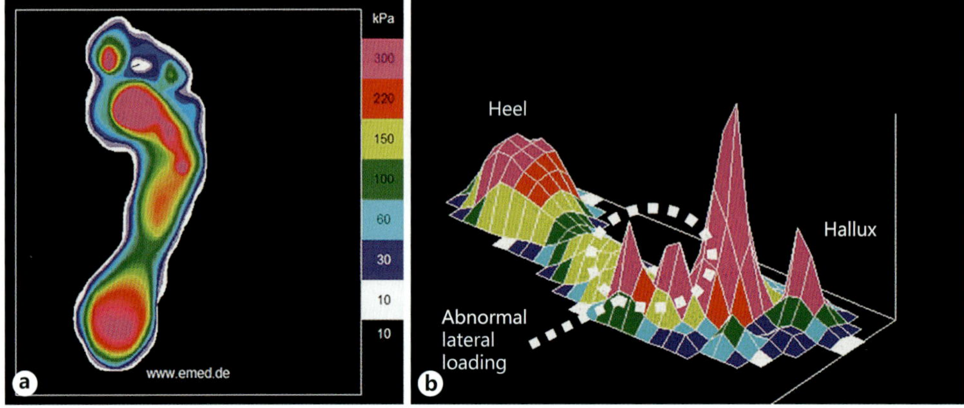

Fig. 3. Peak pressure profile for a diabetic foot. **a** Two-dimensional depiction of plantar pressure; **b** Three-dimensional depiction of plantar pressure (note the abnormal spikes along the lateral forefoot).

Boghossian · Miller · Armstrong

importance. The removal of pressure in the manner of surgically correcting both flexible and rigid abnormalities is essential in healing wounds and preventing their recurrence.

Achilles Tendon Lengthening
Achilles tendon lengthening is an effective method to reduce the recurrence of plantar diabetic neuropathic ulcers of the forefoot in patients with limited ankle dorsiflexory range of motion. The percutaneous procedure involves 3 stab incisions, and can be done with the patient lying prone under local anaesthesia [14]. A 1999 study showed a mean 28% reduction in peak pressures on the plantar aspect of the forefoot following percutaneous Achilles tendon lengthening in diabetic patients who are at high risk for ulcerations of the foot [15]. A subsequent study in 2003 demonstrated that Achilles tendon-lengthening procedures in conjunction with TCC application reduced the recurrence of ulceration from 59 to 15% when compared to TCC applications alone [16].

Surgical Correction of Skeletal Abnormalities
Deformities of the foot's natural osseous architecture are highly linked to development and recurrence of ulcerations; therefore, surgical correction of osseous deformities is often necessary to prolong ulcerative remission [17]. A surgeon must first consider whether digital deformities are a result of either soft tissue contracture or osseous deformity. If the contractures are flexible, tenotomies alone may be preferred to osseous corrections due to their ease of use, short recovery time and ability to provide deformity correction. If the digital abnormalities are rigid, as seen with hallux valgus or limitus, osseous procedures like arthroplasties of the base of the proximal phalanx of the hallux such as a Keller-type procedure with possible reinsertion of the flexor hallucis brevis is recommended to prevent further ulceration [18]. Offloading the first metatarsophalangeal joint can be achieved by either resection of the sesamoids or a dorsiflexion osteotomy at the base of the first metatarsal. By correcting hammertoe deformities of the lesser digits, peak pressures and dangerous shear forces may be mitigated on the distal tips and dorsal joint surfaces. This can be done through a metatarsal head resection, a metatarsal condylectomy or a dorsiflexion osteotomy of the problematic metatarsal. If ulcerations persist to sub-metatarsal heads, single or pan-metatarsal head resections or transmetatarsal amputations may be required for long-term ulcer prevention [19]. The advantage of single or pan-metatarsal head resections is the preservation of the digits, which are lost after transmetatarsal amputations.

Plantar Fat Pad Augmentation
There has been much debate concerning the pathologic consequences of diabetes on the plantar fat pad and its subsequent association with the development of a foot ulcer.

Post-ulcerative soft tissue often remains with significant substance deficit and reduced tissue protection. As plantar pressure is a direct correlate of plantar fat pad thickness, new efforts are being directed towards restoring pre- and post-ulcerative

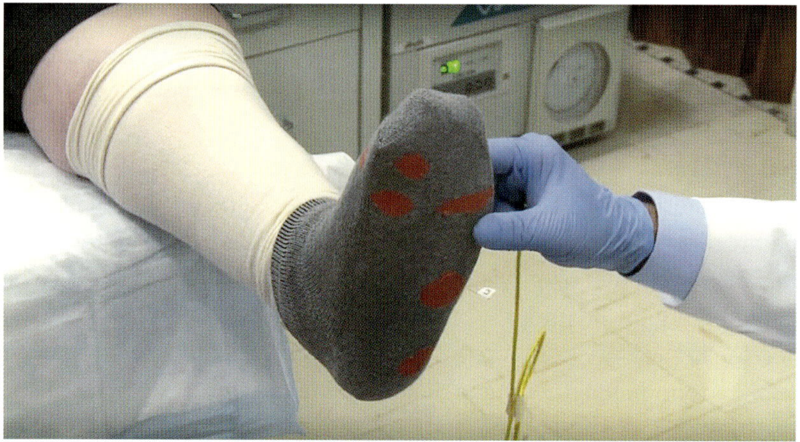

Fig. 4. Smart Sox use fibre optic cables embedded within socks to warn the patient of peaks in plantar pressure. Warning messages are sent to the patient's wristwatch, instructing them to offload areas of high pressure.

soft tissue deficits. Prior reports of silicone injection treatment to add bulk to soft tissue associated with ulceration, or pre-ulceration, have thoroughly indicated its safe utility in the prevention and maintenance of wound remission [20]. Additionally, current efforts are being made to optimize the use of one's own adipocytes to increase soft tissue depth and promote autogenous sourcing of graft material in preventing recurrence of DFUs [21]. Current reports demonstrate efficacy in the injection of autologous abdominal fat into areas of plantar prominence to reduce lesion recurrence or new ulceration formation [21].

Monitoring Strategies and Technological Innovations

Wearables

The emergence of "smart" technologies and wearable electronics paves the way for the integration of both in the context of providing patients and clinicians with objective data about patient health that is easily accessible. Physicians no longer need to rely on the subjective history given by neuropathic patients who lack the ability to sense the deterioration of their own bodies [22]. Such information can now be obtained with the advent of "smart" wearable technologies like SmartSox [23] and other wearables to detect the effect of physical activity on the body (Fig. 4). The success or failure of various treatment regimens instituted for diabetics with neuropathy might correlate with the levels of physical activity undertaken by the patient, as the neuropathic ulcers typically develop due to repetitive stress applied to the feet during weight-bearing [24].

Because shear stresses contribute to the formation of diabetes-related foot ulcers, a 2014 study published in the journal of *Diabetes Science and Technology* evaluated the effect of a custom, novel shear-reducing insole on the thermal response to ambulation and found that significant reductions in forefoot and midfoot temperature increases after walking when using the customizable insole when compared to standard insoles [25].

As constant monitoring paves the way for patient-specific medicine, the implementation and proliferation of three-dimensional printing to personalize exoskeleton suits has found its place in helping paraplegics walk, military personnel carry heavier loads in a more efficient manner, and benefit frail and high-risk diabetics with neuropathy reduce plantar tissue impact and reduce the stress of weight-bearing [26].

These findings, and similar research on customizable, wearable technologies, merit future research on such devices for the prevention of neuropathic ulcers and for prolonging the remission of previous ulceration.

At-Home Monitors

A 2007 study found that those who did not use a system for temperature monitoring system quadrupled their chances of developing foot ulcer recurrence than those who did, emphasizing the major impact this technology could have on global health if implemented ubiquitously [27]. Constant monitoring systems for diabetics will include such technologies that will be integrated into the daily life of the patients via wearable sensors and smart technologies such as "intelligent" insoles or "smart" socks, which can detect and alert both the patient and the physician about the need for possible intervention before ulceration can manifest itself as a neuropathic wound. Some of the earliest known clinical markers for the inflammatory process that occur prior to ulceration include calor, erythema and high peak plantar pressures [28]. The technology behind the "smart" socks, for example, include intelligent textiles that use fibre optics and sensors to monitor pressure, temperature, and joint angles of the feet of neuropathic diabetics who cannot otherwise detect these sensations themselves, and simultaneously measure all 3 parameters to precisely indicate the location on the foot, which is likely to develop an ulcer if left untreated [23].

The Emerging Role of the Multidisciplinary Team

A coordinated team approach has also been shown to decrease the frequency of limb loss in diabetic patients worldwide [29–31]. In the Netherlands, and recently in the United States, the inclusion of podiatrists in a multidisciplinary approach to diabetic foot disease has reduced amputations by 34 and 64%, respectively [32, 33]. Health care teams in Turkey and Thailand report the presence of a strong correlation between teamwork and multidisciplinary protocol in diabetic foot care in reducing rates of amputation [34, 35]. In the United Kingdom, an organized multidisciplinary team (MDT) approach to the diabetic foot has shown sustained reduction in amputation rates [36, 37]. Italian literature also reports a reduction in hospitalization and major limb amputation, thanks to the deployment of an MDT in high-risk patients [38].

While significant data exists to demonstrate the efficacy of multidisciplinary protocol and teamwork in reducing amputations, as yet, there is no data to show definitively that a combination of advanced therapies and care via an MDT leads to shorter healing times. The benefits of an MDT are far reaching, including a focused approach to each patient's particular needs, optimized multifaceted management of patients with diabetes mellitus and enhanced patient surveillance [39]. The International Diabetes Federation recommends that in order to provide comprehensive lower extremity care, an MDT should comprise doctors with specific interest in diabetes, including podiatrists, trained nurses, vascular and surgeons, orthopaedic surgeons, infection specialists, orthotists, social workers and psychologists. These guidelines have been most effective in the United Kingdom where moves to establish a "virtual network" of multispecialty consult services surrounding a core of practitioners are being initiated. In this manner, one clinician acts as a coordinator for multidisciplinary care and referrals. The coordinator may be a podiatrist, a surgeon or another type of clinician with a special interest in diabetes. In some countries, coordinated care may be based within a single clinic [39].

Lasting Comments on Ulcer Remission

In summary, we propose flipping the script, if you will, on our perspective on "wound healing". We propose focussing not on the staccato events that punctuate each acute or chronic event, but rather on the entire score – from the beginning to the end. In this way, our perspective is enhanced, our therapies can be less reactive and we may all find that we are playing together in the same symphony.

References

1 Bloom DE, Cafiero E, Jané-Llopis E, Abrahams-Gessel S, Bloom LR, Fathima S, et al: The global economic burden of noncommunicable diseases [Internet]. Program on the Global Demography of Aging. 2012. https://ideas.repec.org/p/gdm/wpaper/8712.html.

2 American Diabetes Association: Standards of medical care in diabetes – 2014. Diabetes Care 2013; 37:S14–S80.

3 Peters EJ, Armstrong DG, Lavery LA: Risk factors for recurrent diabetic foot ulcers: site matters. Diabetes Care 2007;30:2077–2079.

4 Skrepnek GH, Mills JL, Lavery LA, Armstrong DG: Health Care Service and Outcomes Among an Estimated 6.7 Million Ambulatory Care Diabetic Foot Cases in the U.S. Diabetes Care, 2017.

5 van Netten JJ, Price PE, Lavery LA, Monteiro-Soares M, Rasmussen A, Jubiz Y, et al: Prevention of foot ulcers in the at-risk patient with diabetes: a systematic review. Diabetes Metab Res Rev 2016;32(suppl 1):84–98.

6 Armstrong DG, Boulton AJM, Bus SA: Diabetic foot ulcers and their recurrence. N Engl J Med 2017;376: 2367–2375.

7 Armstrong DG, Mills JL: Toward a change in syntax in diabetic foot care: prevention equals remission. J Am Podiatr Med Assoc 2013;103:161–162.

8 Miller JD, Salloum M, Button A, Giovinco NA, Armstrong DG: How can I maintain my patient with diabetes and history of foot ulcer in remission? Int J Low Extrem Wounds 2014;13:371–377.

Boghossian · Miller · Armstrong

9 Armstrong DG, Boulton AJ: Activity monitors: should we begin dosing activity as we dose a drug? J Am Podiatr Med Assoc 2001;91:152–153.

10 Cavanagh PR, Bus SA: Off-loading the diabetic foot for ulcer prevention and healing. Plast Reconstr Surg 2011;127(suppl 1):248S–256S.

11 Armstrong DG, Peters EJ, Athanasiou KA, Lavery LA: Is there a critical level of plantar foot pressure to identify patients at risk for neuropathic foot ulceration? J Foot Ankle Surg 1998;37:303–307.

12 Najafi B, Grewal GS, Bharara M, Menzies R, Talal TK, Armstrong DG: Can't stand the pressure: the association between unprotected standing, walking, and wound healing in people with diabetes. J Diabetes Sci Technol 2017;11:657–667.

13 Armstrong DG, Boulton AJM, Bus SA: Diabetic foot ulcers and their recurrence. N Engl J Med 2017;376: 2367–2375.

14 Nishimoto GS, Attinger CE, Cooper PS: Lengthening the Achilles tendon for the treatment of diabetic plantar forefoot ulceration. Surg Clin North Am 2003;83:707–726.

15 Armstrong DG, Stacpoole-Shea S, Nguyen H, Harkless LB: Lengthening of the Achilles tendon in diabetic patients who are at high risk for ulceration of the foot. J Bone Joint Surg Am 1999;81:535–538.

16 Mueller MJ, Sinacore DR, Hastings MK, Strube MJ, Johnson JE: Effect of Achilles tendon lengthening on neuropathic plantar ulcers. A randomized clinical trial. J Bone Joint Surg Am 2003;85-A:1436–1445.

17 Armstrong DG, Lavery LA, Stern S, Harkless LB: Is prophylactic diabetic foot surgery dangerous? J Foot Ankle Surg 1996;35:585–589.

18 Armstrong DG, Frykberg RG: Classifying diabetic foot surgery: toward a rational definition. Diabet Med 2003;20:329–331.

19 La Fontaine J, Lavery LA, Hunt NA, Murdoch DP: The role of surgical off-loading to prevent recurrent ulcerations. Int J Low Extrem Wounds 2014;13:320–334.

20 Balkin SW: Injectable silicone and the foot: a 41-year clinical and histologic history. Dermatol Surg 2005; 31:1555–1559; discussion 1560.

21 Luu CA, Larson E, Rankin TM, Pappalardo JL, Slepian MJ, Armstrong DG: Plantar fat grafting and tendon balancing for the diabetic foot ulcer in remission. Plast Reconstr Surg Glob Open 2016;4:e810.

22 Ferber R, Webber T, Everett B, Groenland M: Validation of plantar pressure measurements for a novel in-shoe plantar sensory replacement unit. J Diabetes Sci Technol 2013;7:1167–1175.

23 Najafi B: SmartSox: a smart textile to prevent diabetic foot amputation. Qatar Foundation Annual Research Forum Proceedings, 2013, BIOP 013.

24 Najafi B, Armstrong DG, Mohler J: Novel wearable technology for assessing spontaneous daily physical activity and risk of falling in older adults with diabetes. J Diabetes Sci Technol 2013;7:1147–1160.

25 Wrobel JS, Ammanath P, Le T, Luring C, Wensman J, Grewal GS, et al: A novel shear reduction insole effect on the thermal response to walking stress, balance, and gait. J Diabetes Sci Technol 2014;8:1151–1156.

26 Rankin TM, Giovinco NA, Cucher DJ, Watts G, Hurwitz B, Armstrong DG: Three-dimensional printing surgical instruments: are we there yet? J Surg Res 2014;189:193–197.

27 Lavery LA, Higgins KR, Lanctot DR, Constantinides GP, Zamorano RG, Athanasiou KA, et al: Preventing diabetic foot ulcer recurrence in high-risk patients: use of temperature monitoring as a self-assessment tool. Diabetes Care 2007;30:14–20.

28 Bharara M, Schoess J, Armstrong DG: Coming events cast their shadows before: detecting inflammation in the acute diabetic foot and the foot in remission. Diabetes Metab Res Rev 2012;28(suppl 1): 15–20.

29 Larsson J, Apelqvist J, Agardh CD, Stenström A: Decreasing incidence of major amputation in diabetic patients: a consequence of a multidisciplinary foot care team approach? Diabet Med 1995;12:770–776.

30 Krishnan S, Nash F, Baker N, Fowler D, Rayman G: Reduction in diabetic amputations over 11 years in a defined U.K. population: benefits of multidisciplinary team work and continuous prospective audit. Diabetes Care 2008;31:99–101.

31 Tseng CL, Rajan M, Miller DR, Lafrance JP, Pogach L: Trends in initial lower extremity amputation rates among Veterans Health Administration health care System users from 2000 to 2004. Diabetes Care 2011; 34:1157–1163.

32 van Houtum WH, Rauwerda JA, Ruwaard D, Schaper NC, Bakker K: Reduction in diabetes-related lower-extremity amputations in The Netherlands: 1991–2000. Diabetes Care 2004;27:1042–1046.

33 Sloan FA, Feinglos MN, Grossman DS: Receipt of care and reduction of lower extremity amputations in a nationally representative sample of U.S. elderly. Health Serv Res 2010;45:1740–1762.

34 Aksoy DY, Gürlek A, Cetinkaya Y, Oznur A, Yazici M, Ozgür F, et al: Change in the amputation profile in diabetic foot in a tertiary reference center: efficacy of team working. Exp Clin Endocrinol Diabetes 2004;112:526–530.

35 Rerkasem K, Kosachunhanun N, Tongprasert S, Khwanngern K, Matanasarawoot A, Thongchai C, et al: Reducing lower extremity amputations due to diabetes: the application of diabetic-foot protocol in Chiang Mai University Hospital. Int J Low Extrem Wounds 2008;7:88–92.

36 Edmonds ME, Blundell MP, Morris ME, Thomas EM, Cotton LT, Watkins PJ: Improved survival of the diabetic foot: the role of a specialized foot clinic. Q J Med 1986;60:763–771.

37 Canavan RJ, Unwin NC, Kelly WF, Connolly VM: Diabetes- and nondiabetes-related lower extremity amputation incidence before and after the introduction of better organized diabetes foot care: continuous longitudinal monitoring using a standard method. Diabetes Care 2008;31:459–463.

38 Anichini R, Zecchini F, Cerretini I, Meucci G, Fusilli D, Alviggi L, et al: Improvement of diabetic foot care after the Implementation of the International Consensus on the Diabetic Foot (ICDF): results of a 5-year prospective study. Diabetes Res Clin Pract 2007;75:153–158.

39 Sumpio BE, Armstrong DG, Lavery LA, Andros G: The role of interdisciplinary team approach in the management of the diabetic foot: a joint statement from the Society for Vascular Surgery and the American Podiatric Medical Association. J Am Podiatr Med Assoc 2010;100:309–311.

David G. Armstrong, DPM, MD, PhD
Southwestern Academic Limb Salvage Alliance (SALSA), Department of Surgery
Keck School of Medicine, University of Southern California
1520 San Pablo Street, Suite 4300, Los Angeles, CA 90033 (USA)
E-Mail armstrong@usa.net

Author Index

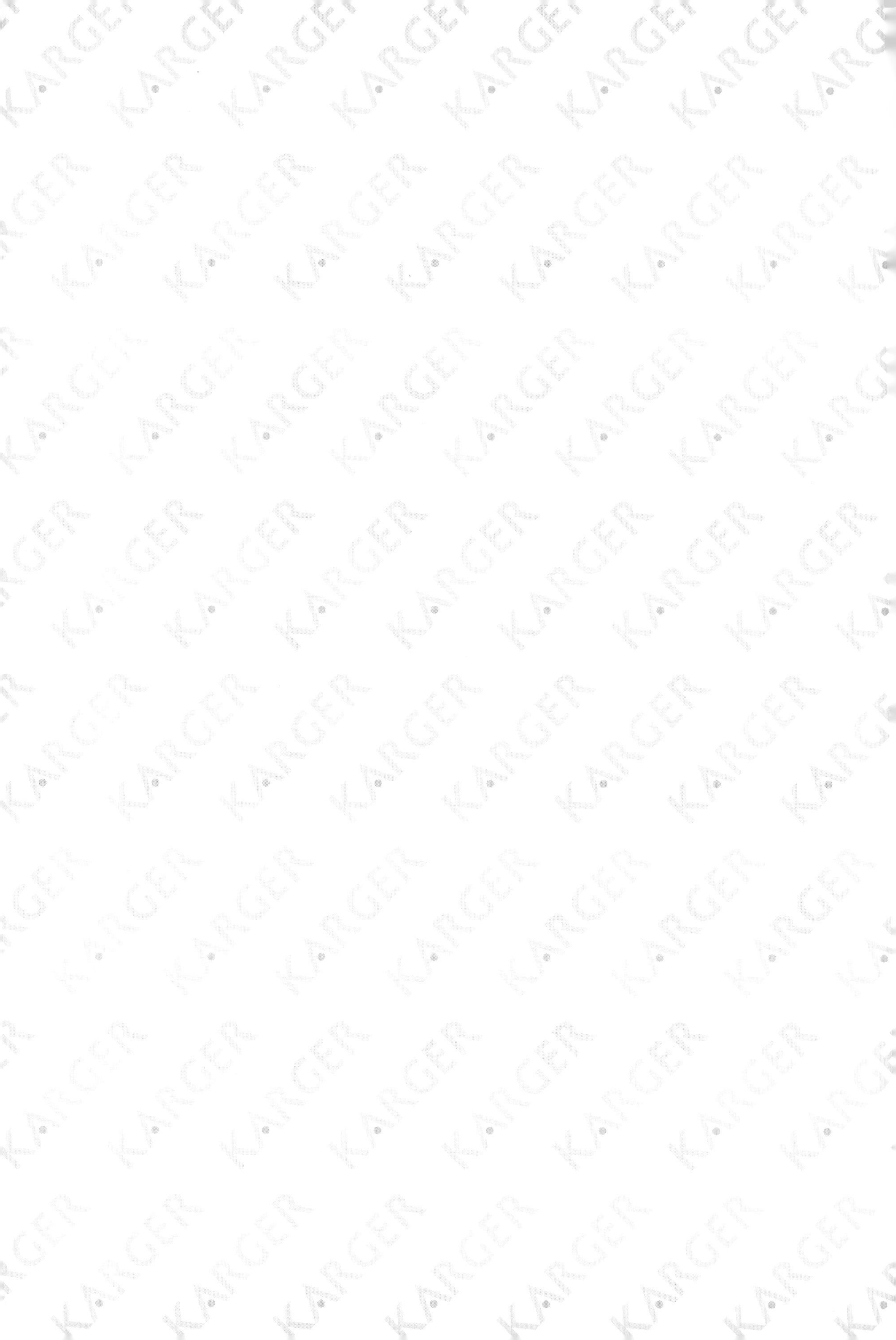